Women's Health

Editors

SARINA SCHRAGER
HEATHER L. PALADINE

PRIMARY CARE:
CLINICS IN OFFICE PRACTICE

www.primarycare.theclinics.com

Consulting Editor
JOEL J. HEIDELBAUGH

June 2025 • Volume 52 • Number 2

ELSEVIER

1600 John F. Kennedy Boulevard ● Suite 1800 ● Philadelphia, Pennsylvania, 19103-2899

http://www.theclinics.com

PRIMARY CARE: CLINICS IN OFFICE PRACTICE Volume 52, Number 2
June 2025 ISSN 0095-4543, ISBN-13: 978-0-443-31756-9

Editor: Taylor Hayes
Developmental Editor: Nitesh Barthwal

Publication information: *Primary Care: Clinics in Office Practice* (ISSN: 0095-4543) is published quarterly by Elsevier, 230 Park Avenue, Suite 800, New York, NY 10169. Periodicals postage paid at New York, NY and additional mailing offices. USA POSTMASTER: Send address changes to Primary Care: Clinics in Office Practice, Elsevier Customer Service Department, 3251 Riverport Lane, Maryland Heights, MO 63043, USA. Months of issue are March, June, September, and December. Subscription prices are $282.00 per year (US individuals), $100.00 (US students), $337.00 (Canadian individuals), $100.00 (Canadian students), $398.00 (international individuals), and $175.00 (international students). For institutional access pricing please contact Customer Service via the contact information below. Foreign air speed delivery is included in all *Clinics* subscription prices. All prices are subject to change without notice. Orders will be billed at individual rate until proof of status is received. Foreign air speed delivery is included in all *Clinics* subscription prices. All prices are subject to change without notice. Orders, claims, and journal inquiries: Please visit our Support Hub page https://service.elsevier.com for assistance.

Reprints. For copies of 100 or more, of articles in this publication, please contact the Commercial Reprints Department, Elsevier Inc., 360 Park Avenue South, New York, NY 10010-1710. Tel. 212-633-3874; Fax: 212-633-3820; E-mail: reprints@elsevier.com.

Primary Care: Clinics in Office Practice is covered in *MEDLINE/PubMed (Index Medicus)* and *EMBASE/Excerpta Medica, Current Contents/Clinical Medicine,* and *ISI/BIOMED.*

Printed in the United States of America.

Contributors

CONSULTING EDITOR

JOEL J. HEIDELBAUGH, MD, FAAFP, FACG
Clinical Professor, Departments of Family Medicine and Urology, Director of Medical Student Education and Clerkship Director, Department of Family Medicine, University of Michigan Medical School, Ann Arbor, Michigan; Ypsilanti Health Center, Ypsilanti, Michigan

EDITORS

SARINA SCHRAGER, MD, MS
Professor, Department of Family Medicine and Community Health, University of Wisconsin, Madison, Wisconsin

HEATHER L. PALADINE, MD, MEd, FAAFP
Assistant Professor, Department of Medicine, Columbia University Irving Medical Center, Center for Family and Community Medicine, New York, New York

AUTHORS

EMILYN ANDERI, MD, MS
Faculty, Family Medicine Residency Program, Department of Family Medicine, Henry Ford Health, Detroit, Michigan

KARINA ATWELL, MD, MPH
Assistant Professor, Department of Family Medicine and Community Health, Family Medicine Residency Program, School of Medicine and Public Health, University of Wisconsin, Madison, Wisconsin

ROBIN BARRY, PhD
Associate Professor, Department of Family Medicine, University of Toledo, Toledo, Ohio

MAYA BASS, MD, MA, FAAFP
Program Director, Cooper/CMSRU Family Medicine Residency, Cooper University Hospital, Assistant Professor, Department of Family Medicine, Cooper Medical School of Rowan University, Camden, New Jersey

JOANNA TURNER BISGROVE, MD, FAAFP
Assistant Professor, Department of Family Medicine, Rush University Medical Center, Chicago, Illinois

LAURA BUJOLD, DO, MS
Assistant Professor, Department of Family Medicine, University of Connecticut School of Medicine, UCONN Family Medicine Residency Program, Hartford, Connecticut

JENSENA CARLSON, MD
Associate Professor, Department of Family Medicine and Community Health, University of Wisconsin School of Medicine and Public Health, Madison, Wisconsin

CHELSEA DANIELS, MD
Staff Physician, Department of Medical Services, Planned Parenthood of South, East and North Florida, Miami, Florida

MONICA DEMASI, MD, FAAFP
Associate Professor of Family Medicine, Providence Family Medicine Residency Program, Portland, Oregon

SHERRI ELDIN, DO, MFA
Communications and Media Consultant, Podcast Host, Creator and Co-Producer, Annals of Family Medicine, Providence, Rhode Island; PGY-1 Department of Family Medicine, Montefiore Medical Center/Albert Einstein College of Medicine, Bronx, New York

CHELSEA FASO, MD
Assistant Professor, Department of Family Medicine and Community Health, Mount Sinai Icahn School of Medicine, New York, New York

MANEESHA FINKLE, LMSW
Counselor, Department of Obstetrics and Gynecology, University of Michigan, Medical Social Worker and Sex Therapist, Center for Sexual Health, Ann Arbor, Michigan

SHERIDAN FINNIE, MD, MPH
PGY-3, Department of Family Medicine, University of North Carolina, Chapel Hill, North Carolina

KRYS FOSTER, MD, MPH, FAAFP
Associate Program Director, Thomas Jefferson University Family Medicine Residency, Thomas Jefferson University Hospital, Clinical Associate Professor, Department of Family and Community Medicine, Sidney Kimmel Medicine College at Thomas Jefferson University, Philadelphia, Pennsylvania

KELITA FOX, MD
Faculty, Department of Family Medicine Residency Program, Henry Ford Health, Detroit, Michigan

AURY V. GARCIA, MD
Assistant Professor of Family Medicine, Department of Internal Medicine, Center for Family and Community Medicine, Columbia University Irving Medical Center/New York Presbyterian Hospital, New York, New York

BRENNA GIBBONS, MD
Assistant Professor, Department of Family Medicine and Community Health, University of Wisconsin, Madison, Wisconsin

ERIN GILLESPIE, MD
Medical Writer and Editor, Integrative Medicine, Internal Medicine, Obesity Medicine, Leap Medical Writing and Editing LLC, Tijeras, New Mexico

HILARY GORTLER, MD, MS
Resident, Division of Family Medicine, Jefferson Einstein Philadelphia Hospital, Philadelphia, Pennsylvania

BETHANY HOWLETT, MD, MHS
Assistant Professor, Department of Family Medicine and Community Health, University of Wisconsin School of Medicine and Public Health, Madison, Wisconsin

NAFEEZA HUSSAIN, MD, MPH
Women's Health Fellow, Department of OBGYN, University of Michigan, Ann Arbor, Michigan

BRIAN P. KENEALY, MD, PhD
Assistant Professor, Department of Family Medicine and Community Health, University of Wisconsin- Madison, Madison, Wisconsin

ANNE KENNARD, DO, FACOG, FACLM
Diplomate ABOIM, Chief, Integrative and Lifestyle Medicine, Faculty, Department of Obstetrics and Gynecology, Marian Regional Medical Center, Santa Maria, California

LAURA KRUGER, MD
Clinical Assistant Professor, Department of Family Medicine, University of Michigan, Ann Arbor, Michigan

EMILY LANDIS, MSPAS
Assistant Professor, Department of Family Medicine, University of Toledo, Toledo, Ohio

RACHEL LEE, MD
Faculty, Family Medicine Residency Program, Department of Family Medicine, Henry Ford Health, Detroit, Michigan

JENNIFER E. LOCHNER, MD
Associate Professor, Department of Family Medicine and Community Health, University of Wisconsin- Madison, Madison, Wisconsin

JULIA LUBSEN, MD
Associate Professor, Department of Family Medicine and Community Health, University of Wisconsin, Madison, Wisconsin

ANDREA ILDIKO MARTONFFY, MD
Associate Professor, Department of Family Medicine and Community Health, University of Wisconsin, Madison, Wisconsin

BRIANNA MARZOLF, DO, MS
Clinical Assistant Professor and Disability Health Fellow, Department of Family Medicine, University of Michigan, Ann Arbor, Michigan

CORAL MATUS, MD
Associate Professor, Departments of Medical Education and Family Medicine, University of Toledo, Toledo, Ohio

REAGAN McKENDREE, MD
Faculty, Department of Family Medicine, Marian Regional Medical Center, Santa Maria, California

WILLIAM E. MICHAEL, MD
Assistant Professor, Department of Family Medicine and Community Health, Associate Program Director, Family Medicine Residency Program, School of Medicine and Public Health, University of Wisconsin, Madison, Wisconsin

KAREN MUCHOWSKI, MD, FAAFP
Family Physician, Graybill Medical Group, Temecula, California

VIKTORIYA OVSEPYAN, MD
Resident Physician, Department of Family Medicine and Community Health, University of Wisconsin School of Medicine and Public Health, UW Madison Family Medicine Residency Program, Madison, Wisconsin

HANNAH ROSENFIELD, MD
Director of Primary Care, Planned Parenthood of Michigan, Clinical Assistant Professor, Departments of OBGYN and Family Medicine, Western Michigan School of Medicine, Kalamazoo, Michigan

TAYLOR ROSS, MD
Faculty Physician, CoxHealth Family Medicine Residency Program, Springfield, Missouri

MARTHA SIMMONS, MD, FAAFP
Core Faculty, Division of Family Medicine, Jefferson Einstein Philadelphia Hospital, Philadelphia, Pennsylvania

JONATHAN SNYDER, MPAS
Assistant Professor, Department of Family Medicine, University of Toledo, Toledo, Ohio

LINDA SPEER, MD
Professor and Chair, Department of Family Medicine, University of Toledo, Toledo, Ohio

YORGOS STRANGAS, MD, MPH
Assistant Professor of Family Medicine, Department of Internal Medicine, Center for Family and Community Medicine, Columbia University Irving Medical Center/New York Presbyterian Hospital, New York, New York

JENNIFER SVARVERUD, DO, FAAFP
Assistant Professor, Department of Family Medicine and Community Health, School of Medicine and Public Health, University of Wisconsin, Family Medicine Residency Program, Madison, Wisconsin

LIBBY WETTERER, MD
Assistant Professor, Department of Family Medicine and Community Health, University of Pennsylvania, Philadelphia, Pennsylvania

Contents

Abnormal uterine bleeding (AUB) is experienced by nearly one-third of patients with a uterus and is commonly addressed in the primary care setting. Abnormal uterine bleeding, defined as deviations from the normal regularity, frequency, heaviness, or duration of flow, may be disruptive to daily life and often leads to secondary complications such as anemia and infertility. Causes and presentations of AUB vary across the lifecycle and the International Federation of Gynecology and Obstetrics System 2 mnemonic PALM-COEIN can assist in understanding both the structural and non-structural etiologies of abnormal uterine bleeding.

As primary care clinicians, it is important to recognize the causes of health disparities in our patients who are women of color in order to advocate and work toward true equity in health outcomes. This article strives to introduce this concept by presenting areas of inequity such as maternal mortality, management of pain, cardiovascular health, and breast cancer outcomes. Lastly, we will introduce a framework and actionable steps that can be taken to counteract the biases known to influence patient care.

This article serves as a resource for primary care providers to ensure equitable reproductive and sexual health care for patients with disabilities. It covers: Ensuring clinic accessibility; screening for abuse in women with disabilities and educating patients and families about safety, consent, healthy relationships, and boundaries; providing sexual health education to patients with disabilities; validating and affirming patients' identities in their roles as sexual beings, partners, and parents;menstrual management; health maintenance screenings tailored for individuals with disabilities.

PRIMARY CARE:
CLINICS IN OFFICE PRACTICE

SERIES OF RELATED INTEREST

Medical Clinics (http://www.medical.theclinics.com)
Physician Assistant Clinics (https://www.physicianassistant.theclinics.com)

THE CLINICS ARE AVAILABLE ONLINE!
Access your subscription at:
www.theclinics.com

Foreword

The Challenges in Reducing Disparities

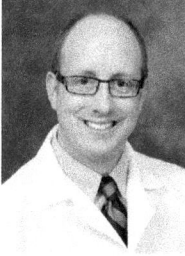

Joel J. Heidelbaugh, MD, FAAFP, FACG
Consulting Editor

Nearly every lecture, nearly every grand rounds presentation, nearly every manuscript, and nearly every patient encounter now include (and should) elements of social determinants of health and posit some strategy toward recognizing and improving health care disparities. While women's health has evolved into a very codified and well-recognized specialty than spans both primary and subspecialty care, the challenges in reducing health care disparities in women still exist and are at risk of being heightened. For example, a woman who presents to the emergency department is still less likely to be recognized as having a cardiovascular disease or acute event compared with a man. This issue of *Primary Care: Clinics of North America* explores a path toward understanding health care disparities through a focus on diverse women.

Pardon the cliché, but we live in very interesting times. As I pen this foreword, there are many uncertainties in our country that may impact the health care delivery and reproductive options for women. This issue of *Primary Care: Clinics of North America* provides a very timely article on the impact of the current political landscape on women's health, as well as materials on reproductive and sexual health of individuals with disabilities, contraception updates, abortion in primary care, and infertility. The remainder of the issue provides evidence-based updates on very commonly encountered elements of women's health, including guidance for management of chronic pain, mental health, and cancer screening. There are novel integrative medicine options for many conditions in women's health, as well as strategies for management of menopausal symptoms and cardiovascular disease.

Dr Sarina Schrager and Dr Heather Paladine are expert clinicians with practices focused on women's health and are also seasoned authors and medical editors. Together, they have crafted a comprehensive array of articles on salient topics in

Prim Care Clin Office Pract 52 (2025) xiii–xiv
https://doi.org/10.1016/j.pop.2025.03.002
0095-4543/25/© 2025 Published by Elsevier Inc.

primarycare.theclinics.com

women's health that will guide primary care clinicians toward delivering a higher level of care, especially in these uncertain times.

Joel J. Heidelbaugh, MD, FAAFP, FACG
Departments of Family Medicine
and Urology
University of Michigan Medical School
Ann Arbor, MI 48103, USA

Ypsilanti Health Center
200 Arnet, Suite 200
Ypsilanti, MI 48198, USA

E-mail address:
jheidel@umich.edu

Preface

A Broader Vision of Women's Health

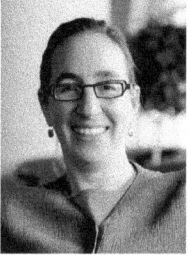

Sarina Schrager, MD, MS   Heather L. Paladine, MD, MEd, FAAFP
Editors

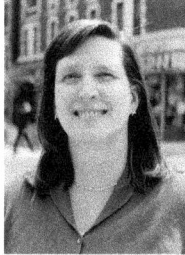

Our goal in editing this *Primary Care: Clinics of North America* issue on Women's Health was to cover common conditions that are unique to women or more common in women, as well as to discuss the impacts of social determinants of health on women's lived experiences. Historically, many medical texts have focused on the male patient as the standard and have not included differences in presentation or treatment in women. Medical conditions that are unique to women are often relegated to one chapter of a textbook or one lecture as part of a course. We believe that this is inadequate coverage for 51% of the US population.

The field of medicine has also focused on gender as a male/female binary and excluded the experiences of people who are transgender and gender nonconforming. Although this issue refers to the health of women, and most studies refer to women, primary care clinicians should be aware that these conditions affect transgender men and gender nonbinary people as well. A recent Pew Foundation survey[1] found that up to 1.6% of the US population identifies as transgender or nonbinary, and this may be as high as 5% of people under age 30. As our goal is to have inclusive practices that care for all individuals, we must be mindful of the needs of transgender/nonbinary patients as well. The articles that we have included attempt to highlight the health care needs of this population as well.

The broad topics included in this issue include both medical issues more common in women and also broader sociocultural issues that impact a woman's life and health, like the pandemic or politics. Many women are the health care steward for their entire family. As such, their own health takes a back seat to the health of their children, their parents, and even their partners. The environment a woman lives in can greatly impact her health. The ability to obtain healthy food or to walk outside without worrying about safety is integrally related to health. What country (or what state) a woman lives in can

Prim Care Clin Office Pract 52 (2025) xv–xvi
https://doi.org/10.1016/j.pop.2025.03.001
0095-4543/25/© 2025 Published by Elsevier Inc.

primarycare.theclinics.com

dictate her ability to obtain reliable contraception or abortion. The COVID-19 pandemic, with its differential levels of new responsibilities, affected women in many cases more than their male partners. Women were the "at-home" parent, monitoring children's schoolwork while also trying to work. It is not a surprise that while career advancement was common for many male workers, the opposite was true for many female workers.

The life-cycle model of women's health incorporates social and environmental factors in addition to biology to define what is happening at any given time during a woman's life. Biological life cycles are predicated on what is happening during the menstrual cycle. But a broader concept includes extrinsic factors as well. For example, a 15-year-old can be seen as an adolescent (with concerns of acne and dysmenorrhea), but if she becomes pregnant, then her health issues move quickly into the reproductive-age cohort. The physiology of the menstrual cycle becomes inherently a guide for a life-cycle model of women's health, but it is not the only factor that impacts health. This collection of articles attempts to cover the broad range of conditions more common in women, but to also provide a tapestry of the numerous issues that can influence a woman's health and her life.

DISCLOSURES

The authors have no conflicts of interest to disclose.

Sarina Schrager, MD, MS
Department of Family Medicine
and Community Health
University of Wisconsin
Madison, WI 53705, USA

Heather L. Paladine, MD, MEd, FAAFP
Department of Medicine
Columbia University Irving Medical Center
Center for Family and
Community Medicine
New York, NY 10032, USA

E-mail addresses:
sbschrag@wisc.edu (S. Schrager)
hlp222@gmail.com (H.L. Paladine)

REFERENCE

1. Pew Research Center. About 5% of young adults say their gender is different from their sex assigned at birth. 2022. Available at: https://www.pewresearch.org/short-reads/2022/06/07/about-5-of-young-adults-in-the-u-s-say-their-gender-is-different-from-their-sex-assigned-at-birth/. Accessed September 1, 2024.

Lifecycle Approach to Abnormal Uterine Bleeding

Bethany Howlett, MD, MHS[a],*, Viktoriya Ovsepyan, MD[b],
Taylor Ross, MD[c], Jensena Carlson, MD[a]

KEYWORDS

- Abnormal uterine bleeding • PALM-COEIN • PCOS • Postmenopausal bleeding

KEY POINTS

- Abnormal Uterine Bleeding (AUB) describes bleeding that deviates from the typical regularity, frequency, heaviness, or duration of flow in a patient's menstrual cycle.
- Sensitivity to the patient's story coupled with a thorough history is essential to prevent misdiagnosis and mitigate barriers to treatment.
- Causes of AUB can be classified using the PALM-COIEN mnemonic.
- The most common causes of AUB include ovulatory and anovulatory patterns.
- Treatment of AUB is based on age and cause and frequently includes hormonal therapy.

INTRODUCTION

Abnormal uterine bleeding (AUB) is experienced by nearly one-third of patients with a uterus and is commonly addressed in the primary care setting (**Fig. 1**). The definition and presentation of AUB varies through the life cycle depending on the expected menstrual patterns of each age group. Generally, AUB is defined as deviations from the normal regularity, frequency, heaviness, or duration of flow.[1,2] The severity of AUB can range from annoyance to emergent; however, it is universally disruptive to daily life and often leads to secondary complications such as anemia and infertility.[3,4] Factors that delay a patient presenting for treatment include lack of knowledge around normal menstrual cycles, fear of discussing a "taboo" subject, and negative experiences with health care professionals.[5,6] In addition to patience in exploring the history, ruling out nonhormonal causes, and performing a physical examination

[a] Department of Family Medicine and Community Health, University of Wisconsin School of Medicine and Public Health, 610 North Whitney Way Suite 200, Madison, WI 53705, USA;
[b] Department of Family Medicine and Community Health, UW Madison Family Medicine Residency Program, University of Wisconsin School of Medicine and Public Health, 610 North Whitney Way Suite 200, Madison, WI 53705, USA; [c] CoxHealth Family Medicine Residency Program, 3800 South National Avenue, Suite 610, Springfield, MO 65807, USA
* Corresponding author.
E-mail address: bethany.howlett@fammed.wisc.edu

Prim Care Clin Office Pract 52 (2025) 181–192
https://doi.org/10.1016/j.pop.2024.12.003
primarycare.theclinics.com
0095-4543/25/© 2025 Elsevier Inc. All rights reserved, including those for text and data mining, AI training, and similar technologies.

Abbreviations	
AUB	abnormal uterine bleeding
CBC	complete blood count
COC	combined oral contraceptive pill
FIGO	International Federation of Gynecology and Obstetrics
hCG	human chorionic gonadotropin
HPO	hypothalamic-pituitary-ovarian axis
HRT	hormone replacement therapy
IUD	intrauterine device
PALM-COEIN	polyps, adenomyosis, leiomyomas, malignancy, coagulopathies, ovulatory dysfunction, endometrial disorders, iatrogenic, and not yet classified
PCOS	polycystic ovary syndrome
PT	prothrombin time
PTT	partial thromboplastin time
TSH	thyroid-stimulating hormone
TVUS	transvaginal ultrasound
US	ultrasound

and appropriate testing, understanding the pathophysiology of the menstrual cycle is key to successfully managing AUB. Abnormal uterine bleeding can be classified into structural and nonstructural etiologies using the International Federation of Gynecology and Obstetrics (FIGO) System 2 acronym PALM-COEIN,[7] described in **Tables 1–3**. The PALM (polyps, adenomyosis, leiomyomas, and malignancy) designation describes structural causes of AUB and the COEIN (coagulopathies, ovulatory dysfunction, endometrial disorders, iatrogenic, and not yet classified) describes nonstructural causes of AUB.

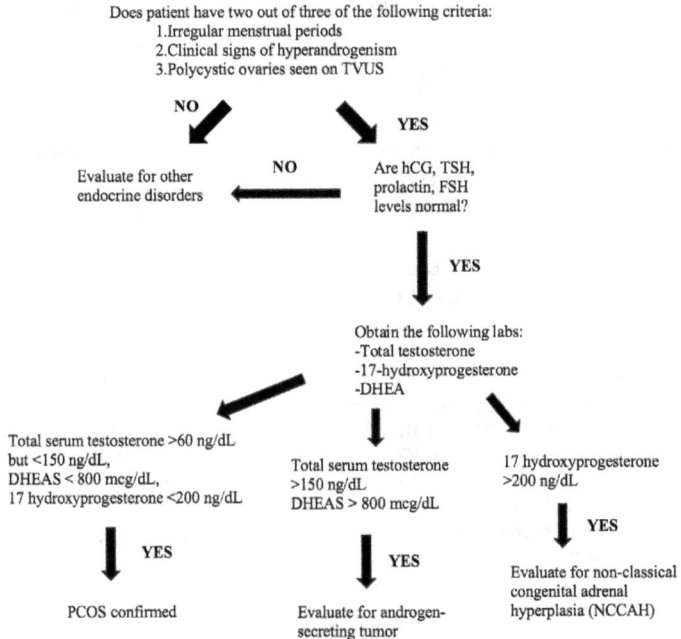

Fig. 1. Evaluation for polycystic ovary syndrome.

Table 1
Abnormal uterine bleeding – polyps, adenomyosis, leiomyomas, malignancy, coagulopathies, ovulatory dysfunction, endometrial disorders, iatrogenic, and not yet classified (PALM COEIN) mnemonic

Differential Diagnosis	Clinical History	Initial Work-Up
PALM (structural causes)		
Polyps	May cause postcoital bleeding, intermenstrual spotting. Cervical polyps may be seen on examination.	Pelvic examination[a] & pelvic ultrasound
Adenomyosis	Heavy menstrual bleeding, painful menses, and chronic pelvic pain may be present. An enlarged, boggy, tender uterus may be felt on examination.	Pelvic examination & US or MRI
Leiomyomas	Heavy or prolonged menstrual bleeding, bulk-related symptoms such as pelvic pressure and pain, and reproductive dysfunction such as infertility or miscarriage may be present. Uterus may feel enlarged on examination.	Pelvic examination & US
Malignancy	Risk factors for endometrial neoplasia include older age and exposure to unopposed estrogen and chronic disease (eg: obesity, anovulation, PCOS, estrogen replacement therapy, tamoxifen, HTN, DM).	Pelvic examination & US, pap smear, endometrial biopsy in patients > 45 y or in patients w/risks for endometrial neoplasia
COEIN (non-structural causes)		
Coagulopathies VWD Thrombocytopenia Platelet function disorders Clotting factor deficiencies	• Family hx of abnormal bleeding or bleeding disorder • Personal hx of heavy menstrual bleeding since menarche, frequent bruising, bleeding gums, epistaxis, postpartum hemorrhage, or bleeding with surgical and dental procedures	CBC, PT/PTT, fibrinogen VWD: VWF Ag, VWF functional assay, Factor 8 activity Platelet function testing – consult hematology
Ovulatory Dysfunction	• Hx of eating disorder	• TSH, prolactin, urine hCG

(continued on next page)

Table 1
(continued)

Differential Diagnosis	Clinical History	Initial Work-Up
Immature HPO axis, Relative energy deficiency in sport, Eating disorder, obesity, primary ovarian insufficiency Endocrine Disorders: PCOS, thyroid disease, adrenal insufficiency, Cushing's, nonclassic CAH, hyperprolactinemia	• Primary ovarian insufficiency: Hot flashes, vaginal dryness, bone loss/osteoporosis • PCOS, nonclassic CAH: hirsutism, excessive acne, male pattern baldness • Cushing's: Resistant HTN, osteoporosis, striae, proximal myopathy	• PCOS: check androgen levels if diagnosis unclear • Primary ovarian insufficiency: check FSH, estradiol • Cushing's: Check cortisol
Endometrial disorders Endometriosis Endometritis	• Family hx of endometriosis • Personal hx of chronic pelvic pain, severe dysmenorrhea, dyspareunia, bowel/bladder dysfunction • Risk factors for pelvic inflammatory disease	Pelvic examination to check for cervical motion tenderness, uterine tenderness, chlamydia/gonorrhea/trichomoniasis laboratorys
Iatrogenic Hormonal contraception, anticoagulants, steroids, antipsychotics, antidepressants, tamoxifen	• Hx of irregular hormonal contraceptive use • Hx of recent contraceptive initiation • Hx of taking SSRIs, TCAs, antipsychotics	Consider pelvic examination or TVUS to ensure IUD is in place
Not yet classified Cesarean scar defect, arteriovenous malformations	• Hx of postmenstrual spotting • AUB refractory to hormonal management	Pelvic US AVM: US w/dopplers

DM, diabetes mellitus; HTN, hypertension; hx, history; SSRI, selective serotonin reuptake inhibitor; VWF, Von Willebrand factor.
^a Pelvic examination should include a speculum and bimanual examination. It's important to examine all potential bleeding sites, including the vagina, cervix, urethra, perineum, and anus. Pelvic examination can be deferred in adolescents if the patient is not sexually active, trauma and infection is not suspected, and response to initial treatment is adequate.

Table 2
Medical management of abnormal uterine bleeding

Drug	Dose	Notes
Acute Bleeding		
Conjugated equine estrogen	2.5 mg orally every 6 h for 21 d or 25 mg IV every 4-6 h for 24 h	Follow treatment with a progestin to provoke withdrawal bleeding; do not use in patients at increased risk of thrombosis
Estrogen-progestin oral contraceptives	1 monophasic pill containing 35 mcg of ethinyl estradiol orally 3 times daily for 7 d	Do not use in patients at increased risk of thrombosis
Norethindrone acetate	5–10 mg one to four times a day for 5–10 d	Used for treatment in patients with contraindications to estrogen
Medroxyprogesterone acetate	10–20 mg three times a day for 5–10 d	Used for treatment in patients with contraindications to estrogen
Tranexamic acid	1300 mg three times daily for up to 5 d	Do not use in patients at increased risk of thrombosis
Chronic Bleeding		
Medroxyprogesterone acetate (Depo Provera)	150 mg IM or 104 mg subq every 13 wk or 5–20 mg pills per day in 1–3 divided doses	Irregular bleeding is common in first 3 mo of using Depo-Provera injection but ~ 50% of patients become amenorrheic after 12 mo of use
Estrogen-progestin oral contraceptives	1 monophasic pill containing 35 mcg of ethinyl estradiol daily	Other routes (transdermal patch, intravaginal ring) are likely also effective
Levonorgestrel	52 mg IUD	Irregular bleeding is common in the first 3 mo of use, but ~ 20% of patients become amenorrheic after 12 mo of use
Norethindrone	5–15 mg per day in 1–3 divided doses	Continuous use is preferred due to increased efficacy and patient adherence
Tranexamic Acid	1300 mg three times daily for up to 5 d during monthly menstruation	Do not use in patients at increased risk of thrombosis
Nonsteroidal antiinflammatory drugs	Naproxen 500 mg orally 2 times daily or ibuprofen 600–800 mg every 6–8 h	Administer only while patient is bleeding; do not use in patients with coagulopathy

Table 3
Abnormal uterine bleeding - differential diagnosis and treatment overview

Most Common Causes of Abnormal Uterine Bleeding	Differential Diagnosis	Treatment
Adolescents		
Anovulation Coagulopathies	Late onset 21 hydroxylase deficiency Hyperprolactinemia Iatrogenic Infection PCOS Pregnancy Restrictive eating disorders Thyroid dysfunction Trauma	Combined oral contraception
Reproductive-age patients		
Ovulatory Dysfunction PCOS	Coagulopathies Hyperprolactinemia Iatrogenic Infection Malignant neoplasm Nonuterine bleeding PCOS Pregnancy Restrictive eating disorders Structural Systemic disease Thyroid dysfunction Trauma	Ovulatory inducing agents Medroxyprogesterone
Perimenopausal patients		
Structural Iatrogenic	Coagulopathies Hyperprolactinemia Infection Malignant neoplasm Nonuterine bleeding Pregnancy Systemic disease Thyroid dysfunction Trauma	Oral contraception
Menopausal patients		
Endometrial cancer Structural	Coagulopathies Hyperprolactinemia Infection Malignant neoplasm Nonuterine bleeding Pregnancy Systemic disease Thyroid dysfunction Trauma	Continuous combined HRT Cyclic HRT

A lifecycle approach to AUB is predicated on the fact that similar bleeding patterns can be caused by different etiologies (sometimes normal and sometimes pathologic) depending on a person's age and menstrual status. For example, anovulation is common in adolescents during the first 18 to 24 months after menses starts, is common in perimenopausal women leading up to the menopausal transition, but is abnormal in reproductive aged women.

Abnormal Uterine Bleeding Assessment Overview

1. Obtain a history of the bleeding using FIGO-AUB system 1: frequency, duration, regularity, flow volume, intermenstrual bleeding, and unscheduled bleeding on hormone therapy. Documenting the volume of menstrual flow is inconsistent and unreliable but often is described as how many tampons or pads a person uses during a day, whether they need to wake up at night to change their tampon or pad, and how often they "overflow" their protection.
2. Obtain a medical, surgical, and medication history.
3. Obtain a family history with a focus on gynecologic malignancy, age of menopause onset, and presence of bleeding disorders.
4. Complete a speculum examination with pap smear (if due) and bimanual examination (to feel for any uterine abnormalities).
5. Consider an endometrial biopsy (if $\geq$45 yrs) after a negative pregnancy test (in women with heavy bleeding or postmenopausal).
6. Consider relevant laboratory tests and imaging:
   a. History of heavy bleeding: complete blood count (CBC), prothrombin time (PT), partial thromboplastin time (PTT), TVUS (transvaginal ultrasound); test for Von Willebrand's disease in adolescents with heavy bleeding.
   b. Human chorionic gonadotropin (hCG).
   c. Anovulation: thyroid-stimulating hormone (TSH), prolactin
7. Consider obstetrician/gynecologist referral if surgical intervention is desired or diagnosis is unclear.

Abnormal uterine bleeding among adolescents

Case: A 15-year-old presents to the clinic with concerns for fatigue. She has been having irregular periods since going through menarche at age 12 and thinks that periods are "normal" in flow. Her BMI is 22 and she is not sexually active.

AUB affects 3% to 20% of reproductive-aged females, with a higher incidence in adolescents.[8]

The mean age of menarche is 12 to 13 year old and typically occurs within 2 to 2.5 years of thelarche.[9] The normal volume of menstruation is 3 to 6 pads or tampons daily.[9] About 34% to 37% of adolescents experience heavy menstrual bleeding, which is defined as menses that last more than 7 days or that requires changing a sanitary product every 1 to 2 hours.[10,11] Bleeding disorders (such as Von Willebrand's disease) should be considered in adolescents with heavy menstrual bleeding. It is normal for adolescents to experience anovulatory cycles for the first 2 to 3 years after menarche, as the hypothalamic-pituitary-ovarian (HPO) axis matures. By year 3 after menarche, 60% to 80% of adolescents report a regular cycle, although it can take up to 5 to 6 years for 95% of adolescents.[9] Among adolescents, nonstructural causes of AUB are more common, with ovulatory dysfunction accounting for 90% of AUB, often due to immaturity of the HPO axis.[9,12,13]

It is reasonable to pursue work-up for AUB among adolescents who have anovulatory cycles lasting more than 2 to 3 years after menarche, or who experience heavy menstrual bleeding that is affecting their quality of life.[9,14] Among patients who are taking a combined oral contraceptive pill (COC), AUB is common in the first 3 to 6 months of use.[15] If menses are cyclic but heavy in volume or duration, clinicians should evaluate for a coagulopathy disorder, especially since research shows that 20% to 53% of adolescents with AUB or heavy menstrual bleeding have an underlying bleeding disorder, compared with 1% to 2% of the general population.[12,16] Structural causes of AUB (such as leiomyomas or adenomyosis) among adolescents are rare, with one study showing that structural causes were seen in only 1.3% of adolescents who received a pelvic ultrasound (US) for evaluation of AUB.[17] Refer to **Table 1** for details.

Treatment of AUB in adolescents is based on the effect of symptoms on a person's daily life. Watchful waiting in someone with anovulation (after exclusion of secondary causes such as thyroid dysfunction and pregnancy) is appropriate. Many adolescents elect to use some type of hormonal contraception which can regulate their menstrual bleeding as well as provide contraception.

Case Conclusion: On further history the patient discloses periods lasting 8 days with at least 3 to 4 days where she experiences 7 saturated "heavy" tampons with leakage. You want to screen for relative energy deficiency in sport (which is the new name for the female athlete triad). The patient is not exercising outside of her swim team practices, has not lost weight, and demonstrates a healthy body image. Evaluation for coagulopathy is normal and CBC demonstrates mild iron deficiency anemia. She elects to initiate combined oral contraceptives and an iron supplement with plan to follow up in 3 months.

Abnormal uterine bleeding among reproductive-age patients

Case: A 28-year-old presents to the clinic with irregular menstrual cycles since coming off her COC 3 months ago with the goal of conception. She reports that she was initially started on COCs as a teenager for irregular bleeding.

Similar to adolescents, ovulatory dysfunction is the most common cause of AUB in reproductive-age patients. However, among adults, the most common cause of ovulatory dysfunction is polycystic ovary syndrome (PCOS). PCOS is one of the most common endocrine disorders among women, affecting 5% to 10% of reproductive-age patients.[18] PCOS is primarily a clinical diagnosis, based on the presence of at least 2 of the 3 Rotterdam criteria: oligo or anovulation, clinical evidence of hyperandrogenism, and polycystic ovaries on ultrasound. Women with PCOS typically have fewer than 9 menstrual periods in a year or no menstrual period for 3 or more consecutive months, with irregular menses typically beginning in teenage years. Patients also typically have clinical signs of hyperandrogenism, including hirsutism (excess hair growth on chin, upper lip, midsternum, periareolar area, along linea alba of lower abdomen), acne, and male-pattern hair loss. About 40% to 85% of patients with PCOS are also overweight.[19] The pathophysiology of PCOS is complex and includes genetic and environmental factors that contribute to insulin resistance, hormonal imbalance, and chronic low grade inflammation which impair folliculogenesis and increase the risk of developing comorbidities such as cardiovascular disease, dyslipidemia, fatty liver, and obstructive sleep apnea. PCOS is a clinical diagnosis but further testing to exclude a pathologic cause of increased testosterone or dehydroepiandrosterone is indicated if symptoms have accelerated or are new. In that case, evaluation to rule out adrenal or ovarian causes of masculinizing hormones is important. See **Table 1** for details.

Treatment of a person with PCOS depends on their reproductive goals. In people who do not want to get pregnant, use of hormonal contraception (COCs) can help regulate menstrual cycles as well as improve some symptoms of hyperandrogenism. The use of hormonal intrauterine devices (IUDs) may also be beneficial in managing abnormal uterine bleeding. People with PCOS will often have unopposed estrogen due to anovulation. It is important to provide interventions to protect the endometrium (such as a progestin IUD, a COC, or cyclic progesterone withdrawal). People should have withdrawal bleeds at least 4 times a year. For people who want to conceive, treatment with ovulation induction with clomiphene or letrozole may be indicated.

Hormonal contraceptives are a common cause of iatrogenic (PALM-COIEN) AUB in this age group. AUB is common in the first 3 to 6 months after starting a combined oral contraceptive pill and approximately 35% of patients who have a levonorgestrel IUD placed experience frequent or prolonged bleeding the first 3 months, although bleeding decreases within 12 months for 90% of patients.[20] Among patients with the Nexplanon progestin subcutaneous implant, AUB may occur for up to 23% users and is less likely to improve with time.[21] The depo-medroxyprogesterone acetate injection may cause longer menses in the first 3 months in 26% of patients, but similar to the IUD, AUB improves by 12 months for about 85% of patients.[22,23]

Case Conclusion: The patient reports that she has also struggled with acne and excessive facial hair. Her BMI is 31 and vital signs are otherwise normal. Laboratorys including hCG, TSH, prolactin and follicle stimulating hormone (FSH) are normal. She meets criteria for PCOS. She has normal lipids, HgAIC, and her pelvic ultrasound demonstrates multiple cysts around the periphery of her ovaries. You discuss starting her on metformin and ovulation induction (letrozole or clomiphene) and suggest referral to a reproductive endocrinologist if she is not pregnant in 6 to 12 months.

Abnormal uterine bleeding among perimenopausal patients

Case: A 48-year-old presents to the clinic with recent intermenstrual bleeding over the last year. She had been using a progestin IUD for contraception for most of her post-childbearing life but this was removed about 3 years ago after her divorce. She is getting a period every 2 weeks.

Perimenopause is often a time of irregular bleeding for those with a uterus. Anovulatory bleeding secondary to the onset of menopause is a common cause of abnormal uterine bleeding in the perimenopausal period, which begins at age 47 on average.[24] The menopausal transition begins with a persistent difference of 7 days or more in the length of cycles or skipped cycles.[24] In the late stages, menses may be spaced out 60 or more days and is associated with vasomotor symptoms.[24]

Perimenopause is diagnosed reliably based on symptoms, including changes in menstruation and vasomotor symptoms, but should be treated as a diagnosis of exclusion when assessing AUB. Menopause is diagnosed as amenorrhea for 12 consecutive months. FSH levels vary widely for those in perimenopause or combined hormonal contraceptives; for this reason, FSH is not recommended as a screening test for menopause.[24] FSH may be used to assess menopause status and the need for continued contraception in those who are over 50 years, amenorrheic, and on progesterone-only contraceptives for more than 6 weeks.[19] If the FSH is greater than 30 nmol/L, the patient should remain on contraceptives for 1 year and then menopause is assumed.

Structural lesions (PALM) are common during the perimenopausal period, although nonstructural (COEIN) causes of abnormal bleeding are also important to consider. Leiomyomas are more common as people age, for example, coagulopathies and the associated abnormal uterine bleeding continue in perimenopausal individuals. Providers should assess pregnancy risk in all people who present with abnormal bleeding. Medications such as hormonal contraceptives, therapeutic anticoagulation, Non-steroidal anti-inflammatory drugs, ginkgo, ginseng, motherwort, dopamine agonists, and estrogen modulators can trigger bleeding. Follicular phase dark bleeding may point toward a cesarean scar defect (CSD) in patients with relevant surgical history.[25] Heavy cyclic bleeding should prompt suspicion for coagulopathies, leiomyoma, adenomyosis, and other endometrial disorders. Evaluation for heavy cyclic bleeding includes CBC, hCG, a pelvic ultrasound to look for structural abnormalities, and commonly an endometrial biopsy.

Irregular periods secondary to anovulatory cycles of perimenopause may be challenging to differentiate from intermenstrual bleeding suspicious for malignancy, hyperplasia, or other structural etiology. Due to this, endometrial biopsy is the first-line test for patients older than 45 years experiencing abnormal uterine bleeding. Transvaginal ultrasound is useful for identifying structural issues such as polyps, adenomyosis, leiomyomas, and cesarean scar defects. However, due to the varying thickness of the endometrial stripe in cycling individuals, TVUS cannot definitiely rule out malignancy.

Case Conclusion: The patient reports that her mother and older sister went through menopause around age 50, and there is no family history of endometrial cancer. She does report night sweats and fatigue. Her CBC, TSH, and urine hCG were normal and TVUS did not show uterine fibroids. With shared decision making, you elect to forgo an endometrial biopsy as it is likely she is in perimenopause. She elects to have a progesterone IUD replaced to help manage bleeding symptoms for the foreseeable future.

Postmenopausal bleeding

Case: A 75-year-old with a history of depression, anxiety, hypothyroidism, and hypertension presents to clinic with uterine bleeding after 25 years without cycles.

AUB after menopause is defined as bleeding that occurs 1 year after amenorrhea resulting from loss of follicular activity. Vaginal atrophy is the most common cause of AUB in this age group, with polyps being the second most common cause.[26] Leiomyomas tend to regress in size during menopause without estrogen and progesterone, although new fibroids may still occur. Around 10% of women with abnormal bleeding will have endometrial cancer, with bleeding as the primary presentation in 95% of cases.[27] Coagulopathies again persist into this age and may be exacerbated by anticoagulation for other medical conditions. People receiving hormone therapy to manage menopausal symptoms commonly experience uterine bleeding. Bleeding occurs in around 50% of these individuals and resolves around 6 months after initiation.[27]

In postmenopausal individuals, transvaginal ultrasound has a 99% negative predictive value for endometrial cancer if the endometrial thickness of 4 mm or less.[28] Endometrial sampling could be considered if abnormalities are identified or the endometrial stripe is thickened. When endometrial sampling is negative for hyperplasia or cancer but symptoms remain, a referral for hysteroscopy or dilation and curettage is recommended.[27]

Case Conclusion: The patient does have a history of hormone replacement therapy (HRT) use during perimenopause. She has a TSH at goal for treatment and mild iron deficiency anemia. TVUS demonstrates an endometrial thickness of 3 mm with an 8 mm submucosal leiomyoma. An endometrial biopsy is negative. Following a discussion of risks and benefits, the patient elects to follow up in clinic for routine care and will call if further bleeding recurs.

SUMMARY

It is essential that clinicians approach the patient presenting with AUB systematically with a thorough and open approach. Given the patterns associated with AUB within each life cycle, familiarizing one's self with common causes, differential diagnoses, and treatments can facilitate patient care. Determination about further laboratory testing, imaging, and procedural intervention are determined by patient age and history and guided by the differential represented by the PALM-COEIN mnemonic. Nonstructural AUB is most frequently managed with hormonal therapies.

CLINICS CARE POINTS

- Abnormal uterine bleeding (AUB) is the preferred nomenclature for bleeding that deviates from the typical regularity, frequency, heaviness, or duration of flow in a patient's menstrual cycle.
- Sensitivity to the patient's story coupled with a thorough history is essential to prevent misdiagnosis and mitigate barriers to treatment.
- Causes of AUB can be classified using the PALM-COIEN mnemonic.
- The most common causes of AUB include ovulatory and anovulatory patterns.
- Treatment of AUB is based on age and cause, although frequently includes hormonal therapy.

DISCLOSURE

The authors have nothing to disclose.

REFERENCES

1. Wong M, Crnobrnja B, Liberale V, et al. The natural history of endometrial polyps. Hum Reprod 2017;32(2):340–5.
2. Upson K, Missmer SA. Epidemiology of adenomyosis. Semin Reprod Med 2020; 38(2–03):89–107.
3. Wise LA, Laughlin-Tommaso SK. Epidemiology of uterine fibroids: from menarche to menopause. Clin Obstet Gynecol 2016;59(1):2–24.
4. Ghosh S, Naftalin J, Imrie R, et al. Natural history of uterine fibroids: a radiological perspective. Curr Obstet Gynecol Rep 2018;7(3):117–21.
5. SEERExplorer. Corpus and Uterus. SEER incidence age-adjusted incidence rates, 2017-2021. Available at: https://seer.cancer.gov/statistics-network/explorer/. Accessed June 22, 2024.
6. SEERExplorer. Cervix Uteri. SEER incidence Age-Adjusted Incidence Rates, 2017-2021. https://seer.cancer.gov/statistics-network/explorer/. Accessed June 22, 2024.
7. Munro MG. Practical aspects of the two FIGO systems for management of abnormal uterine bleeding in the reproductive years. Best Pract Res Clin Obstet Gynaecol 2017;40:3–22.
8. Munro MG, Critchley HOD, Fraser IS, FIGO Menstrual Disorders Committee. The two FIGO systems for normal and abnormal uterine bleeding symptoms and classification of causes of abnormal uterine bleeding in the reproductive years: 2018 revisions. Int J Gynaecol Obstet 2018;143:393–408.
9. Kabra R, Fisher M. Abnormal uterine bleeding in adolescents. Curr Probl Pediatr Adolesc Health Care 2022;52(5):101185.
10. Pike M, Chopek A, Young NL, et al. Quality of life in adolescents with heavy menstrual bleeding: validation of the adolescent menstrual bleeding questionnaire (aMBQ). Res Pract Thromb Haemost 2021;5(7):e12615.
11. Menstruation in girls and adolescents: using the menstrual cycle as a vital sign. Committee Opinion No. 651. American College of Obstetricians and Gynecologists. Obstet Gynecol 2015;126:e143–6.
12. Emans SJH, Laufer MR, DiVasta AD, et al. Goldstein's pediatric & adolescent Gynecology. 7th edition. Lippincott Williams & Wilkins, (PA): Wolters Kluwer; 2020.

13. Slap GB. Menstrual disorders in adolescence. Best Pract Res Clin Obstet Gynaecol 2003;17(1):75–92.

14. Haamid F, Sass AE, Dietrich JE. Heavy menstrual bleeding in adolescents. J Pediatr Adolesc Gynecol 2017;30(3):335–40. https://doi.org/10.1016/j.jpag.2017.01.002 [published correction appears in J Pediatr Adolesc Gynecol. 2017 Dec;30(6): 665. doi: 10.1016/j.jpag.2017.06.004].

15. Schrager S, Fox K, Lee R. Abnormal uterine bleeding associated with hormonal contraception. Am Fam Physician 2024;109(2):161–6.

16. ACOG Committee Opinion No. 785: screening and management of bleeding disorders in adolescents with heavy menstrual bleeding. Obstet Gynecol 2019; 134(3):e71–83.

17. Pecchioli Y, Oyewumi L, Allen LM, et al. The utility of routine ultrasound in the diagnosis and management of adolescents with abnormal uterine bleeding. J Pediatr Adolesc Gynecol 2017;30(2):239–42.

18. Munro MG, Critchley H, Fraser IS. Research and clinical management for women with abnormal uterine bleeding in the reproductive years: more than PALM-COEIN. BJOG 2017;124(2):185–9.

19. Wouk N, Helton M. Abnormal uterine bleeding in premenopausal women. Am Fam Physician 2019;99(7):435–43.

20. Friedlander E, Kaneshiro B. Therapeutic options for unscheduled bleeding associated with long-acting reversible contraception. Obstet Gyne- col Clin North Am 2015;42(4):593–603.

21. Mansour D, Korver T, Marintcheva-Petrova M, et al. The effects of Implanon on menstrual bleeding patterns. Eur J Contracept Reprod Health Care 2008;13(suppl 1): 13–28.

22. Berenson AB, Odom SD, Breitkopf CR, et al. Physiologic and psychologic symptoms associated with use of injectable contraception and 20 microg oral contraceptive pills. Am J Obstet Gynecol 2008;199(4):351.e1-12.

23. Munro MG, Critchley HO, Broder MS, et al. FIGO classification system (PALM-COEIN) for causes of abnormal uterine bleeding in nongravid women of reproductive age. Int J Gynaecol Obstet 2011;113(1):3–13.

24. Delamater L, Santoro N. Management of the perimenopause. Clin Obstet Gynecol 2018;61(3):419–32.

25. Jain V, Munro MG, Critchley HOD. Contemporary evaluation of women and girls with abnormal uterine bleeding: FIGO Systems 1 and 2. Int J Gynaecol Obstet 2023; 162(Suppl 2):29–42.

26. Marnach ML, Laughlin-Tommaso SK. Evaluation and management of abnormal uterine bleeding. Mayo Clin Proc 2019;94(2):326–35. https://doi.org/10.1016/j.mayocp. 2018.12.012.

27. Sakna NA, Elgendi M, Salama MH, et al. Diagnostic accuracy of endometrial sampling tests for detecting endometrial cancer: a systematic review and meta-analysis. BMJ Open 2023;13(6):e072124.

28. Smith PP, O'Connor S, Gupta J, et al. Recurrent postmenopausal bleeding: a prospective cohort study. J Minim Invasive Gynecol 2014;21(5):799–803.

Understanding Health Care Disparities

A Focus on Diverse Women

Maya Bass, MD, MA[a,b],*, Krys Foster, MD, MPH[c,d]

KEYWORDS

- Women's health • Health disparities • Cardiovascular health • Maternal mortality
- Breast cancer disparities • Reproductive justice • Implicit bias

KEY POINTS

- Racial Bias and Racism are linked to health disparities in communities of color.
- For Women, these inequalities are especially evident: that is, maternal mortality, management of pain, cardiovascular health, and breast cancer outcomes.
- As Primary care clinicians, it is critical that we recognize the causes of these health disparities and use an intersectionality framework to advocate and work toward true equity in health outcomes for our patients of color.

INTRODUCTION

There is a stark difference in mortality and morbidity experienced by women of color (WOC) in America. We suggest that you reflect on your own identity and how it, as well as your lived experiences, including your medical education, may affect the way that this information impacts you as you read this article. **Table 1** below defines key terms essential for your review of subsequent sections of the article.

Healthcare Disparities

The United States is increasingly diverse. Approximately 42% of the population belongs to a racial or ethnic minority according to the 2020 US Census.[3] Despite

---

[a] Cooper/CMSRU Family Medicine Residency, Cooper University Hospital; [b] Department of Family Medicine, Cooper Medical School of Rowan University, 101 Haddon Avenue, Suite 204, Camden, NJ 08103, USA; [c] Thomas Jefferson University Family Medicine Residency, Thomas Jefferson University Hospital; [d] Department of Family and Community Medicine, Sidney Kimmel Medicine College at Thomas Jefferson University, 1015 Walnut Street, Suite 401, Philadelphia, PA 19107, USA
* Corresponding author. Department of Family Medicine, Cooper Medical School of Rowan University, 101 Haddon Avenue, Suite 204, Camden, NJ 08103.
E-mail address: Bass-Maya@Cooperhealth.edu
Twitter: @MayaBassMD; @DrKFosterMD

Prim Care Clin Office Pract 52 (2025) 193–203
https://doi.org/10.1016/j.pop.2024.12.004
primarycare.theclinics.com

Abbreviations	
BW	Black women
L/H	Latinx/Hispanic
MI	myocardial infarction
MM	maternal mortality
NH	non-Hispanic
NIH	National Institutes of Health
PCOS	polycystic ovarian syndrome
WOC	women of color

many health indicators improving, certain minority groups bear a disproportionate burden of avoidable disease, death and disability compared to nonminority populations. For instance, in 2017, the life expectancy at birth of a non-Hispanic (NH) Black woman was only 77.9 years, compared to 81.0 years for an NH White woman (**Fig. 1**).[4]

The Historical Basis for Health Inequities in the United States

In order to address health inequities, clinicians should review the timeline of policies and events that occurred, and consider why we, as a health care system, have not earned the trust of communities of color. There is a complex history that contributes to mistrust among many populations when engaging with health care systems.

Medical harm
Examples of ethically unjustified studies and research misconduct are covered later in this text (eg, The US Public Health Service untreated syphilis study at Tuskegee, and use of the cancer cells of Henrietta Lacks without the patient's or family's knowledge or consent), but highlight the legacy of broken trust between Americans, particularly Black Americans, and the medical establishment.

Lack of representation in medical research
The lack of adequate representation of women, especially WOC, in clinical trials limits medical understanding and contributes to health inequities and social injustice.[5]

In 1977, the Federal Drug Administration issued guidelines excluding reproductive-age women from early-phase clinical research unless they faced life-threatening conditions in response to birth defects caused by prior research on thalidomide. This further reduced poor representation and lead to diagnoses and treatments based on male-only trials.[6] For example, The New England Journal of Medicine's 1989 study establishing that aspirin reduced the risk of myocardial infarction (MI) was based on 22,071 participants but notably, no women.[7] Additionally, the landmark Framingham

Table 1 Important definitions	
Health Inequities	Differences in health outcomes that are *systematic, avoidable, and unjust*[1] arise from systematic discrimination or exclusion due to societal barriers, are often *patterned*, and are not caused by patients.
Implicit (or unconscious) Bias	*The automatic activation of stereotypes derived from common cultural experiences, which may override deliberate thought and influence one's judgment in unintentional and unrecognized ways and may affect communication behaviors and treatment decisions.*[2]
Social Determinants of Health	*The conditions in the environments where people are born, live, learn, work, play, worship, and age that affect a wide range of health, functioning, and quality-of-life outcomes and risks.*[1]

Health Disparities in Women in the US
Created with Data from Chin et al, 2021

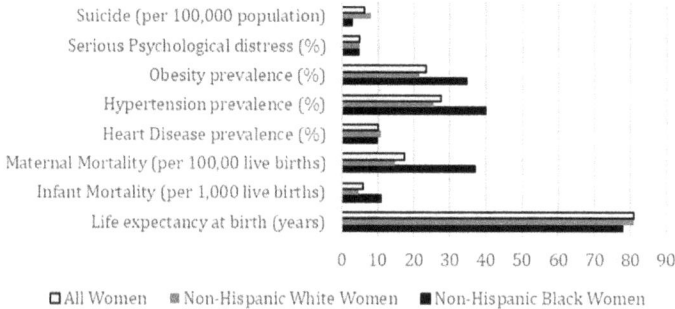

Suicide (per 100,000 population)
Serious Psychological distress (%)
Obesity prevalence (%)
Hypertension prevalence (%)
Heart Disease prevalence (%)
Maternal Mortality (per 100,00 live births)
Infant Mortality (per 1,000 live births)
Life expectancy at birth (years)

0   10   20   30   40   50   60   70   80   90

☐ All Women   ■ Non-Hispanic White Women   ■ Non-Hispanic Black Women

Fig. 1. Health disparities in US women.[4]

Heart Study, initially lacked racial diversity, which limited the applicability of its findings to non-White populations.[8]

The 1985 US Public Health Service Task Force concluded that the *historical lack of research focus on women's health concerns has compromised the quality of health information available to women, as well as the health care they receive.*[9] In response, federal agencies established policies for including women and minorities in clinical research.[10] In 1993, the National Institutes of Health (NIH) mandated their inclusion and required NIH-funded research to analyze differences in effects.[11] While these mandates have somewhat improved participant demographics, continued efforts are needed.[12]

Reproductive coercion

Reproductive coercion, state or societal sanctioned as well as within a relationship or family, has been linked to poor mental health, increased sexually transmitted disease among other issues.[13] This history of reproductive coercion begins with slavery. The decision of when to conceive, when not to, with whom, and whether to parent that child was within the purview of the slave owner. Since then, it has taken other forms. Dr Marion Sims performed procedures without anesthesia on WOC in slavery (**Fig. 2**). The *Mississippi appendectomy*, removal of uterus or tubal ligation without consent, was done on thousands of women from the 1920s to 1970s.[14] The first birth control was tested without informed consent on women in Puerto Rico. The Family Planning Act led to sterilization of 25% of reproductive age indigenous women in the 1970s.[15]

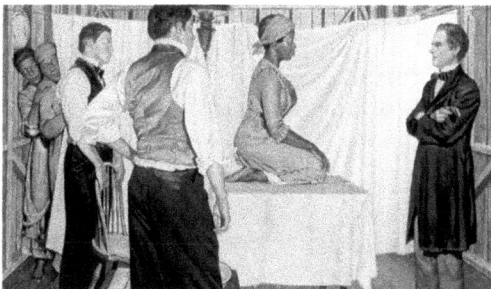

Fig. 2. Dr Marion Sims.

Disparities in Women's Health

Maternal mortality

Maternal mortality (MM) in the United States continues to be significantly higher than any other similarly high resource country.[16] Recent data cites that 80% of these deaths are preventable.[17] The Centers for Disease Control and Prevention data shows that the rate of death is disproportionately higher in Black women (BW). This disparity is persistent even in BW with higher education, access to prenatal care, and younger age and has persisted despite improvements seen in rates of MM of White women.[18] This inequity has been maintained overtime (**Fig. 3**).[19]

Bias shows up in care of peripartum diverse women.[16] From 1988 to 1999, rates of preeclampsia, preterm labor, and other maternal morbidities were not significantly different between racial groups. However, BW were 2 to 3 times more likely to die secondary to these complications than their white counterparts. With no biological or pathologic reason, one must consider the gap due, at least in part, to bias of the clinician and systemic racism.[20]

Mitigating the inequity must be done at both the microlevel and macrolevel. Clinicians need to recognize internal biases when managing patients who are WOC. On a macro level, policies should aim to decrease barriers to care, healthy food, and safe communities while providing resources for healthy lifestyles and paid leave.[21] California's strategic plan is an example of state policy change created to decrease disparities by providing BW within their state with increased support during the peripartum period.[22]

Management of pain

Clinicians disproportionately underestimate, undertreat, or dismiss pain suffered by women, people of color, and those with lower socioeconomic status, even when patients undergo similar medical procedures or present with similar findings.[23,24]

One study demonstrated that women with acute abdominal pain in emergency departments were less likely to receive analgesia, including opioids, and waited longer for pain relief compared to men, even after controlling for factors like age and pain score.[25] Research indicates that women's pain is often not taken as seriously as men's. This may explain why, despite reports of significant discomfort and studied pain relief methods, procedures like intrauterine device insertions are frequently done without anesthesia other than non-steroidal anti-inflammatory drugs.[26,27]

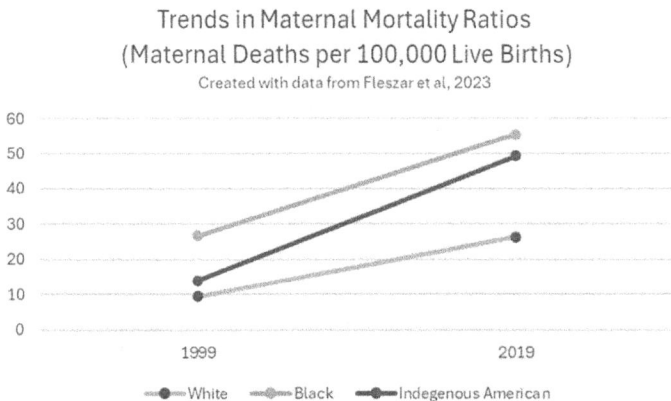

Trends in Maternal Mortality Ratios
(Maternal Deaths per 100,000 Live Births)
Created with data from Fleszar et al, 2023

Fig. 3. Racial disparity trends in MM.[19]

Further disparities in pain treatment persist, with Black and Latinx/Hispanic (L/H) patients often undertreated compared to White patients.[28,29] A study found that many medical learners believed in biological differences, such as *Black people's skin is thicker than White people's*. Those holding such beliefs rated Black patients' pain lower and made less accurate treatment recommendations.[30] In a study of post-partum pain, despite higher pain scores, WOC received fewer inpatient opioid doses and were less likely to get an opioid prescription at discharge. The differences in pain management were not due to less perceived pain.[31]

Addressing pain is subjective and thus challenging. Using objective findings and guidelines can help reduce subjective bias and prevent discriminatory care.[32]

Cardiovascular disease

There is a well-established gap between the care of women versus men in treatment and prevention of cardiovascular disease and it is widened when cardiovascular outcomes are compared between NH white women and WOC. A BW is over 30% more likely to die of cardiovascular disease than an NH White woman. This risk is more evident when you exclude women over 65 and are consistent across different aspects of cardiovascular morbidity and mortality (**Fig. 4**).[33,34] Management of cardiovascular disease in women is reviewed in a later chapter.

The stereotypical presentation of MI is the male presentation—chest pressure, diaphoresis-, and radiation to the left arm. It is not described as what is typically seen in females—nausea, anxiety, and radiation to the jaw.[35] Women experience longer time from presentation to catheterization, decreased treatment including revascularization and cardiac rehabilitation (**Fig. 5**), and decreased rates of patients being on guideline-directed treatment regimens including statins, anticoagulation, and aspirin.[36,37] The Cleveland Clinic use of standardized protocols improved some disparities.[38]

Cardiovascular calculators are based on a population that was mostly white men and do not account for independent cardiovascular risk factors that are uniquely fe-male such as preeclampsia, gestational diabetes, gestational hypertension, polycystic ovarian syndrome (PCOS) nor ones that are more common in females—depression and inflammatory bowel disease.[39,40] Studies have shown that preeclampsia or PCOS alone increases risk of cardiovascular events by 2-fold.[40,41]

2019 Death Attributed to high blood pressure:
Rates per 100,000 people
(Data Source: Tsao et al, 2022)

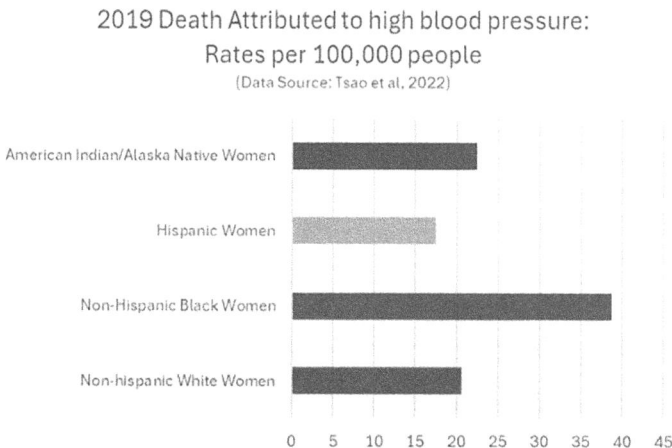

Fig. 4. Disparities in cardiovascular mortality.[34]

Rates of Revascularization Following Acute
Coronary Syndrome by Sex Assigned at Birth
Created with data from UDell et al, 2017

Rates of Revascularization Following Acute
Coronary Syndrome by Race
Created with data from Rodriguez et al 2015

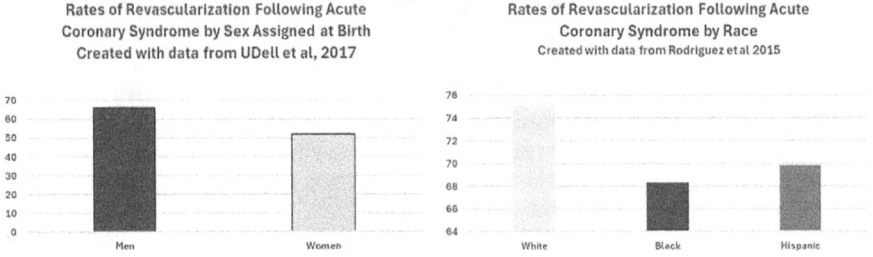

Fig. 5. Rates of revascularization by gender and race.[36,37]

Breast cancer

Although breast cancer (BC) rates are highest in white individuals, WOC have higher risk for BC specific mortality. The poor mortality rate in BW is independent of subtype, disease stage and socioeconomic status. Research has identified that WOC experience limited access to high quality care, higher risk for more aggressive subtypes, lower treatment adherence, and more advanced stage at diagnosis.[42] **Fig. 6** gives one example of racial inequity. Delays in initiation of adjuvant therapy, especially of greater than 90 days are associated with poorer prognosis.[43]

INTERSECTIONALITY

Intersectionality (**Fig. 7**) is *the complex, cumulative way in which the effects of multiple forms of discrimination (such as racism, sexism, and classism) combine, overlap, or intersect especially in the experiences of marginalized individuals or groups.*[44] The framework highlights how aspects of a person's identity combine (eg, socioeconomic status, sexuality, religion, disability, etc.) and how power and oppression impact their experiences, health, and well-being. Multiple forms of disadvantages may further compound and perpetuate health inequities among WOC.[45] For example, racial disparities in cardiovascular risk during the perinatal period for BW have been well documented as having some of the worst outcomes.[46] US immigrant BW who lived in the United States for greater than 10 years have a higher risk of preeclampsia than newcomer BW, suggesting that the adaptation of immigrants to the United States may play a role in those outcomes.[47]

Epidemiologic studies have also identified the L/H paradox, where L/H populations have health outcomes comparable to or better than NH White counterparts, despite

Odds Ratio of > 90 day Delay in Initiation of
Adjuvant Therapy
Created with data from Green et al, 2018

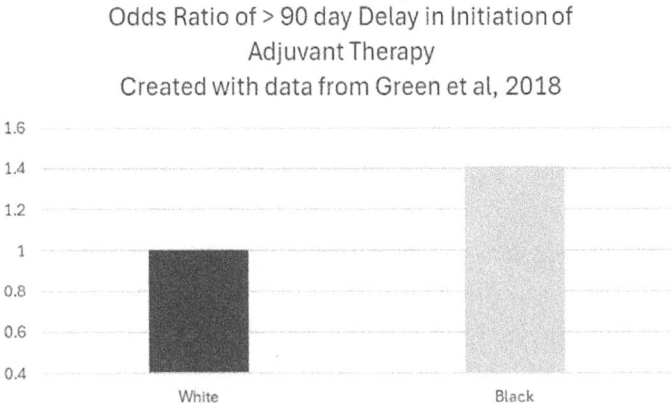

Fig. 6. Difference in delay of care by race.[43]

Intersectionality

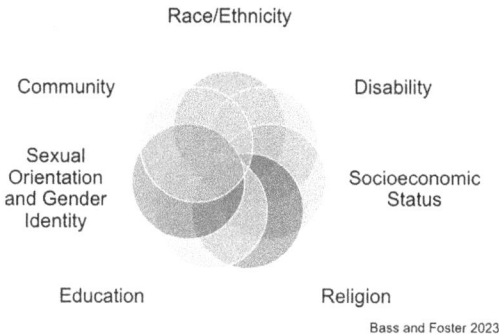

Race/Ethnicity

Community

Disability

Sexual
Orientation
and Gender
Identity

Socioeconomic
Status

Education

Religion

Bass and Foster 2023

Fig. 7. Intersectionality. (*Image courtesy* Dr Maya Bass, MD, MA, FAAFP and Dr Krys Foster, MD, MPH, FAAFP.)

lower income, education, and poor access to care. These suggest the influence of other intersectional experiences.[48] For example, compared with those who are born outside the United States, US-born L/H populations have higher rates of obesity, hypertension, smoking, heart disease, and cancer.[49] Current data suggests diminishing effects or nonexistence of the L/H paradox, highlighting the need for systematic exploration of factors contributing to L/H health.[50]

COGNITIVE BIAS IN PATIENT CARE

Health professionals' cognitive biases, including confirmation, anchoring, and outcomes bias, complicate racial and gender biases, leading to errors.[51] Recent studies have also found that physicians' use of different linguistic mechanisms is influenced by patients' race and gender, which can skew subsequent assessments.[2,52,53]

It is crucial to identify such language, remain mindful, and use alternative descriptions in clinical settings. A word cloud with terms commonly contributing to bias in medical encounters can be seen below (**Fig. 8**).

DISCUSSION AND RECOMMENDATIONS

Given the evidence, clinicians must make changes to their practice to better serve patients of all genders, races, and ethnicities.

Clinicians need to take time to explore their own implicit biases. This can be done using the Harvard Implicit Association Test available here: https://implicit.harvard.edu/implicit/takeatest.html.[54] Evidence has also shown that mindfulness strategies

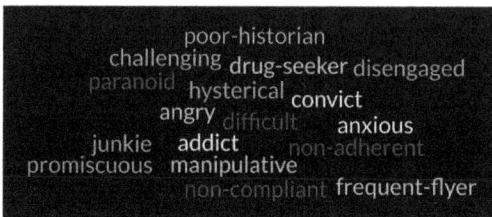

poor-historian
challenging drug-seeker disengaged
paranoid hysterical convict
angry difficult anxious
junkie addict non-adherent
promiscuous manipulative
non-compliant frequent-flyer

Fig. 8. Examples of pejorative language used in medical encounters.

E	N	R	I	C	H
• Engage your thoughts	• Notice assumptions	• Recognize other's perspectives	• Integrate into diverse work and social groups	• Challenge prejudices	• Hold space for diverse opinions

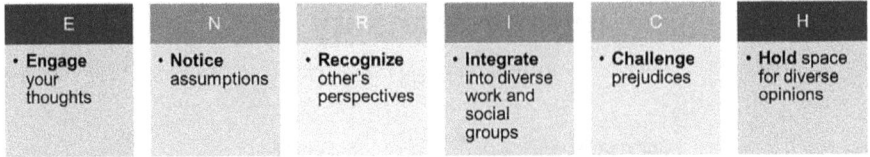

Fig. 9. Enrich framework.

can be used to explore and combat unconsciously held biases.[55] In every patient encounter, acknowledge the influence of bias and advocate for patients. Outside of the patient encounter, seek further training to better understand these inequities. Collaborate in research to improve health disparities. The goal is to recognize how a patient's intersectional identities may affect their risk factors. The model below can be used to guide daily practice (**Fig. 9**).

National medical organizations have recognized that other factors, including racism, are linked to health disparities.[56–58] Membership and advocacy through national organizations allows for change on a larger scale.

SUMMARY

Health disparities exist in women, especially WOC, likely due to a combination of medical harm done to communities of color throughout US history, compounded by implicit bias and the intersection of social determinants of health and other aspects of a patient's identity. In order to improve these health inequities, clinicians need to play an active role.

CLINICS CARE POINTS

- Take time to assess your own bias.
- Familiarize yourself with the historical impact on WOC.
- Recognize the underdiagnoses and barriers to screening experienced by WOC.
- Consider standardized protocols, based on research including diverse populations, to diminish the impact of bias.
- Use the Intersectionality framework to make adjustments when determining management.
- Advocate for change within daily practice and in national organizations.

DISCLOSURES

The authors have nothing to disclose.

REFERENCES

1. Healthy people 2030. Available at: https://health.gov/healthypeople. Accessed December 21, 2022.
2. Goddu AP, O'Conor KJ, Lanzkron S, et al. Do words matter? Stigmatizing language and the transmission of bias in the medical record. J Gen Intern Med 2018;33(5):685–91.
3. U.S. Census Bureau. 2020 U.S. population more racially and ethnically diverse than in 2010. Available at: https://www.census.gov/library/stories/2021/08/2020-united-states-population-more-racially-ethnically-diverse-than-2010.html. Accessed July 6, 2024.

4. Chinn JJ, Martin IK, Redmond N. Health equity among BW in the US. J Womens Health (Larchmt) 2021;30(2):212–9.
5. Bierer BE, Meloney LG, Ahmed HR, et al. Advancing the inclusion of underrepresented women in clinical research. Cell Rep Med 2022;3(4):100553. Published March 7, 2022.
6. Association of American Medical Colleges (AAMC). Why we know so little about women's health. Available at: https://www.aamc.org/news/why-we-know-so-little-about-women-s-health#: ~ :text=Womenwerealreadypoorlyrepresented,2clinicaltrials unlessthey. Accessed July 30, 2024.
7. Steering Committee of the Physicians' Health Study Research Group. Final report on the aspirin component of the ongoing Physicians' Health Study. N Engl J Med 1989;321(3):129–35.
8. Framingham Heart Study. History. Available at: https://www.framingh amheartstudy.org/fhs-about/history/. Accessed July 30, 2024.
9. National Center for Biotechnology Information (NCBI). Women's participation in clinical studies - women and health research. Available at: https://www.ncbi. nlm.nih.gov/books/NBK236535/. Accessed July 30, 2024.
10. Bibbins-Domingo K, Helman A, editors. Improving representation in clinical trials and research: building research equity for women and underrepresented groups - appendix B, Key trends in demographic diversity in clinical trials. Washington (DC): National Academies Press (US); 2022.
11. Office of Research on Women's Health (ORWH). History of women's participation in clinical research. Available at: https://orwh.od.nih.gov/toolkit/recruitment/ history. Accessed July 11, 2024.
12. Chen MS, Lara PN, Dang JHT, et al. Twenty years post-NIH Revitalization Act: enhancing minority participation in clinical trials (EMPaCT): laying the groundwork for improving minority clinical trial accrual: renewing the case for enhancing minority participation in cancer clinical trials. Cancer 2014;120 Suppl 7(07): 1091–6.
13. Tarzia L, Hegarty K. A conceptual re-evaluation of reproductive coercion: centering intent, fear and control. Reprod Health 2021;18:87.
14. Roberts DE. Killing the Black Body: Race, Reproduction, and the Meaning of Liberty. New York: Pantheon Books; 1997.
15. Ross LJ, Solinger R. Reproductive justice: an introduction. 1st edition. Oakland (CA): University of California Press; 2017. Available at: http://www.jstor.org/ stable/10.1525/j.ctv1wxsth.
16. 2023 National Healthcare Quality and Disparities Report. Content last reviewed May 2024. Agency for Healthcare Research and Quality, Rockville (MD). Available at: https://www.ahrq.gov/research/findings/nhqrdr/nhqdr23/index.html.
17. Trost SL, Beauregard JL, Smoots AN, et al. Preventing pregnancy-related mental health deaths: insights from 14 US maternal mortality review committees, 2008-17. Health Aff (Millwood) 2021;40(10):1551–9.
18. CDC. CDC infographic: racial/ethnic disparities in pregnancy-related deaths — US, 2007–2016. February 2020. Available at: https://www.cdc.gov/reproductivehealth/ maternal-mortality/disparities-pregnancy-related-deaths/infographic.html.
19. Fleszar LG, Bryant AS, Johnson CO, et al. Trends in state-level maternal mortality by racial and ethnic group in the US. JAMA 2023;330(1):52–61.
20. Tucker MJ, Berg CJ, Callaghan WM, et al. The Black-White disparity in pregnancy-related mortality from 5 conditions: differences in prevalence and case-fatality rates. Am J Publ Health 2007;97(2):247–51.

21. Office of the surgeon general (OSG). The surgeon general's call to action to improve maternal health. US department of health and human services. 2020. Available at: https://www.ncbi.nlm.nih.gov/books/NBK568218.

22. California Department of Public Health. Maternal mortality. Available at: https://www.cdph.ca.gov/Programs/CFH/DMCAH/Pages/Health-Topics/Maternal-Mortality.aspx. Accessed August 6, 2024.

23. Bonham VL. Race, ethnicity, and pain treatment: striving to understand the causes and solutions to the disparities in pain treatment. J Law Med Ethics 2001;28(1):52–68.

24. Wang ML, Jacobs O. From awareness to action: pathways to equity in pain management. Health Equity 2023;7(1):416–8.

25. Chen EH, Shofer FS, Dean AJ, et al. Gender disparity in analgesic treatment of emergency department patients with acute abdominal pain. Acad Emerg Med 2008;15(5):414–8.

26. Maguire K, Morrell K, Westhoff C, et al. Accuracy of providers' assessment of pain during intrauterine device insertion. Contraception 2014;89(1):22–4.

27. How women are educating others about 'excruciating' IUD procedures. The Washington Post. Available at: https://www.washingtonpost.com/wellness/2024/03/25/tiktok-iud-birth-control-pain/. Accessed July 30, 2024.

28. Cintron A, Morrison RS. Pain and ethnicity in the US: a systematic review. J Palliat Med 2006;9(6):1454–73.

29. Anderson KO, Green CR, Payne R. Racial and ethnic disparities in pain: causes and consequences of unequal care. J Pain 2009;10(12):1187–204.

30. Hoffman KM, Trawalter S, Axt JR, et al. Racial bias in pain assessment and treatment recommendations, and false beliefs about biological differences between Blacks and Whites. Proc Natl Acad Sci USA 2016;113(16):4296–301.

31. Badreldin N, Grobman WA, Yee LM. Racial disparities in postpartum pain management. Obstet Gynecol 2019;134(6):1147–53.

32. Harbell MW, Maloney J, Anderson MA, et al. Addressing bias in acute postoperative pain management. Curr Pain Headache Rep 2023;27(9):407–15.

33. Post WS, Watson KE, Hansen S, et al. Racial and ethnic differences in all-cause and cardiovascular disease mortality: the MESA study. Circulation 2022;146(3):229–39.

34. Tsao CW, Aday AW, Almarzooq ZI, et al. Heart disease and stroke statistics—2022 update: a report from the American Heart Association. Circulation 2022;145(8):e153–639.

35. Al Hamid A, Beckett R, Wilson M, et al. Gender bias in diagnosis, prevention, and treatment of cardiovascular diseases: a systematic review. Cureus 2024;16(2):e54264.

36. Udell JA, Koh M, Qiu F, et al. Outcomes of women and men with acute coronary syndrome treated with and without percutaneous coronary revascularization. J Am Heart Assoc 2017;6(1):e004319.

37. Rodriguez F, Foody JM, Wang Y, et al. Young Hispanic women experience higher in-hospital mortality following an acute MI. J Am Heart Assoc 2015;4(9):e002089.

38. Holtzman JN, Kaur G, Hansen B, et al. Sex differences in the management of atherosclerotic cardiovascular disease. Atherosclerosis 2023;384:117268.

39. Matheny M, McPheeters ML, Glasser A, et al. Systematic review of cardiovascular disease risk assessment tools [Internet]. Rockville (MD): Agency for Healthcare Research and Quality (US); 2011. Report No.: 11-05155-EF-1.

40. Inversetti A, Pivato CA, Cristodoro M, et al. Update on long-term cardiovascular risk after pre-eclampsia: a systematic review and meta-analysis. Eur Heart J Qual Care Clin Outcomes 2024;10(1):4–13.

41. Wekker V, van Dammen L, Koning A, et al. Long-term cardiometabolic disease risk in women with PCOS: a systematic review and meta-analysis. Hum Reprod Update 2020;26(6):942–60.

42. Zavala VA, Bracci PM, Carethers JM, et al. Cancer health disparities in racial/ethnic minorities in the US. Br J Cancer 2021;124(2):315–32.

43. Green AK, Aviki EM, Matsoukas K, et al. Racial disparities in chemotherapy administration for early-stage BC: a systematic review and meta-analysis. BC Res Treat 2018;172(2):247–63.

44. Merriam-Webster. Intersectionality definition & meaning. Available at: https://www.merriam-webster.com/dictionary/intersectionality. Accessed July 6, 2024.

45. Vohra-Gupta S, Petruzzi L, Jones C, et al. An intersectional approach to understanding barriers to healthcare for women. J Community Health 2023;48(1):89–98.

46. MacDorman MF, Thoma M, Declercq E, et al. Racial and ethnic disparities in maternal mortality in the US using enhanced vital records, 2016-2017. Am J Publ Health 2021;111(9):1673–81.

47. Baiden D, Parry M, Nerenberg K, et al. Connecting the dots: structural racism, intersectionality, and cardiovascular health outcomes for African, Caribbean, and Black mothers. Health Equity 2022;6(1):402–5.

48. Hayes-Bautista DE, Bryant M, Yudell M, et al. Office of Management and Budget racial/ethnic categories in mortality research: a framework for including the voices of racialized communities. Am J Publ Health 2021;111(S2):S133–40.

49. Dominguez K, Penman-Aguilar A, Chang M-H, et al, CDC. Vital signs: leading causes of death, prevalence of diseases and risk factors, and use of health services among Hispanics in the US - 2009-2013. MMWR Morb Mortal Wkly Rep 2015;64(17):469–78.

50. Montanez-Valverde R, McCauley J, Isasi R, et al, SouthEast Enrollment Center Investigators, All of us Research Program Demonstration Projects Subcommittee. Revisiting the latino epidemiologic paradox: an analysis of data from the all of us research program. J Gen Intern Med 2022;37(15):4013–4.

51. Doherty TS, Carroll AE. Believing in overcoming cognitive biases. AMA J Ethics 2020;22(9):E773–8.

52. Blair IV, Steiner JF, Fairclough DL, et al. Clinicians' implicit ethnic/racial bias and perceptions of care among Black and Latino patients. Ann Fam Med 2013;11(1):43–52.

53. Sun M, Oliwa T, Peek ME, et al. Negative patient descriptors: documenting racial bias in the electronic health record. Health Aff 2022;41(2):203–11.

54. Greenwald AG, McGhee DE, Schwartz JL. Implicit association test (IAT) [database record]. PsycTESTS 1998. https://doi.org/10.1037/t00770-000.

55. Burgess DJ, Beach MC, Saha S. Mindfulness practice: a promising approach to reducing the effects of clinician implicit bias on patients. Patient Educ Counsel 2017;100(2):372–6.

56. American Academy of Family Physicians. Institutional racism in the health care system. Available at: https://www.aafp.org/about/policies/all/institutional-racism.html. Accessed July 11, 2024.

57. American College of Obstetricians and Gynecologists. Health care disparities. Available at: https://www.acog.org/topics/health-care-disparities. Accessed July 11, 2024.

58. American College of Physicians. Racial health disparities, prejudice and violence. Available at: https://www.acponline.org/advocacy/where-we-stand/racial-health-disparities-prejudice-and-violence. Accessed July 11, 2024.

Reproductive and Sexual Health of Individuals with Disabilities

Brianna Marzolf, DO, MS[a],*, Maneesha Finkle, LMSW[b],
Laura Kruger, MD[a], Sherri Eldin, DO, MFA[c,d],
Nafeeza Hussain, MD, MPH[e]

KEY WORDS

- Disability • Disparity • Accommodation • Abuse • Education • Screening
- Health maintenance • Preventative care

KEY POINTS

- Clinicians should adopt a universal design approach to create an inclusive clinic environment that accommodates the needs of all patients.
- Adults with intellectual or developmental disabilities face high abuse risks and should be routinely screened, especially with behavior changes, while receiving ongoing education on relationships, boundaries, consent, and safety.
- Clinicians should affirm patients' sexual identities by fostering a safe, nonjudgmental environment, using inclusive language, normalizing sexual desires, and addressing challenges related to sexual activity.
- Clinicians should consider offering menstrual suppression if it aligns with the patient's goals, such as contraception, prevention of anemia, and reduction of cyclical behavioral changes or catamenial seizures.
- People with disabilities face disparities in routine health maintenance screenings. Clinicians should select the most accessible screening methods for each patient and their family or caregivers.

[a] Department of Family Medicine, University of Michigan, 1018 Fuller Street, Ann Arbor, MI 48104-1213, USA; [b] Department of Obstetrics & Gynecology, University of Michigan, Center for Sexual Health, 4260 Plymouth Road, Ann Arbor, MI 48109, USA; [c] Annals of Family Medicine Editorial Office, Department of Family Medicine, Warren Alpert Medical School, Brown University, Providence, RI 02912; [d] Department of Family & Social Medicine Montefiore Medical Center, 3544 Jerome Avenue, Bronx, NY 10467, USA; [e] Department of OBGYN, University of Michigan, 7300 Dexter Ann Arbor Road #110, Dexter, MI 48130, USA
* Corresponding author.
E-mail address: briannamarzolf@gmail.com

Prim Care Clin Office Pract 52 (2025) 205–221
https://doi.org/10.1016/j.pop.2024.12.005   primarycare.theclinics.com
0095-4543/25/© 2025 Elsevier Inc. All rights reserved, including those for text and data mining, AI training, and similar technologies.

Abbreviations	
AAP	American Academy of Pediatrics
ASL	American Sign Language
COC	combined oral contraceptive
DHH	deaf or hard of hearing
DMPA	depot medroxyprogesterone acetate
DS	Down syndrome
IDD	intellectual or developmental disability
STI	sexually transmitted infection
PWD	persons with a disability or disabilities
VTE	venous thromboembolism

REPRODUCTIVE AND SEXUAL HEALTH OF INDIVIDUALS WITH DISABILITIES

A total of 61 million Americans live with a disability (1 in 4 people). Unfortunately, many do not receive equitable reproductive and sexual health care.[1] A 2021 report found that 60% of physicians report an inability to provide the same quality of care to persons with disabilities and those without disabilities.[2] Persons with a disability or disabilities (PWD) experience disparities in screening and preventative services, cancer diagnosis and treatment, reproductive and pregnancy care, communication with health care professionals, and overall satisfaction with care.[2]

This article covers key topics that all clinicians should be familiar with when caring for individuals with various types of disabilities (physical, sensory, intellectual, and others). This volume is focused on women's health; however, patients may be trans women, trans men, nonbinary, agender, or have other gender identities[3]; therefore, the authors use inclusive, gender-neutral language throughout this article.

Accessibility

Only half of physicians strongly agree that they welcome PWD into their practice.[2] To create an inclusive environment that provides accommodations for patients with specific needs, we suggest a universal design approach. **Table 1** highlights recommendations and suggested implementation strategies to create an accessible, inclusive clinic environment.

Screening for Abuse

Adults with IDD are 2.5 to 10 times more likely to experience abuse than those without IDD[8] and often face repeated incidents of abuse.[9] When abuse occurs, individuals with IDD may display behaviors that are harmful or dangerous to themselves, others, or the environment[10] such as self-injury, aggression, outbursts of anger, and irritability. Therefore, abuse should be on the differential when a person with IDD presents with a new or changed behavior.

Providers should routinely screen individuals with IDD for abuse (physical, sexual, exploitation, neglect) by asking questions such as

- *"Is anyone hurting you?"*
- *"Is anyone mean to you?"*
- *"Has anyone touched your body without your permission?" (If so, where?)*

It is best to ask these questions when the patient is alone. If the patient has any known comfort aids, be sure that they have those items present with them. Screening for abuse can provide a segue into education about sexual health and healthy relationships/boundaries, discussed in detail later.

Table 1
Actionable steps to ensure accessible, inclusive clinic environment for individuals with disabilities

	Recommendation	Implementation
Preparing for a Visit	• Assess whether the patient will require any accommodations or support.	• Implement the use of standardized screening questionnaires for all patients prior to their visit that address the need for disability-specific accommodations.[4]
	• Implement clinic-based protocols to ensure needed accommodations are provided.	• Display accommodation and communication needs in a visible area in the patient's chart. Ensure documentation is clear and accessible to other members of care team[4] by updating the patient storyboard in the electronic medical record and documenting the preferred communication strategies on the problem list.
	• Ensure equitable access to care.	• This requires extended visit times for patients with intellectual/developmental disabilities (IDD), or those who are deaf or hard of hearing (DHH) requiring ASL interpreters.
		• Offer virtual or in-home visits, when possible, as transportation is often a barrier for PWD.[5]
	• Train and diversify health care team to meet patient needs.	• Hire doctors and staff with disabilities. Train all staff, including front desk, medical assistants, and call center representatives on disability health topics including ableism, stigma, discrimination, and accessibility.
Medical Equipment	• Ensure clinic is accessible for patients with physical disabilities.	• Wheelchair-accessible scales, height adjustable examination table, barrier-free examination table.
		• Provide space for patient using wheelchair and care provider to be comfortable in the examination room. Use larger examination rooms/procedure rooms if necessary.
	• Ensure clinic is accessible for patients who are deaf or hard of hearing (DHH).	• Examination rooms should be well lit without any visual obstacles (eg, laptop) obstructing the providers face or lips.[4]
		• Use masks with a clear window to allow lip-reading.
		• Use visual alerts to notify patient when someone knocks on door.[4]
		• Use live transcription/closed captions for all virtual visits.
	• Ensure clinic is accessible for patients with intellectual or developmental disability (IDD).	• Minimize time in waiting room by rooming early if possible.
		• A sensory kit with noise-canceling headphones and weighed blanket is useful.
		• Use patients visual support aids if present.

(continued on next page)

Table 1
(continued)

Recommendation	Implementation
During the Visit	
• Use patient-centered communication.	• Ask patients for the language that they use to refer to themselves and their bodies. This may be in reference to sexual orientation, gender identity and pronouns, their anatomic parts, and their disabilities but may expand further. For patients with IDD[6].
	• Introduce yourself to the patient first and communicate directly with patient.
	• Assume better receptive than expressive language.
	• Allow time for processing (up to 10 s).
	• Use meaningful gestures.
	• Explain using words, actions, or pictures what you are going to do before you do it.
	• Avoid abstract language or concepts ("Is your throat on fire?").
• Be flexible to meet patient needs.	• Modify examination to meet patient needs (see **Fig. 2**, alternative positions for pelvic examination).
	• For patient with IDD, medical assistant can defer vitals if patient is uncomfortable. Provider may be able to obtain vitals later in visit or may not be able to complete a physical examination at all. Visits simply for rapport building are worthwhile.
After the Visit	
• Thoroughly discuss the plan of care.	• Engage the patient and others as indicated (caregiver) when discussing treatment options to ensure that the recommended plan is within patients' goals of care, and logistically possible.
	• Use teach back/teach to goal method.
• Provide clear after-visit summary.	• Simplify patient handouts and educational materials in general using health literacy principles.[4]
	• Incorporate pictures/graphics.
	• Ensure that after-visit summary materials are adapted to the patient's reading level or video comprehension level. Easyhealth.org.uk has easy-read materials about common health conditions.[7]

Safety and Consent

Safety and consent are important concepts for all vulnerable individuals to understand. While there is an expectation that all PWD will have the support of an identified safety person, crimes committed are frequently by those with whom patients feel safe.[8] Discussing safety and consent provides patients with the tools necessary to make informed decisions and accurately report an adverse event if necessary. Providers should ensure that patients understand consent (**Box 1**).

No, Go, and Tell can effectively educate individuals aged 3 years and up about self-protection and abuse reporting[11] by explaining body parts and who is allowed to touch them (**Box 2**). "No" teaches individuals to use their words or actions to stop unwanted behavior or leave a situation. "Go" encourages individuals to escape or run away if they are in danger. "Tell" instructs individuals to report any issues to a trusted adult, caregiver, or support person.

Healthy Relationships and Boundaries

A healthy relationship is one that feels safe, respects boundaries, and is collaborative. Understanding the nature of a healthy relationship is important for PWD to ensure physical and emotional safety. A tool called Circles[12] can be used by any member of the health care team to teach people with IDD and their families about different relationship structures and support continuing education around boundaries at home.

Circles is performed by creating a visual, using concentric circles, to outline different relationship structures and contexts (**Fig. 1**). The person who is learning is in the center of the circle, the people closest to this individual outside of that circle, acquaintances outside of that circle, and strangers outside of that circle.

Creating this visual helps foster conversation about the role that various individuals play in a patient's life, and how their role influences appropriate boundaries. For example, with the patient's consent, only those in the innermost circle—closest to the patient—should hug them. Acquaintances might support a patient, but it would not be appropriate for them to hug or touch the patient in any other way.

Sexual Health Education

Sexual health education is essential for PWD to understand their bodies and establish appropriate boundaries to prevent abuse. Sexual health education should be introduced early, before puberty, and frequently revisited at well visits.

Physicians should ask patients how they learn best—whether through visual aids, listening, reading, or other methods. Visual aids and videos can be particularly

---

Box 1
Providers should ensure that patients understand consent by the following

- Ask if the patient can identify their private areas using accurate anatomic terms.
- Ask if anyone has touched these areas and discuss scenarios where touching might be necessary for hygiene or medical reasons (eg, caregivers, parents, aides, partners).
- Explain that the patient must give permission for anyone to touch them, including during medical visits and examinations.
- Ask what the patient would do if someone touched them without permission.
- Ask who the patient trusts to report concerns about their safety.

Box 2
No, go, and tell to explain body parts and touch[10]

Here is how No, Go, and Tell can be used to explain body parts and touch:
1. *No*: Teach patients that they have the right to say "no" to any unwanted touch. Emphasize that their personal boundaries must always be respected, and they have the right to refuse any touch or action that makes them uncomfortable.
2. *Go*: Explain that if someone touches them inappropriately, they should move away or get out of the situation. This helps them understand that they can take action to protect themselves.
3. *Tell*: Encourage patients to inform a trusted person if someone touches them inappropriately. This could be a caregiver, family member, or another trusted adult. Make sure that they understand the importance of communicating any concerns or uncomfortable experiences.

---

beneficial. Resources like Amaze.org[13] and Teachers Pay Teachers[14] offer helpful tools for various learning styles.

Consent is a crucial component of sexual health education. Providers should verify that patients understand consent (see **Box 1**) before conducting any sensitive

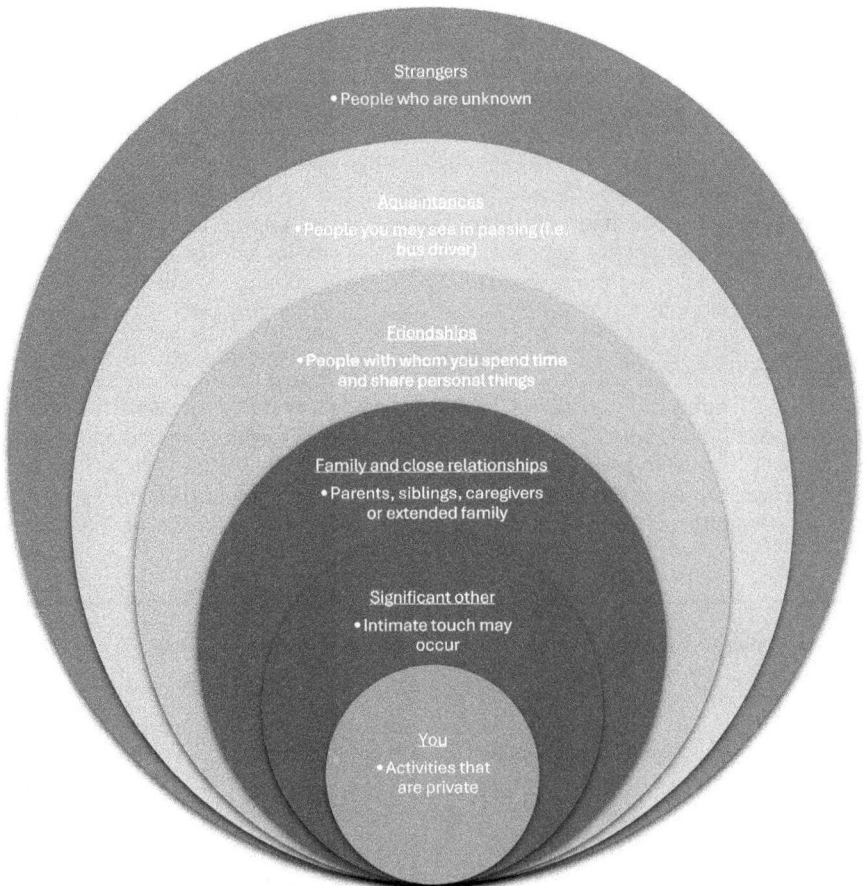

Fig. 1. Circles—understanding relationship structures and context for individuals with IDD.

examinations. Visual aids can help clarify what will be done during these examinations, supporting the patient's comprehension and comfort.

Validate and Affirm Patient Sexuality

PWD have a history of being regarded as nonsexual beings. Women with disabilities have also reported feeling that their roles as lovers, partners, and mothers are unrecognized or ignored by clinicians.[2] When these identities are acknowledged, clinicians may still minimize or deny patients' experiences.[15]

Clinicians can validate and affirm patients by doing the following.

Create a safe, nonjudgmental environment and relationship

Many PWD, particularly those in marginalized populations who have faced discrimination and adverse experiences, feel unsafe communicating about sexuality or intimacy with their health care providers. It is important to show patients that their experience with you will be different.

- Begin by ensuring that patients may ask any questions they may have, that no question or topic is off-limits.
- If a caregiver is present, give the patient an opportunity to speak privately with the provider.
- Let the patient know that you are there to help them find solutions to their challenges. Come from a place of respect.
- Do not force anything outside of their comfort zone. Meet the patient "where they are!"

Use inclusive language

a. Do not make assumptions. Ask patients for the language/vocabulary that they use to refer to themselves and their bodies. This may be in reference to sexual orientation, gender identity and pronouns, their anatomic parts, and their disabilities but may expand further.

b. Use preface statements when approaching a topic that can be perceived as sensitive and provide your rationale for asking them. For example, "I'm going to ask you some questions that may be a bit sensitive and am doing so because I want to be respectful and understand your specific needs."

Normalize sex, sexual desires, sexual/body exploration, and masturbation

PWD of all types are commonly infantilized, and their identities as sexual beings are seen within that context by those around them, including health care professionals and families/caregivers. Sexuality and masturbation are healthy and natural parts of the human experience, regardless of an individual's disability status. If patients want to explore this part of their identity, providers should encourage them to do so in safe and healthy ways, free of shame. Masturbation should be done in a private setting with body-safe tools and proper hygiene to avoid harm. Understanding sexual health and masturbation is important for the purpose of having the ability to consent, maintain safety, understand boundaries, and explore one's own pleasure.[16]

Address common physical challenges related to sexual activity

1. Limited mobility
   a. Disability-related limitations may include difficulty or inability to get into and maintain any number of sexual positions. Providers should help patients explore creative options, including assistive devices like pillows or other supportive tools such as swings or hammocks.

2. Decreased sex drive/libido and/or the struggle or inability to orgasm
   a. Etiology may be due to emotional or psychiatric concerns, but adverse medication effects should not be overlooked and may be a concurrent cause. A comprehensive medication list review should be performed. Regardless of cause, difficulties reaching orgasm can lead to emotional distress. Providers should offer support and consider referrals to occupational therapists or behavioral health specialists for additional assistance.

Menstrual Management

Approximately 10% of women of childbearing age have a disability.[17] To best support the reproductive and sexual health of these patients, providers must consider several factors including the life stage of the person with a disability, relationship status and expectations, desires for the future (eg, marriage, family planning, healthy aging), and support systems.

Menstruation often poses challenges for PWD including difficulties with menstrual hygiene, cyclical mood changes, catamenial epilepsy, caregiver burden, and desire for contraception.[18] Physicians should implement similar strategies used for those without disabilities when discussing menstrual cycle management.[19]

When managing menstrual care for individuals with IDD, it is crucial to prioritize and respect patient autonomy, given the historic context of forced sterilization in the United States.[20] Menstrual suppression should be considered if menstrual cycles are creating difficulties in the patient's life, as determined by the patient, caregivers, and family. Menstrual suppression offers several benefits, including preventing anemia, improving hygiene and cleanliness, and reducing cyclical behavioral changes or catamenial seizures.[21]

Historic discrimination based on racism and ableism has led to unequal contraceptive prescribing practices that continue today. Individuals with IDD are less likely to receive long-acting reversible contraception or oral contraceptive pills and more likely to be offered no contraception or surgical sterilization.[20] PWD should have access to the same menstrual management options as those without disabilities.[22] **Table 2** can be used by providers to guide discussions on menstrual management with patients and families.[19] Given the many safe and effective nonsurgical options available, the risks and costs of surgical sterilization generally outweigh the benefits, and hysterectomy or tubal ligation should only be considered after all other options have been thoroughly explored.[20]

Health Maintenance Screenings in Persons with Disabilities

PWD are more frequently diagnosed with cancer but are less likely to be screened compared to the general population.[31–33] When diagnosed, they often present at a more advanced stage, with nearly half showing stage IV cancer.[34] Women with severe disabilities are particularly under-screened.[35] Barriers to screening include limited provider knowledge, physical obstacles such as transportation and accessible equipment, health insurance challenges, and sociodemographic factors.[36,37]

Breast cancer screening

Patients with complex activity limitations are more likely to be diagnosed with breast cancer but are less likely to be screened.[32] Patients with IDD alone have a similar incidence of breast cancer but are screened less. The CDC reports that 72% of women aged over 40 years have had a mammogram in the past 2 years,[38] compared to only 17% of women with IDD.[39] This disparity likely contributes to the higher likelihood of late-stage cancer diagnosis[34] and increased mortality rates among people with IDD.[38,40]

Table 2
Methods for menstrual management in people with disabilities[19]

Category	Method	Benefits	Interactions with Antiepileptic Drugs	Cautions
NSAIDS	Oral as needed	Reduced flow and pain	No	Gastrointestinal
Estrogen and Progestin				Estrogen-containing hormones increase the risk of venous thrombotic events (VTEs). *For patients with limited mobility:* • Assess family history for inherited thrombophilia • Consider using low-dose estrogen combined with first- or second-generation progestins, norethindrone or levonorgestrel associated with lower VTE risk[19,23]
	Combined oral contraceptive (COC)	• Can be used continuously to limit bleeding[19] • Complete amenorrhea is reported in 62% of individuals[19] • Formulations are available that can be chewed, crushed, or administered via G-tube[19]	Yes	• Consider scheduled withdrawal bleed every 3–4 mo if complete amenorrhea is not achieved to limit unpredictable breakthrough bleeding[24]
	Patch	• Can be used continuously by changing patch weekly • Similar breakthrough bleeding patterns as COC[25]	Yes	• Inadvertent removal of patch; consider placing on back or buttocks
	Ring	• Leaving ring in for 28 d at a time can provide continuous hormones in an off-label use[24]	Yes	• Dexterity/privacy with insertion • When used continuously, 8% amenorrhea rate[26]
Progesterone Only		• Lower VTE risk than estrogen-containing products		

(continued on next page)

Table 2
(continued)

Category	Method	Benefits	Interactions with Antiepileptic Drugs	Cautions
	Progesterone only pills	• If attempting to achieve amenorrhea, use medroxyprogesterone (10–40 mg) or norethindrone (5–15 mg).[19]	Yes	• Irregular bleeding
	Depot medroxyprogesterone acetate (DMPA)	• High amenorrhea rate	No	• Weight gain: Average 13 pounds in 4 y[19] • Decreased bone density: PWD often have several risk factors for early osteoporosis at baseline.[27] Bone density loss appears reversible after stopping DMPA (however, no data on teens with limited mobility)[28] • Subcutaneous (SubQ) injection every 3 mo may be a barrier if transportation issues
	Implant	• Insertion once every 5 y	No	• Irregular bleeding/spotting is common • Low amenorrhea rate (13% after 1 y)[29] • Procedure to insert and remove requires patient cooperation
	Levonorgestrel intrauterine device	• Insertion once every 8 y[30]	No	• May require anesthesia for insertion and removal • Initial irregular bleeding
Surgical	Endometrial ablation		No	• Amenorrhea rates low • Does not universally prevent pregnancy • Legal and ethical issues
	Hysterectomy	• Amenorrhea	No	• Legal and ethical issues of permanent sterilization

Recommendations
- Follow current breast cancer screening recommendations based on age group and breast density.
  - Traditional mammography may be uncomfortable or intolerable for some patients. Breast ultrasound or breast MRI can be considered, recognizing there are limitations with each modality.
- For patients with IDD, we recommend explaining the mammogram process and importance to patients and their caregivers. It is helpful to provide reading materials, like the Easy Read Breast Cancer Screening Guide created by the NHS.[41]
- The breast examination is typically performed with the patient supine but can be modified to be upright or semi-upright to improve patient comfort and limit needs for transfers.
- When ordering breast imaging:
  - Providers can specifically request multiple technicians be present to assist with patient positioning and education.
  - Ensure that mammography equipment can accommodate wheelchairs and has adjustable height features.

Cervical cancer/sexual health screening
Abstinence from sexual activity should not be assumed; PWD are as likely to be sexually active as their peers without disabilities.[42] Women with IDD are at high risk of sexual abuse[8] and may have difficulty recognizing or communicating such incidents. Women with physical and intellectual disabilities have a higher prevalence of sexually transmitted infections (STIs) compared to persons without disabilities but are significantly less likely to be screened.[43] Women with physical disabilities are more likely to be diagnosed with cervical cancer but are less likely to be screened.[32] Women with IDD are less likely to know about cervical cancer screenings.[44]

Recommendations
- All persons with a cervix should be offered cervical cancer screening and screening for STIs per guidelines for the general population.
  - Clinicians may want to consider discussing the pelvic examination and performing a pelvic examination at separate visits to allow patients time to prepare/process.
  - Use accessible equipment such as adjustable-height examination tables, leg supports, additional pillows, and assistants for patient positioning. **Fig. 2** reviews alternative positions for pelvic examinations that may be more comfortable.[45,46] Some patients may be able to tolerate an external examination or bimanual examination but may not be able to tolerate a speculum examination.
  - There is strong evidence that blind sampling or patient self-sampling is comparable to clinician-collected samples for primary human papillomavirus (HPV)-based screening.[47] Blind sampling or patient sampling may not be appropriate in all situations (eg, such as in a symptomatic patient) but can be offered to those who cannot tolerate a speculum examination and/or as part of a trauma-informed approach to screening.
  - If a patient is unable to tolerate a pelvic examination or blind sampling with accommodations or if direct visualization is needed, a pelvic examination under anesthesia may be considered. Care should be taken to coordinate this procedure with other procedures under sedation (eg, colonoscopy, dental cleanings, G-tube exchange, and Baclofen pump replacement) to maximize efficiency and minimize risk.

Description	Example
Diamond-Shaped or Frog-Legged In this position, the patient lies on their back with their knees bent and the plantar surfaces of their feet together. This position does not require stirrups. Additionally, the patient must feel comfortable and balanced laying on their back for this position to be successful.	
V-Shape In this position, the patient lies on their back with their legs extended. The legs should be spread to opposite sides of the table. This position may require that an assistant holds up the patient's legs for support. Alternatively, the patient may use this position and place one foot in the stirrup while the other leg remains extended. This position does not require stirrups, but they may be used. Additionally, the patient must feel comfortable and balanced laying on their back for this position to be successful.	
M-Shape In this position, the patient lies on their back with their knees bent and feet placed on the exam table close to their buttocks. This position does not require stirrups. Additionally, the patient must feel comfortable and balanced laying on their back for this position to be successful.	
Stirrups In this position, the patient lies on their back near the edge of the table. The patient's legs should be supported under the knee using obstetrical stirrups. This position requires stirrups and provides patients more support than the traditional lithotomy position. To make this position more comfortable, padding can be added to the stirrups.	
Knee-to-chest In this position, the patient lies on the side with both knees bent. The top leg should be brought close to the patient's chest. Alternatively, the patient may lie on their back with one leg extended. The other leg should be bent at the knee and brought close to the patient's chest. This position does not require stirrups. Additionally, the patient must feel comfortable and balanced laying on their side for this position to be successful.	

Fig. 2. Alternative pelvic examination positions.[45,46] For the first 3 positions shown in the table, consider using the speculum upside down to improve patient comfort and enhance provider mechanics. (The original artwork for the figure, first published in 2024 by Barbara et al,[45] was adapted by Julie Downs, BSN, RN from Ferreyra S, Hughes K. Table Manners: A Guide to the Pelvic Examination for Disabled Women and Health Care Providers (1982).[46] Used with permission from both authors.)

- *STI screening*: Ask patients about the types of sex in which they engage to determine whether STI testing should be completed via vaginal, anorectal, and/or pharyngeal sampling.

Colorectal cancer screening
As PWD live longer, their risk for colorectal cancer and other cancers also increases. However, they are less likely to be screened for colorectal cancer.[31] Patients with IDD

specifically are more likely to present with more advanced disease,[31] which in turn can make management more challenging for both patients and caregivers.

Recommendations
- Follow current screening guidelines for all patients based on age, family history, and comorbidities (eg, inflammatory bowel disease and genetic cancer syndromes).
- Noninvasive tests such as fecal occult blood test or Cologuard should be considered for patients who are appropriate candidates, particularly for those who may have challenges with undergoing colonoscopy prep and/or sedation.
- If colonoscopy is needed, consider coordinating with other examinations/services under anesthesia (eg, dentistry and pelvic examination).

Osteoporosis screening
Osteoporosis and osteoporotic fractures are more common and occur at a younger age in people with IDD compared to the general population,[48] yet they are less frequently screened.[49] People with IDD often have more than 2 risk factors for early osteoporosis[27] including long-term use of medications such as anticonvulsants, glucocorticoids, injectable depo progesterone, vitamin D deficiency, prolactinemia, immobility, low weight or obesity, hypothyroidism, early menopause, profound or multiple disabilities, and certain genetic syndromes. Similarly, physical disabilities, including spinal cord injury and cerebral palsy, are associated with significant bone loss[50] and increased mortality risk from nontraumatic fractures.[51]

Recommendations
- Prevention:
  - Promote regular physical activity, weight-bearing exercise, adequate dietary or supplemental intake of calcium and Vitamin D (unless contraindicated such as in Williams syndrome) and implement fall risk reduction measures including optimizing vision.
- Screening:
  - Men and women with IDD should be screened for osteoporosis starting at the age of 40 to 45 years.[52,53] Screening should be repeated every 2 years as needed if results would change clinical management or if significant changes in bone density are expected.
  - Immobility should be considered a risk factor prompting consideration of early osteoporosis screening in patients with physical disabilities.
  - Consult with a radiologist regarding alternative methods (such as forearm-only measurements) if a patient cannot be assessed using typical bone mineral density testing.
  - For patients with Down syndrome (DS):
- Use shared decision-making to determine when to screen and encourage prevention as earlier.
  - Evidence is inadequate regarding when to screen for osteoporosis and how to interpret bone mineral density values in patients with DS.[54] Patients with DS have higher rates of esophageal dysmotility and are at greater risk of esophageal ulceration secondary to bisphosphonate treatment.[55] Recommend discussion with endocrinology before treating osteoporosis in a patient with DS.[52]
- All adults with DS who sustain a fragility fracture should be evaluated for secondary causes of osteoporosis, including hyperthyroidism, celiac disease, vitamin D deficiency, hyperparathyroidism, and medications associated with adverse effects on bone health.[54]

CLINICS CARE POINTS

- *Abuse screening*: People with IDD face a heightened risk of abuse, making routine screening essential, especially when new behaviors like aggression or self-injury arise. Ask direct, simple questions privately, such as "Is anyone hurting you?"
- *Consent*: Ensure that patients can identify trusted individuals for reporting abuse and recognize appropriate versus inappropriate touch. Tools like "No, Go, and Tell" can help teach self-protection and reporting procedures.
- Healthy relationships and boundaries: Educate patients about boundaries using the Circles model, which helps visualize different relationship types and emphasizes appropriate physical contact.
- *Sexual health*: Start sexual health education before puberty, covering anatomy, consent, and healthy sexual behaviors. Normalize discussions about sexual desires and masturbation. Visual aids enhance understanding.
- *Validate and affirm patient sexuality*: Avoid assumptions and foster a nonjudgmental space for exploring sexuality. Address barriers such as limited mobility or medication-induced sexual dysfunction. Utilizing assistive devices like pillows can enhance comfort, and referrals to occupational therapy can improve sexual experiences.
- *Menstrual management*: Consider menstrual suppression for individuals who face difficulties with menstrual hygiene, experience-related health issues, or need contraception. Prioritize autonomy and informed consent. For individuals with IDD, risks of surgical sterilization outweigh benefits, making hysterectomy or tubal ligation a last resort after exploring all other options.
- *Cancer and health screenings*: Follow standard guidelines for breast, cervical, and colorectal cancer, but adapt approaches to encourage completion. Offer the most accessible methods for each patient and their caregivers, clearly explain procedures, and use visual aids. Consider requesting extra technicians or utilizing support staff to coordinate multiple procedures under anesthesia to reduce barriers to care.
- *Osteoporosis*: For people with IDD, begin screening for osteoporosis at the age of 40 to 45 years. For patients with DS, use shared decision-making to determine when to screen. Consider immobility a risk factor for early screening in people with physical disabilities.

DECLARATION OF ARTIFICIAL INTELLIGENCE (AI) AND AI-ASSISTED TECHNOLOGIES IN THE WRITING PROCESS

During the preparation of this work, the authors used Chat GPT to improve readability and language. After using this tool/service, the authors reviewed and edited the content as needed and take full responsibility for the content of the publication.

DISCLOSURE

The authors declare that there are no personal, financial, or competing interests that could be perceived as influencing the content of this work.

FUNDING

Dr Marzolf received funding from the Agency for Healthcare Research and Quality (T32 HS000053).

REFERENCES

1. CDC. Disability impacts all of us infographic | CDC. Centers for Disease Control and Prevention; 2024. Available at: https://www.cdc.gov/ncbddd/disabilityandhealth/infographic-disability-impacts-all.html. Accessed August 30, 2024.

2. Iezzoni LI, Rao SR, Ressalam J, et al. Physicians' perceptions of people with disability and their health care. Health Aff 2021;40(2):297–306. https://doi.org/10.1377/hlthaff.2020.01452.

3. Practices B. A gender-inclusive language guide for gynecologists. Empowered Women's Health. Available at: https://www.volusonclub.net/empowered-womens-health/a-gender-inclusive-language-guide-for-gynecologists/. Accessed August 30, 2024.

4. McKee M, James TG, Helm KVT, et al. Reframing our health care system for patients with hearing loss. J Speech Lang Hear Res 2022;65(10):3633–45.

5. Brucker DL, Rollins NG. Trips to medical care among persons with disabilities: evidence from the 2009 national household travel survey. Disabil Health J 2016;9(3):539–43.

6. Communicate CARE – ddpcp. Available at: https://ddprimarycare.surreyplace.ca/tools-2/general-health/communicating-effectively/. Accessed August 30, 2024.

7. Common Health Conditions. Easy health. Available at: https://www.easyhealth.org.uk/pages/common-health-conditions. Accessed August 30, 2024.

8. Crime against persons with disabilities, 2009-2015 - statistical tables | Bureau of Justice Statistics. Available at: https://bjs.ojp.gov/library/publications/crime-against-persons-disabilities-2009-2015-statistical-tables. Accessed August 30, 2024.

9. Sobsey D, Doe T. Patterns of sexual abuse and assault. Sex Disabil 1991;9(3):243–59.

10. Howlin P, Clements J. Is it possible to assess the impact of abuse on children with pervasive developmental disorders? J Autism Dev Disord 1995;25(4):337–54.

11. Five safety rules to teach your child before they Start school. Child Abuse Prevention Service; 2022. Available at: https://www.caps.org.au/our-newsletter/five-safety-rules-to-teach-your-child-before-they-start-school. Accessed August 30, 2024.

12. Circles complete. Stanfield. Available at: https://stanfield.com/product/circles-complete/. Accessed August 30, 2024.

13. Amaze - age appropriate puberty and sex education videos. amaze. Available at: https://amaze.org/. Accessed August 30, 2024.

14. Teaching resources & Lesson plans | TPT. Available at: https://www.teacherspayteachers.com/. Accessed August 30, 2024.

15. Dillaway H, Marzolf B, Fritz H, et al. Experiences of reproductive and sexual health and health care among women with disabilities. In: Ussher BM, Chrisler JC, Perz J, editors. Routledge international handbook of women's sexual and reproductive health. London: Routledge; 2019. p. 569–80.

16. Silverberg C, Kaufman M, Odette F, et al. Masturbation and sexual abuse, the ultimate guide to sex and disability: for all of us who live with disabilities, chronic pain, and illness. San Francisco (CA): Cleis Press Inc.; 2003.

17. World report on disability. Available at: https://www.who.int/publications/i/item/9789241564182. Accessed June 30, 2024.

18. Zacharin M, Savasi I, Grover S. The impact of menstruation in adolescents with disabilities related to cerebral palsy. Arch Dis Child 2010;95(7):526–30.

19. Quint E, OBrien R, et al. Menstrual management for adolescents with disabilities. Pediatrics 2016;138(1):e20160295.

20. Fletcher J, Yee H, Ong B, et al. Centering disability visibility in reproductive health care: dismantling barriers to achieve reproductive equity. Womens Health (Lond Engl) 2023;19:17455057231197166. https://doi.org/10.1177/17455057231197166.

21. Frank S, Tyson NA. A clinical approach to catamenial epilepsy: a review. Perm J 2020;24:1–3.

22. Atkinson E, Bennet MJ, Dudley J, et al. "Consensus statement: menstrual and contraceptive management in women with an intellectual disability". Aust N Z J Obstet Gynaecol 2003;43(2):109–10.

23. Lidegaard Ø, Nielsen LH, Skovlund CW, et al. Risk of venous thromboembolism from use of oral contraceptives containing different progestogens and oestrogen doses: Danish cohort study, 2001-9. BMJ 2011;343:d6423.

24. Jacobson JC, Likis FE, Murphy PA. Extended and continuous combined contraceptive regimens for menstrual suppression. J Midwifery Wom Health 2012;57(6): 585–92.

25. Stewart FH, Kaunitz AM, Laguardia KD, et al. Extended use of transdermal norelgestromin/ethinyl estradiol: a randomized trial. Obstet Gynecol 2005;105(6): 1389–96.

26. Sulak PJ, Smith V, Coffee A, et al. Frequency and management of breakthrough bleeding with continuous use of the transvaginal contraceptive ring: a randomized controlled trial. Obstet Gynecol 2008;112(3):563–71.

27. Srikanth R, Cassidy G, Joiner C, et al. Osteoporosis in people with intellectual disabilities: a review and a brief study of risk factors for osteoporosis in a community sample of people with intellectual disabilities. J Intellect Disabil Res 2011;55(1): 53–62.

28. Bachrach LK, Sills IN. Section on Endocrinology. Clinical report—bone densitometry in children and adolescents. Pediatrics 2011;127(1):189–94.

29. Hubacher D, Lopez L, Steiner MJ, et al. Menstrual pattern changes from levonorgestrel subdermal implants and DMPA: systematic review and evidence-based comparisons. Contraception 2009;80(2):113–8.

30. Paradise SL, Landis CA, Klein DA. Evidence-based contraception: common questions and answers. Am Fam Physician 2022;106(3):251–9.

31. Willis D, Samalin E, Satgé D. Colorectal cancer in people with intellectual disabilities. Oncology 2018;95(6):323–36.

32. Iezzoni LI, Rao SR, Agaronnik ND, et al. Associations between disability and breast or cervical cancers, accounting for screening disparities. Med Care 2021;59(2): 139–47.

33. Liu Q, Adami HO, Reichenberg A, et al. Cancer risk in individuals with intellectual disability in Sweden: a population-based cohort study. PLoS Med 2021;18(10): e1003840.

34. Heslop P, Cook A, Sullivan B, et al. Cancer in deceased adults with intellectual disabilities: English population-based study using linked data from three sources. BMJ Open 2022;12(3):e056974.

35. Horner-Johnson W, Dobbertin K, Andresen EM, et al. Breast and cervical cancer screening disparities associated with disability severity. Wom Health Issues 2014; 24(1):e147–53.

36. Ramjan L, Cotton A, Algoso M, et al. Barriers to breast and cervical cancer screening for women with physical disability: a review. Women Health 2016;56(2):141–56.

37. Chan DNS, Law BMH, So WKW, et al. Factors associated with cervical cancer screening utilisation by people with physical disabilities: a systematic review. Health Pol 2022;126(10):1039–50.

38. Arana-Chicas E, Kioumarsi A, Carroll-Scott A, et al. Barriers and facilitators to mammography among women with intellectual disabilities: a qualitative approach. Disabil Soc 2020;35(8):1290–314.

39. National Core Indicators. Chart generator. 2014–15. "National association of state directors of developmental disabilities services and human services research

institute.". 2018. from the National Core Indicators Website: Available at: http://www.nationalcoreindicators.org/charts/.

40. Cuypers M, Schalk BWM, Boonman AJN, et al. Cancer-related mortality among people with intellectual disabilities: a nationwide population-based cohort study. Cancer 2022;128(6):1267–74.

41. Breast screening: easy guide. GOV.UK. 2023. Available at: https://www.gov.uk/government/publications/breast-screening-information-for-women-with-learning-disabilities. Accessed August 30, 2024.

42. Cheng MM, Udry JR. Sexual behaviors of physically disabled adolescents in the United States. J Adolesc Health 2002;31(1):48–58.

43. O'Brien K, Woolford S, Dobson C, et al. 39. Do adolescents with disabilities have lower rates of STI screening than non-disabled peers? J Pediatr Adolesc Gynecol 2024;37(2):255.

44. Parish SL, Swaine JG, Luken K, et al. Cervical and breast cancer-screening knowledge of women with developmental disabilities. Intellect Dev Disabil 2012;50(2): 79–91.

45. Barbera JP, Cichon B, Ankam N, et al. Equitable care for patients with disabilities. Obstet Gynecol 2024;143(4):475–83.

46. Ferreyra S, Hughes K. Table manners: a guide to the pelvic examination for disabled women and health care providers. San Francisco (CA): Sex Education for Disabled People; 1982.

47. Harper DM, Bettcher CM, Young AP. It is time to switch to primary HPV screening for cervical cancer. Am Fam Physician 2024;109(1):8–9C. Available at: https://www.aafp.org/pubs/afp/issues/2024/0100/editorial-hpv-screening-cervical-cancer.html.

48. Frighi V, Smith M, Andrews TM, et al. Incidence of fractures in people with intellectual disabilities over the life course: a retrospective matched cohort study. EClinicalMedicine 2022;52:101656.

49. Dreyfus D, Lauer E, Wilkinson J. Characteristics associated with bone mineral density screening in adults with intellectual disabilities. J Am Board Fam Med 2014;27(1):104–14.

50. Strategies to maintain bone health with SCI | MSKTC. Available at: https://msktc.org/sci/factsheets/bone-loss-after-spinal-cord-injury. Accessed August 30, 2024.

51. Whitney DG, Bell S, Hurvitz EA, et al. The mortality burden of non-trauma fracture for adults with cerebral palsy. Bone Reports 2020;13:100725.

52. Sullivan WF, Diepstra H, Heng J, et al. Primary care of adults with intellectual and developmental disabilities: 2018 Canadian consensus guidelines. Can Fam Physician 2018;64(4):254–79.

53. Wilkinson JE, Culpepper L, Cerreto M. Screening tests for adults with intellectual disabilities. J Am Board Fam Med 2007;20(4):399–407.

54. Tsou AY, Bulova P, Capone G, et al. Medical care of adults with down syndrome: a clinical guideline. JAMA 2020;324(15):1543–56.

55. McKelvey KD, Fowler TW, Akel NS, et al. Low bone turnover and low bone density in a cohort of adults with Down syndrome. Osteoporosis Int 2012;24(4):1333–8.

Impact of Politics on Women's Health

Chelsea Daniels, MD[a],*, Joanna Turner Bisgrove, MD[b],
Sheridan Finnie, MD, MPH[c]

KEYWORDS

- Political and social determinants of health • Women's health movement
- Abortion and access-to-care bans • Maternity care desert • Physician retention

KEY POINTS

- Women, particularly marginalized women, historically and presently face increased barriers to routine medical care.
- The 3 political determinants of health are voting, government, and policy; together, these create the social determinants that exacerbate health inequities.
- Overall health outcomes, especially those for women and children, are worse in states with access-to-care bans.
- Legislative and judicial decisions regarding women's health care directly affect residency applications and physician retention.
- Physician advocacy for patients' access to equitable care is a powerful tool in the health care landscape.

INTRODUCTION

Among the many imperatives of modern-day primary care clinicians is to understand the historical context and modern-day political determinants of health that influence the positionality and lived experiences of their patients. One constant, dating back to the beginning of record keeping itself, is the drive for control over marginalized groups through political, socio-cultural, moral, and religious means.[1] The oppression of women, particularly Black, brown, indigenous, disabled, and queer women, by limiting economic and political power, autonomy over one's body, and choice in life's

[a] Department of Medical Services, Planned Parenthood of South, East and North Florida, 585 NW 161st Street, Suite 200, Miami, FL 33169, USA; [b] Department of Family Medicine, Rush University Medical Center, Chicago, IL, USA; [c] PGY-3, Department of Family Medicine, University of North Carolina, Chapel Hill, NC, USA
* Corresponding author.
E-mail address: chelseadaniels1114@gmail.com

Prim Care Clin Office Pract 52 (2025) 223–231
https://doi.org/10.1016/j.pop.2024.12.006
0095-4543/25/© 2025 Elsevier Inc. All rights reserved, including those for text and data mining, AI training, and similar technologies.

Abbreviations	
AAMC	American Association of Medical Colleges
AMA	American Medical Association

pursuits, has wide-ranging roots across time and culture.[2–4] This system of power and oppression is often exercised through expressly political means and for expressly political gains, and has far-reaching consequences over nearly every aspect of women's lives, including the provision of women's health care.

Formalized political control over women can be traced back centuries. In the 1700s, for example, governments began to develop a political rationale that conceived of "populations" as entities to be managed by the state.[5] This concept effectively catapulted the traditional regulation of women's bodies to a legally sanctioned necessity in service of birth rates and fertility.[5,6] Michael Foucalt, a French philosopher and historian, coined the term "biopolitics" to describe this practice and ideology, defining it as the political mandate for a government to "to ensure, sustain, and multiply life".[5]

Another lasting legacy of the intrusion of politics into women's health is the construct of biology as destiny. This construct proliferated in colonial America and found its foothold in "natural truths" created by those in power to maintain systems of oppression. One "natural truth," the "racial construction of whiteness," rose to prominence in the United States, as well as biological gender differences grounded in the belief that women were innately inferior due to their reproductive physiology.[7,8] This nineteenth century "logic of difference" held that white, middle class women were delicate, less intelligent than men, and unsuitable for the public sphere. Even worse, the qualities attributed to women of color emphasized their racial difference over concepts of feminity, allowing for stereotypes of "bestial, promiscuous" Black women to foment and consequently provide justification for the enslavement, rape, and mistreatment of women of color.[8,9] These socially constructed differences imparted easy logic for ongoing oppression, and inevitably led to coercion and control across multiple spheres of women's lives. Unsurprisingly, women's health was and is no exception.

Definitions	
Political determinants of health	Voting, governmental, and policy decisions that determine how systems are structured, resources are distributed, and power is administered. These decisions create the social conditions that drive health disparities.[10]
Social determinants of health	Non-medical factors, including the conditions in which people are born, grow, work, and live, that affect health outcomes. Includes broader forces and systems that shape everyday life conditions.
Autonomy	The capacity and ability to make an informed, uncoerced decision.
Self-determination	A person's ability to make choices and manage their own life and health care decisions.
Coverture	Common law concept in which a married woman is included in her husband's legal status and therefore lacks independent legal rights, such as the right to own land, the right to her own bank account, and the right to vote.
Eugenics	The practice or advocacy of controlled, selective breeding of human populations to alter a population's genetic composition.
Maternity care desert	A county where there is a lack of maternity care services and/or barriers to access.

POLITICS, POLICY, AND POWER
Political Determinants of Health

There are 3 primary categories of political determinants of health: voting, government, and policy.[10] The uneven distribution of political power across these 3 spheres lays the groundwork for health inequities that have existed in the United States since its inception and persist to this day.[10]

For example, the inability of women to participate in all 3 spheres of the aforementioned political determinants of health—voting, government, and policy—in the early days of the United States severely limited their ability to control their own health. Preventing women from accessing any means of political power was justified by the legal doctrine of coverture, which prohibited women, particularly married women, from having their own legal and political identity.[11] Coverture also reinforced the notion of biology as destiny: because women were traditionally viewed as remaining in the home to raise children, policies were rarely crafted with women's needs in mind. Today, though women have left the home and entered the workforce in droves, the vestiges of coverture linger in myriad ways. For instance, the lack of universal paid family leave reflects the long-held view that women remain in the home and therefore do not need protected or paid time to care for children or other family members.[11]

At the same time, the predominantly male medical profession did not research women's health and therefore understood little about how women's bodies functioned. Most women sought care from non-physician health practitioners, the ranks of which were primarily made up of women. However, with the formation of the then exclusively white male American Medical Association (AMA) in 1847, physicians sought to "professionalize" medical practice. One of the first acts of the AMA in their work to "elevate" physicians above other societal healers was to advocate for nationwide restrictions on abortion. Their movement gained widespread political traction, and ultimately consigned women's health to the shadows.[12] An additional consequence of this movement was that women were also discouraged from becoming physicians.

The effects of this have reverberated for generations. The American Association of Medical Colleges (AAMC) previously noted that women did not start applying to medical school at even close to the same rates as men until 2003, and men continue to far outpace women in the upper levels of medical leadership.[13] A consequence of this phenomenon is that there have been relatively few women in the medical field to champion women's health-based research. As recently as the year 2020, only 10.8% of NIH research funding was allocated to women's health research.[14] The consequences of this are severe: women are underrepresented in clinical trials, meaning that medications are frequently less effective for women.[14] Additionally, the lack of overall research into women's health, as compared to men's health, means that women spend 25% more of their lives in poorer health than men.[14]

Women of color have faced additional barriers in achieving autonomy and self-determination over their bodies throughout history. The story of Henrietta Lacks is a commonly cited example of how women, particularly women of color, have been prohibited from making their own choices, highlighting how physicians have historically ignored principles of informed consent. In 1951, Lacks died of cervical cancer, mere months after presenting to the Johns Hopkins Hospital with vaginal bleeding. Without consent, her doctors collected and studied her cervical cells, finding that they thrived in the laboratory environment; her cells, named the HeLa line, have since underpinned a substantial amount of medical research. Lacks and her family never consented to the use of her cells for research, and have never received compensation for said use.[15]

Court rulings further reflect the lack of autonomy women have over their bodies. In the 1927 case *Buck v Bell*, the Supreme Court upheld a Virginia statute allowing the state to sterilize institutionalized people it considered genetically unfit, paving the way for 30 additional states to enforce such laws. Coming at the height of the Eugenics movement, the ruling led to an estimated 60,000 people in the United States being forcibly sterilized between the 1920s and the 1970s.[16]

The Women's Health Movement and Roe v Wade

Starting in the 1960s, the tide began to change with the second wave of the Women's Health Movement, a nationwide grassroots movement for women to gain control of their reproductive rights.[17] An early success of the Women's Health Movement was the Supreme Court ruling in *Griswold v Connecticut* (1965), which struck down the Comstock Act's ban on contraceptives and ruled that the law violated a couple's right to make private decisions.[18]

A primary aim of the Women's Health Movement was to legalize abortion. In the 1960s, approximately 1 million illegal abortions were performed yearly. Nearly one-third of women obtaining illegal abortions suffered complications requiring hospital admission, and 500 to 1000 women died annually as a result. With *Roe v Wade* (1973), the US Supreme Court ruled that laws banning abortion were a violation of the 14th Amendment's implicit guarantee of the right to privacy, thereby making all US laws banning abortion unconstitutional.[19]

Importantly, both *Griswold* and *Roe* were based on the right to privacy, a right that is not explicitly guaranteed in the 14th Amendment, but rather extrapolates from the right to liberty and due process. Furthermore, neither case was predicated on the equal protection clause of the 14th Amendment.[20] For this reason, *Roe* not only became vulnerable to future court decisions that could reverse its precedent, but it also ignited an anti-abortion and anti-women's health fervor in the decades after its passage. In the subsequent 50 years post-*Roe*, the anti-abortion movement successfully lobbied for a range of policies restricting abortion, including waiting periods and gestational age restrictions. Their goal was always the overturning of *Roe*, and their long-time efforts culminated in *Dobbs v Jackson* in June 2022.[20]

Rather than settling the legal question, *Dobbs v Jackson*'s reversal of *Roe v Wade* sparked a patchwork of state laws surrounding women's health, shown in **Fig. 1** from The Guttmacher Institute. Furthermore, since the US Supreme Court overturned *Roe* with the *Dobbs* decision, more and more data unequivocally demonstrate that the impacts on medical training and physician access are severe and worsening.

DISCUSSION
Impact on Medical Training and Physician Access

According to the AAMC, the number of overall applications by graduating medical students to residency programs in states with complete abortion bans decreased by 4.2% from the 2022 to 2023 cycle to the 2023 to 2024 cycle, compared to a 0.6% decrease in the overall number of applications in states without abortion bans during that same time period.[21] For specialities that are most directly affected by bans that restrict access to care, this trend is starker. For example, Obstetrics and Gynecology residencies in complete ban states saw a decrease in total applications by 6.7% from the 2022 to 2023 cycle to the 2023 to 2024 cycle, compared to an increase of 0.4% in states without access-to-care bans.[21] In Family Medicine, the trends were similar: applications decreased by 5.2% in complete ban states,

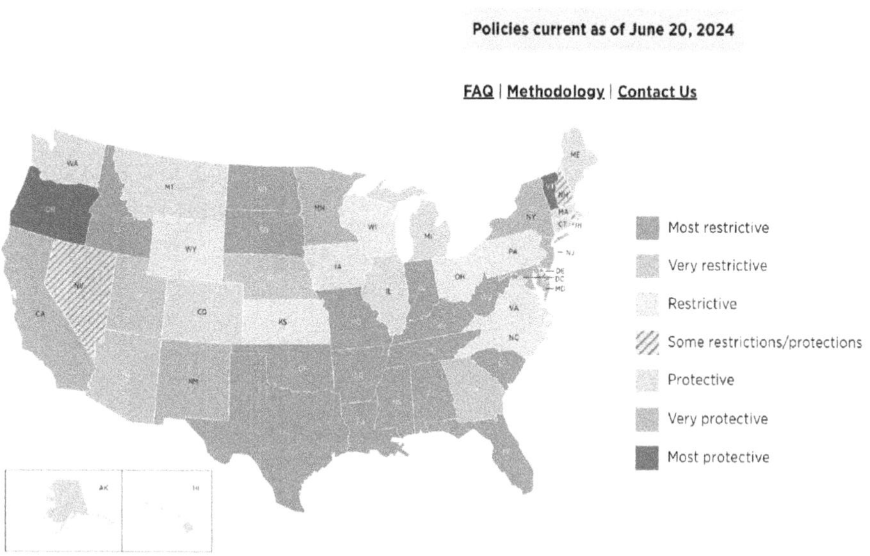

Fig. 1. Policies and Access after Roe. Note: Map lines delineate study areas and do not necessarily depict accepted national boundaries. (Guttmacher Institute, Interactive Map: US Abortion Policies and Access After Roe, March 5, 2025, https://states.guttmacher.org/policies.)

compared to 3.4% in non-ban states.[21] And in Pediatrics (Peds), the findings were the most devastating: applications in complete ban states decreased by 17.3%, compared to an 8.8% decrease in non-ban states.[21] Further complicating the picture is that most states with abortion bans also have bans on transgender care for those under the age of 18 years.[22]

These patterns highlight the tremendous effect of access-to-care bans on residency application decisions, particularly in those specialties whose scope includes the provision of reproductive health care and family planning (**Fig. 2**).

Moreover, physicians, as a whole, are less likely to seek employment in states with care restrictions, to better align with both their career goals and personal lives. A 2022 study illustrates this point by finding that 11% of physicians and residents endorsed either having an abortion themselves or having partners that had abortions, and that same study found that 15% of medical students reported that either they or their partners had an abortion at some point during training.[23] These data demonstrate that access-to-care bans shape career decisions for physicians in various ways.

SPECIAL CONSIDERATIONS AND POPULATIONS

Another result of access-to-care restrictions is the disproportionate impact wrought on marginalized communities, particularly those that are predominantly Black and brown, LGBTQ, living in poverty, and/or in rural or geographically isolated areas.[24] For example, by the end of 2022, 39% of counties in states with abortion bans were considered maternity care deserts, compared to 25% in non-ban states.[25] One well-documented driver of this trend is the lack of maternal care providers in ban states compared to non-ban states.[25] Maternal mortality rates are 62% higher in ban-states compared to non-ban states and are increasing "nearly twice as fast" in ban states compared to non-ban states.[25]

Percent Change in Residency Applications
2022-2023 Cycle vs 2023-2024 Cycle

◼ Abortion Banned   ◼ Abortion Legal

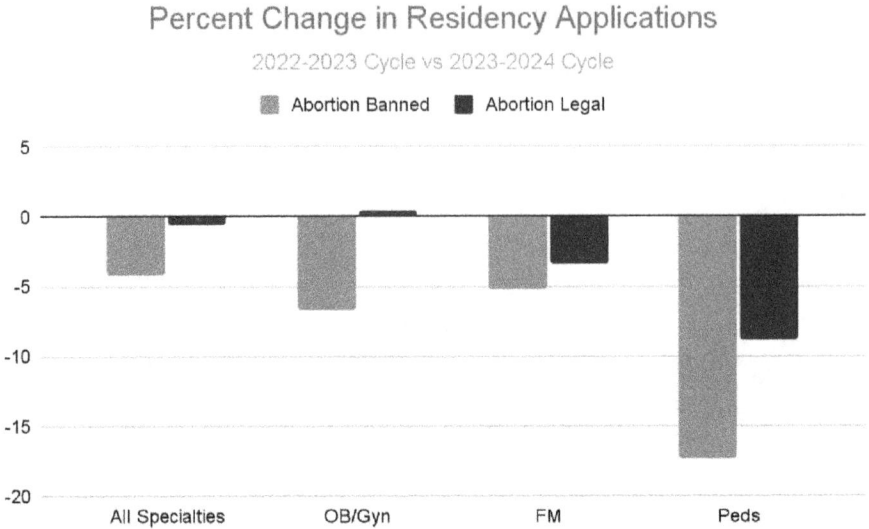

Fig. 2. Percent change in residency applications.

Furthermore, due to deeply entrenched wealth and geographic inequity, ban states are more likely to have populations that are uninsured and rural, a known risk factor for maternity care disparities.[25] Ban states also perform worse in other health-related outcomes, including neonatal mortality, premature death, and access to preventative/primary care.[25] A prime example of the increasing disparity is a recent study published in the JAMA Pediatrics that showed that the infant death rate rose 12.9% in Texas the year after its abortion ban was implemented, compared to a 1.8% increase in infant deaths in the rest of the country.[26] Living in a state that completely or partially bans any element of access to care has the potential to affect the overall health of a state's population.[25]

Compounding these inequities, the communities most likely to be affected by access-to-care bans are those who are already the most vulnerable and subject to poor health outcomes. One result of structural racism in the United States that outcomes in maternal care commonly exist along racial lines. For example, Black women die due to pregnancy-related complications at rates of up to four times higher than their white counterparts.[27,28] And per the Guttmacher Institute, over half of reproductive-aged Black women in the United States live in states with abortion restrictions, and Black women make up greater than 56% of the reproductive-aged population in those states.[29] As a result, Black women are uniquely targeted by bans that restrict access to care.

SUMMARY

A long line of legislative and judicial decisions have laid the groundwork for today's systemic disparities in women's health care. It is easy to become overwhelmed by the sheer volume of ever-changing legislation that impacts patient care. However, it is also vitally important to understand the laws and policies that directly affect clinical practice, especially in primary care. Primary care doctors see patients from a range of backgrounds who present for a range of reasons. And though not every primary care physician provides women's health services, fluency in the modern-day politics of women's health is key.

Primary care doctors are uniquely positioned to provide scientifically backed, compassionate, and person-centered women's health education, at a time when misinformation abounds. Physicians are already anecdotally reporting a massive uptick in patients "coming in with misconceptions about birth control fueled by influencers and political commentators".[30]

However, health care providers must provide their patients with supportive and evidence-based care. Patients may be uncertain and questioning, often as they attempt to synthesize disparate and conflicting information from social media algorithms, political pundits, and elected representatives. The clinic visit, though, can be a remarkable opportunity to dispel medical myths, encourage patient autonomy, and present factual, guideline-driven information about women's health.

In order to do so, it is crucial to recognize that the struggle between the forced control of women's bodies and the denial of knowledge and decision-making power by women regarding their bodies continues to be immensely relevant to the practice of primary care. Health professionals today must therefore understand the ways society, politics, and health collide in the past and the present.

CLINICS CARE POINTS

- *Opportunities for advocacy:* for the primary care clinician looking to support evidence-based guidelines and ethical principles of care through advocacy.
  - Advocate using AAFP's *Speak Out* tool: https://aafp.org/advocacy/fight/speak-out.html
  - Engage through ACOG's *Get Involved* advocacy toolkit: https://www.acog.org/advocacy/get-involved
  - ACOG's toolkit also has a specific focus on abortion advocacy and information: https://www.acog.org/advocacy/abortion-is-essential
  - Join your local Reproductive Health Access Project (RHAP) chapter: https://www.reproductiveaccess.org/

- *Stay up-to-date in the ever-changing landscape:* the oft-quoted adage that the PCP does not need to know every medical fact but rather where to find it rings true for the quickly changing legal and political landscape surrounding health care.
  - *Policy Resource Hub for Reproductive Health* through Lawyers for Good has the most updated, state-by-state information on local abortion laws. It is updated daily and offers a bi-weekly newsletter: https://rhlap.lawyersforgoodgovernment.org/
  - *Guttmacher Institute* is a reputable source for data, reports, and research regarding reproductive rights and abortion in the United States and globally. Explore state policies, track legislation, and even build a personal graph or map: https://www.guttmacher.org/united-states/abortion
  - Find specific legal advice for abortion providers through the Abortion Defense Network: https://abortiondefensenetwork.org/
  - The Repro Legal Helpline also has a direct number to call for legal advice: 1-844-868-2812

- *Educational resources:* for those looking to bolster their women's health knowledge and skill set.
  a. *Innovating Education in Reproductive Health* boasts several short, open access courses in topics ranging from contraception, first trimester abortion, and early pregnancy loss: https://www.innovating-education.org/
  b. AAFP offers a *Women's Health Online CME Self Study Package:* https://www.aafp.org/cme/self-study.html#:~:text=Designedtohelpfamilyphysicians,everystageofherlife

DISCLOSURE

The authors have nothing to disclose.

REFERENCES

1. Shannon G, Morgan R, Zeinali Z, et al. Intersectional insights into racism and health: not just a question of identity. Lancet 2022;400(10368):2125–36. PMID: 36502850.
2. Hubbard R. The politics of women's biology. New Brunswick, N.J.: Rutgers University Press; 1990.
3. Coen-Sanchez K, Ebenso B, El-Mowafi IM, et al. Repercussions of overturning Roe v. Wade for women across systems and beyond borders. Reprod Health 2022;19(1):184.
4. Boston Women's Health Book Collective. Women and their bodies: a course. Boston (MA): Boston Women's Health Collective: New England Free Press; 1970.
5. Foucault M. The History of Sexuality, Volume 1: An Introduction. New York City (NY): Vintage Books; 1990.
6. Purdy L. Women's reproductive autonomy: medicalisation and beyond. J Med Ethics 2006;32(5):287–91.
7. Whittle KL, Inhorn MC. Rethinking difference: a feminist reframing of gender/race/class for the improvement of women's health research. Int J Health Serv 2001; 31(1):147–65.
8. Carver T. Gender, . Political concepts. Manchester, England: Manchester University Press; 2018. https://doi.org/10.7765/9781526137562.00018. Retrieved June 26, 2024.
9. Wills H. Women in the history of science. UCL press. 2023. Available at: https://www.uclpress.co.uk/products/211143.
10. Dawes D. The political determinants of health. Baltimore (MD): Johns Hopkins University Press; 2020.
11. Allgor A. Coverture - the word you probably don't know but should. National Women's History Museum; 2014. Available at: www.womenshistory.org/articles/coverture-word-you-probably-dont-know-should.
12. Johnson R. A movement for change: horatio Robinson Storer and physicians' crusade against abortion. James Madison Undergraduate Research Journal 2017;4(1):13–23. Available at: http://commons.lib.jmu.edu/jmurj/vol4/iss1/2.
13. American Association of Medical Colleges. "2018-2019: the state of women in academic medicine: exploring pathways to equity.". Available at: https://www.aamc.org/data-reports/data/2018-2019-state-women-academic-medicine-exploring-pathways-equity.
14. McKinsey Health Institute. Closing the women's health gap: a $1 trillion opportunity to improve lives and economies. World Economic Forum 2024.
15. Editorial. Henrietta Lacks: science must right a historical wrong. Nature 2020;585.
16. Disability Justice. The right to self determination: freedom from involuntary sterilization. Available at: https://disabilityjustice.org/right-to-self-determination-freedom-from-involuntary-sterilization/. Accessed June 18, 2024.
17. Nichols FH. "History of the women's health movement in the 20th century.". J Obstet Gynecol Neonatal Nurs 2000;v29(1):56–64.
18. Wex Definitions Team. "Griswold v Connecticut." legal information Institute at cornell law school. 2022. Available at: https://www.law.cornell.edu/wex/griswold_v_connecticut_(1965).
19. National Archives. "14th amendment to the US constitution." National Archives. Available at: https://www.archives.gov/milestone-documents/14th-amendment. Accessed June 18, 2024.

20. Ruth B. Ginsburg, some thoughts on autonomy and equality in relation to Roe v. Wade. 63 N.C. L. Rev 1985;375.
21. Orgera K, Grover A. States with abortion bans see continued decrease in U.S. MD senior residency applicants. Washington, DC: AAMC; 2024. https://doi.org/10.15 766/rai_dnhob2ma.
22. Human Rights Campaign. Map: attacks on gender affirming care by state. Available at: https://www.hrc.org/resources/attacks-on-gender-affirming-care-by-state-map. Accessed August 16, 2024.
23. Levy MS, Arora VM, Talib H, et al. Abortion among physicians. Obstet Gynecol 2022;139(5):910–2. MED 38, 2419–2423 (2023).
24. March of Dimes, Nowhere to go: maternity care deserts throughout the U.S.: 2020 report (March of Dimes, 2020).
25. E Declercq et al., The U.S. Maternal health divide: the limited maternal health services and worse outcomes of states proposing New abortion restrictions (commonwealth fund, 2022). https://doi.org/10.26099/z7dz-8211.
26. Gemmill A, Margerison CE, Stuart EA, et al. Infant deaths after Texas' 2021 ban on abortion in early pregnancy. JAMA Pediatr 2024;178(8):784–91.
27. Trost SL, Beauregard J, Njie F, et al. Pregnancy-related deaths: data FFarom maternal mortality review committees in 36 US states, 2017-2019. Centers for Disease Control and Prevention, US Department of Health and Human Services; 2022.
28. Howell EA. Reducing disparities in severe maternal morbidity and mortality. Clin Obstet Gynecol 2018;61(2):387–99.
29. Sully EA, Biddlecom A, Darroch JE, et al. Adding it up: investing in sexual and reproductive health 2019. New York: Guttmacher Institute; 2020. Available at: https://www.guttmacher.org/report/adding-it-up-investing-in-sexual-reproductive-health-2019.
30. Weber L, Mahli S. "Women are getting off birth control amid misinformation explosion." the Washington post. 2024. Available at: https://www.washingtonpost.com/health/2024/03/21/stopping-birth-control-misinformation/.

Cancer Screening in Women

Brian P. Kenealy, MD, PhD*, Jennifer E. Lochner, MD

KEYWORDS

- Breast cancer screening • Cervical cancer screening • Colon cancer screening
- Lung cancer screening • Ovarian cancer screening

KEY POINTS

- Women aged 40 to 74 years who are of average risk should be offered breast cancer screening with mammography every 2 years.
- Women aged 21 to 65 years should be offered cervical cancer screening every 3 to 5 years via cervical cytology alone, human papillomavirus testing alone, or co-testing.
- Women aged 45 to 75 years who are of average risk should be offered colon cancer screening via a stool-based test every 1 to 3 years or via a direct visualization-based test every 5 to 10 years.
- Women who are aged 50 to 80, have a 20 pack-year smoking history and either smoke, or have quit within the past 15 years, should be offered lung cancer screening with annual low-dose computed tomography.
- Ovarian cancer screening is not recommended for average risk women.

INTRODUCTION

Globally, cancer is second only to cardiovascular disease as the leading cause of death in women.[1,2] In the United States, cancer continues to account for approximately 20.5% of deaths in women.[3] With an aging global population, the crude cancer death rate rose by approximately 21% since 1990.[1] Although overall incidence rates continue to rise, global age-standardized rates of cancer deaths have decreased by approximately 15%, suggesting improvement in cancer screening, diagnosis, and treatment efforts.[1]

Cancer screening programs remain essential tools in early detection and diagnosis of cancer. Mathematical modeling suggests that increased screening increases early detection and decreases cancer mortality[4,5]; although, the degree of impact is perhaps debatable.[6,7] In recognition of the importance of screening efforts on early cancer detection, Healthy People 2030 initiatives prioritize increasing cancer screening rates.[8] This article reviews current issues regarding US cancer screening

Department of Family Medicine and Community Health, University of Wisconsin- Madison, 610 North Whitney Way Suite 200, Madison, WI 53705, USA
* Corresponding author.
E-mail address: brian.kenealy@fammed.wisc.edu

Prim Care Clin Office Pract 52 (2025) 233–248
https://doi.org/10.1016/j.pop.2024.12.007   **primarycare.theclinics.com**
0095-4543/25/© 2024 Elsevier Inc. All rights reserved, including those for text and data mining, AI training, and similar technologies.

Abbreviations	
ACG	American College of Gastroenterology
ACOG	American College of Obstetricians and Gynecologists
ACR	American College of Radiology
ACS	American Cancer Society
CRC	Colorectal cancer
CT	computed tomography
FDA	US Food and Drug Administration
FIT	fecal immunochemical test
HPV	human papillomavirus
LDCT	low dose CT
NCCN	National Comprehensive Cancer Network
SBI	Society of Breast Imaging
sDNA-FIT	stool DNA-FIT
TVUS	transvaginal ultrasound
USPSTF	United States Preventive Services Task Force

guidelines in women for breast, cervical, colorectal, lung, and ovarian cancers with attention toward cancer-specific special populations and differences in screening rates and outcomes in minoritized communities.

Breast Cancer Screening

Background
Breast cancer is the second most common type of cancer next to skin cancer and has the second highest mortality next to lung cancer in women (**Table 1**). Since 1999, the incidence of breast cancer has been stable, with approximately 130 cases per 100,000 women annually.[9] Breast cancer mortality rates have dropped over this

Table 1
Pre-pandemic (2019) cancer incidence and mortality rates in the US female population[a,b]

Cancer Type	2019 Incidence (# Cases)	Incidence Rate (per 100,000)	2019 Mortality (# Cases)	Mortality Rate (per 100,000)
All	899,200	432.6	283,722	125.9
Breast	271,950	133.6	42,280	19.4
Lung	113,928	50.6	64,743	28.1
Colorectal	69,068	32.8	24,222	10.8
Uterine	61,110	28.5	11,556	5.1
Melanomas	37,750	19.1	2797	1.3
Thyroid	34,370	19.8	1090	0.5
Non-Hodgkin's lymphoma	33,414	15.7	8792	3.9
Pancreas	27,107	12.1	22,153	9.6
Kidney	25,982	12.5	4795	2.1
Leukemias	22,650	11.1	9743	4.4
Ovarian	20,466	10	13,445	6
Bladder	18,639	8.3	4740	2
Oral cavity/pharynx	14,148	6.7	3117	1.4
Cervical	13,322	7.8	4152	2.2

[a] Abstracted from publicly available data, see ref.[9]
[b] At time of writing, data available up to 2022; however, pre-pandemic data chosen due to COVID-19 pandemic effects that are beyond scope of the article.

period, with the age-adjusted death rate decreasing from 26.6 per 100,000 to 19.4 per 100,000 women. This change has stabilized the number of individuals dying from breast cancer to around 40 to 42,000 women a year.[9]

Current mammography technology is associated with a 41% reduction in mortality and a 25% reduction in rates of advanced breast cancers at time of diagnosis.[10] Sensitivity of screening mammography worsens with increased density of breast tissue (98% sensitive in fatty breast tissue vs 30%–48% in extremely dense tissue).[11] Additionally, women with dense breasts are more likely to develop breast cancer.[12–14] As of September 2024, breast density is required to be reported to patients and ordering clinicians after mammography.[15] Adjunctive imaging with MRI or ultrasound shows a small increase in detection rates in individuals with dense breast tissue; however, it is also associated with increased false positive and biopsy rates, and mortality benefit has yet to be demonstrated.[12,15–17] While this issue remains a concern, consensus among guideline organizations has not been reached regarding the use of adjunctive imaging in average risk women with dense breast tissue (**Table 2**).

Breast cancer screening rates in the United States are stable with 76.4% of women aged 50 to 75 years receiving recommended screening (2019).[18] Screening rates increase with affluence (<200% federal poverty level, 68.3%, >200% 79.6%) and higher educational achievement (less than high school, 69.4%; high school 73.2%; above high school 79.0%).[18]

Screening recommendations
Screening recommendations for breast cancer are based on risk factors and age. Average risk women are healthy women without additional genetic, radiation exposure, or family history-related risk factors.

Average risk. As detailed in **Table 2**, with the 2024 United States Preventive Services Task Force (USPSTF) update,[12] the major screening recommendations for average risk individuals are now nearly all aligned to start screening with mammography at the age of 40 years.[12,13,15,16,19,20] Among the major guideline organizations (USPSTF, American Cancer Society [ACS], American College of Obstetricians and Gynecologists [ACOG], National Comprehensive Cancer Network [NCCN], American College of Radiology [ACR], and the Society of Breast Imaging [SBI]), there is still heterogeneity regarding frequency of screening. For most average risk women, there is room for an individualized approach to screen yearly versus biennially based on age, patient preferences, breast density, and availability of advanced imaging modalities. All organizations recommend continuing screening until the age of 75 years and continuing beyond 75 years to be individualized based on health and life expectancy of at least 10 years.

Moderate risk. Moderate risk women are those with a family history of breast cancer at age greater than 40 years without a known genetic predisposition syndrome to cancer. The most recent ACR guidelines recommend risk assessment by the age of 30 years for all women.[20] Risk assessment tools such as the Tyrer Cuzick model or BOADICEA/CanRisk are available to help patients and clinicians further risk stratify and determine whether high risk recommendations should be followed.[15,21] For women older than 35 years of age, the modified Gail model is an option to assess 5 year risk.[15] The NCCN suggests following high-risk recommendations for those with greater than 20% lifetime risk or greater than 1.7% 5 year risk of invasive breast cancer.[15] For most organizations, recommendations do not change in moderate risk women from average risk women.

Table 2
Breast cancer screening guidelines for women with low-to-moderate risk[a]

Organization	Modality	Start (age, years)	Frequency (years)	End (Age)	Breast Tissue Density
ACS 2015	Mammography	45 option at 40	1 (40–54) then 2 (≥55)	Continue past 75 if life expectancy >10 y	Not discussed
ACOG 2017	Mammography + offer clinical breast examination starting age 25 years	40	1 (40–54) then 2 (≥55)	75 or longer with shared decision making	Recommend against (ACOG #625)
NCCN 2023	Mammography + tomosynthesis	40	1	Not specified	Consider supplemental imaging for heterogenous or extremely dense tissue
USPSTF 2024	Mammography ± tomosynthesis	40	2	75 (insufficient evidence past 75)	Insufficient evidence for supplemental imaging
ACR/SBI 2021	Mammography + offer risk assessment by age of 30 years	40	1	Continue past 75 unless severe comorbidities	Insufficient evidence, however, based on ACR appropriateness criteria: consider supplemental imaging based on density and risk

[a] For details, see Refs.[12,13,15,16,19,20]

High risk. High risk women are those with a family history of first-degree relatives at a young age, prior chest radiation, and/or known genetic predispositions. Most organizations recommend yearly screening for women in this category beginning at the age of 30 years with yearly mammography and breast MRI.[12,13,15,16,19,20] If there are known family history of specific genetic markers, such as BRCA1 and 2, family members should also consider genetic counseling.[12]

Disparities
Racial disparities in breast cancer mortality persist. Despite the non-Hispanic black population having the highest overall screening rates (79% in 2019, 82% in 2021), this population continues to have the highest breast cancer mortality rate (40% higher risk compared to a non-Hispanic white population).[12] Reasons are multifaceted, complex, and linked to social determinants of health which are worse in minoritized and lower resourced communities.[12]

Cervical Cancer Screening

Background
Cervical cancer is the 14th most common type of cancer in US women (see **Table 1**). The annual incidence and mortality rates of cervical cancer have remained stable since 2012 through 2019 at around 7.8 per 100,000 new cases and around 2.2 per 100,000 deaths. Rates of screening in the United States are high (>80% in 2019) but vary by age, ethnicity/race, socioeconomic, education, and geographic location.[22] Screening rates are lower in minoritized racial and ethnic groups, rural residents, sexual and gender minorities, those with limited English proficiency, and with mental health conditions. Infection with a high-risk strain of human papillomavirus (HPV) is associated with nearly all cases of cervical cancer. Transmission of HPV occurs through sexual intercourse. Since the approval of the first HPV vaccine in 2006, studies show promising results in the youngest birth cohorts who are vaccinated, with 65% to 88% estimated reduction in cervical cancer incidence rates.[23,24] HPV vaccination rates have approached approximately 70% of US girls.

Screening recommendations
As summarized in **Table 3**, most guideline organizations recommend routine screening with every 3 year Pap smear starting at age 21 years up to age 30 years. At age 30 years and above, the USPSTF recommends continued screening with every 3 year Pap, or Pap with HPV co-testing every 5 years until the age of 65 years.[25] The ACS recommends HPV only testing every 5 years starting at age 25 years through 65 years as another option.[26] Screening is recommended regardless of HPV vaccination status. Women who have a hysterectomy with removal of the cervix, and who do not have a history of cervical intraepithelial neoplasia grade 2 or 3 or cervical cancer do not need continued cervical cancer screening. Women above the age of 65 years should only be screened if they have not received adequate prior screening, defined as 3 consecutive negative cytology results or 2 consecutive negative co-testing results within the prior 10 years, with the most recent test having occurred in the past 5 years. Women with a precancerous cervical lesion (CIN 2 or greater) should continue screening for at least 20 years after treatment or spontaneous regression of the lesion. A new sexual partner after the age of 65 years is not an indication to re-start cervical cancer screening in a person who otherwise meets criteria to stop screening.[25,26]

Disparities
The incidence and mortality rate for cervical cancer in the United States is higher in non-Hispanic black, American Indian/Alaska native, and Hispanic women than for

Table 3
Cervical cancer screening guidelines[a]

Population	USPSTF-2018 (Endorsed by ACOG, ASCCP)	ACS – 2021 (Endorsed by ASCCP)
Age 21–24 y	Pap test q 3 y	No screening
Age 25–29 y	Pap test q 3 y	HPV test q 5 y or Pap + HPV co-testing q 5 y or Pap test q 3 y
Age 30–65 y	Pap test q 3 y or Pap + HPV co-testing q 5 y	HPV test q 5 y or Pap + HPV co-testing q 5 y or Pap test q 3 y
Age >65 y	No screening unless inadequate prior screening or within 20 y of identification of a precancerous lesion	No screening unless inadequate prior screening or within 20 y of identification of a precancerous lesion

[a] For details, see ref.[25,26]

non-Hispanic white women. Women without health insurance and who live in geographically isolated areas also have higher cervical cancer mortality than the US average. Lower screening rates, inadequate follow-up and differences in treatment seem to be the causes of these differences.[25]

Colorectal Cancer Screening

Background
Colorectal cancer (CRC) is the third most common cancer diagnosed in women and the third leading cause of cancer death in US women (see **Table 1**). The age-adjusted rate of new CRC diagnoses in US women has fallen from 48 per 100,000 in 1999 to 32.8 per 100,000 in 2019.[9] In comparison, this rate for US men from 2019 was 42.7 per 100,000. Due to the aging of the US population, since 2012 the absolute number of new CRC diagnoses each year is rising with over 68,000 new cases reported in 2019. Annual rates of age-adjusted CRC deaths have been declining in women in the United States (17.8 per 100,000 in 1999–10.8 in 2019); an achievement thought due to increased screening rates and the development of more effective treatments for colon cancer.[9]

Though there are demonstrable improvements in rates of cancer diagnosis and death, more detailed analyses show that these improvements are primarily due to decreases in CRC rates in adults age 65 years and older. In people under age 65 years, CRC incidence is rising, with the fastest rate of rise seen in individuals under age 50 years. It is now estimated that over 10% of all new CRC cases will be identified in individuals less than 50 years old.[27] Lifestyle (low physical activity, smoking, high red meat, fat, and alcohol consumption) and obesity are estimated to contribute to over half of all cases of CRC.[28,29] In 2022, the age-adjusted rate of US women age 50 to 75 years who reported being up to date on CRC screening was 73.3% (72.7–74) based on data from the Behavioral Risk Factor Surveillance System. This is higher than the rate for men which was 70.9% (70.2–71.6) in the same survey.[9]

Screening recommendations
CRC screening is recommended for average risk adults age 45 to 75 years according to all major US health care organizations (**Table 4**).[30–34] Multiple options exist for CRC screening (**Table 5**). The American College of Gastroenterology (ACG) recommends fecal immunochemical test (FIT) or colonoscopy as the tests with the best evidence of benefit.[33] For those unable or unwilling to have one of these tests performed on the recommended schedule, multitarget stool DNA-FIT (sDNA-FIT) test, computed tomography (CT) colonography, and flexible sigmoidoscopy are other options (see **Table 5**). In 2024, the US Food and Drug Administration (FDA) approved a cell-free DNA blood test to screen for CRC.[35] The major US health care organizations have yet to recommend this test. To achieve the benefits of screening, abnormal results from any of the non-colonoscopy tests must be followed up with a colonoscopy. While there are risks and benefits to each screening modality for any individual patient, the best screening test for CRC is the one that the patient will complete.

Screening in high-risk populations
Those with above-average risk for colon cancer include individuals with a family history of colon cancer (in one first-degree relative under the age of 60 years, or 2 or more first-degree relatives at any age) and those with a prior history of CRC or adenomas. Women diagnosed with uterine or ovarian cancer before the age of 50 years are also at increased risk of CRC. Weak evidence suggests that for those with a family history, screening should begin at the age of 40 years, or 10 years before the age of the youngest family member at their age of diagnosis.[30–33] Other individuals with above

Table 4
CRC screening guidelines for individuals with average-risk [a]

Population	USPSTF - 2021	ACS – 2018	US Multi-Society Task Force (ACG, AGA, ASGE) - 2022
Age 45–49 y	Screen all grade B	Screen all	Screen all, weak recommendation, low quality
Age 50–75 y	Screen all grade A	Screen all	Screen all, strong recommendation, high quality
Age 76–85 y	Selectively screen (fewer comorbid conditions and longer life expectancy) grade C	Selectively screen (fewer comorbid conditions and longer life expectancy)	Individualized decision, weak recommendation, low quality
Age >86 y	Do not screen	Do not screen	Do not screen

AGA, American Gastroenterological Society; ASGE, American Society for Gastroenterological Endoscopy.
[a] For details, see Refs.[30-32]

Table 5
CRC screening options[a]

Modality	Frequency (years)	Sensitivity (%)	Specificity (%)	Evidence of Efficacy	Other Considerations
Stool-based tests					
FIT	1	74 for CRC	94 for CRC	• Single large cohort study shows decreased CRC mortality	• Ease of use/collection • Requires yearly adherence; benefit seen after multiple tests • Abnormal tests require colonoscopy follow-up and associated risks
sDNA-FIT	1–3	93 for CRC	85 for CRC	• Lacking evidence for effect on CRC mortality • Compared to FIT: improved sensitivity but worse specificity (higher false positive rate) • Modeling for every 3 y testing does not provide favorable balance of benefits vs harms over other stool-based strategies	• Ease of use/collection • Requires adherence; benefit seen after multiple tests • Abnormal tests require colonoscopy follow up and associated risks
Direct visualization tests					
Colonoscopy	10	18–100 for CRC; 89–95 for adenomas ≥10 mm	89 for adenomas ≥10 mm	• Cohort studies show decreased CRC mortality • Risk of bleeding/perforation and risks increase with age	• Benefits of screening and diagnosis in single examination and longer screening interval • Requires bowel preparation, sedation, additional transportation

(continued on next page)

Table 5
(continued)

Modality	Frequency (years)	Sensitivity (%)	Specificity (%)	Evidence of Efficacy	Other Considerations
CT colonography	5	86–100 for CRC; 89 for adenomas ≥10 mm	94% for Adenomas ≥10 mm	• Lacking evidence for effect on CRC mortality • Extracolonic incidental findings common (1.3%–11.4%), limited evidence of benefits or harms	• Abnormal test requires colonoscopy follow up and associated risks • Requires bowel preparation, but no sedation or additional transportation
Flexible Sigmoidoscopy	5	90–100 for distal CRC	83–94 for proximal advanced neoplasms	• Randomized clinical trials show decreased CRC mortality • Risk of bleeding/perforation smaller than colonoscopy • Modeling predicts fewer life-years gained alone compared to other strategies or in combination with stool-based testing	• Abnormal test require colonoscopy follow up and associated risks • Availability declining in USA

[a] *Adapted from Refs.*[30,34]

average risk include those with a personal history of inflammatory bowel disease or a hereditary cancer syndrome such as familial adenomatous polyposis or Lynch syndrome (hereditary non-polyposis colon cancer). These individuals benefit from the involvement of a gastroenterologist in their care.

Disparities

Non-Hispanic black women experience higher rates of CRC than any other racial or ethnic group in the United States.[33] Mortality is also higher for non-Hispanic black women compared to non-Hispanic white women. It is likely that disparities in screening, follow up, and access to treatment underlie these differences.

Lung Cancer Screening

Background

Lung cancer is the second most common cancer and the leading cause of cancer death in women in the United States (see **Table 1**). In 2019, the age-adjusted rate of new lung cancer diagnoses in US women was 50.6 per 100,000, down from a peak of 57 per 100,000 in 2005.[9] Due to an aging US population, the absolute number of new diagnoses of lung cancer in US women has steadily risen with 112,928 cases reported in 2019.[9] The age-adjusted mortality rate for lung cancer in US women was 28.1 per 100,000 in 2019, down from 41.6 in 2002. Lung cancer often has a poor prognosis with a 5 year relative survival rate of 26% reported in 2019. Cancers diagnosed at an earlier stage are more amenable to treatment and have a better prognosis. Smoking tobacco is the key risk factor for lung cancer and the risk is dose dependent. Age is also associated with an increased risk of lung cancer. According to a report from the American Lung Association, only 5.8% of eligible persons in the United States were screened for lung cancer in 2021.[36] This is well below the screening rates for other routinely recommended cancer screening.

Screening recommendations

In 2013, the USPSTF and the ACS released the first recommendations for lung cancer screening. They both recommended annual screening with low dose CT (LDCT) for patients aged 55 to 80 years with 30 pack-years smoking who were current smokers or who had quit within the past 15 years.[37,38] This was based largely on the National Lung Cancer Screening Trial which reported a relative risk reduction in lung cancer mortality of 20% in the intervention group.[39] Updated screening recommendations are found in **Table 6**. The USPSTF lowered the age at which to begin screening to 50 years, decreased the pack-years of smoking threshold to 20, but kept the "years since quit (YSQ)" criteria.[37] Likewise, the ACS recently lowered the age at which to begin screening from 55 to 50 years of age but also eliminated the YSQ criteria; instead, recommending screening anyone in that age group with a 20 pack-year smoking history.[38] Their rationale is based on modeling that showed decreased lung cancer mortality with removal of the YSQ criteria, with an estimated number needed to screen

Table 6 Lung cancer screening guidelines[a]		
Population	**USPSTF - 2021**	**ACS - 2023**
Age 50–80 y	Screen current or former (quit within past 15 y) smokers with $\geq$ 20 pack-year history, grade B	Screen current or former smokers who have a $\geq$ 20 pack-year history

[a] For details, see Refs.[37,38]

of 39 to save one life.[38] These changes ultimately increased the number of women and members of minoritized racial and ethnic groups eligible for screening. These groups appear to be at higher risk of developing lung cancer with less lifetime tobacco exposure.

Disparities

Rates of new lung cancer diagnoses in US women vary based on race and ethnicity. The highest rates are in non-Hispanic white women, followed by American Indian and Alaska native, non-Hispanic black, Asian and Pacific islander, and Hispanic women.[9] Lower socioeconomic status is also associated with higher lung cancer incidence, correlating with a higher prevalence of smoking among these individuals.[40] Notably, tobacco companies have a history of aggressively marketing their products in communities with a lower socioeconomic profile.[41]

Controversies/challenges

A concern with LDCT screening is the potential harms associated with the detection and subsequent evaluation of non-specific lung nodules and other incidental findings. A 2023 study found that 33.8% of all participants in LDCT screening had a significant incidental finding that required follow up.[42] Clinicians should counsel patients about this possibility as part of the shared decision making prior to starting screening. Smoking cessation is the intervention most likely to lead to improved health outcomes in patients who smoke. Patients who smoke should receive tobacco cessation counseling as part of the shared decision-making conversation about screening. Lung cancer screening is not a substitute for quitting smoking.

Ovarian Cancer Screening

Background

Ovarian cancer is the eleventh most common cause of cancer in the United States (see **Table 1**). The incidence and mortality rates of ovarian cancer have steadily declined to about 10 per 100,000 new cases and around 6 per 100,000 deaths. This is a decrease by about 40% and 33%, respectively, from 1975 data when the incidence rates were about 16 per 100,000 and death rates of 9 per 100,000. Most ovarian cancers are diagnosed later in life and at a later stage. The mortality burden of ovarian cancer is high with approximately one third to half of women dying from their disease.[9]

Screening recommendations

Guideline organizations recommend against screening average risk women for ovarian cancer.[43,44] Transvaginal ultrasound (TVUS) and CA-125 blood marker testing have been studied separately and in combination as screening modalities and fail to show reductions in ovarian cancer mortality; however, ACOG recommends women who are high risk due to a hereditary cancer syndrome such as BRCA 1 or 2 to undergo screening with TVUS and CA-125.[44] Studies of this approach have been non-randomized and not designed to prove a survival or mortality benefit.[45] The USPSTF recommends those with significant family history be referred to genetic counseling.[43]

Disparities

According to the US Cancer Statistics Working Group, the incidence of ovarian cancer was highest in non-Hispanic American Indian and Alaska native women (11.4/100,000 women) and non-Hispanic white women (11.0/100,000 women).[9,46] A 2019 study found an 18% higher risk of mortality among non-Hispanic black patients with ovarian cancer compared to non-Hispanic white patients.[47]

Special Populations

Cancer screening in transgender people

Clinicians should offer transgender individuals cancer screening according to usual guidelines for the pertinent organs present in their bodies. In particular, transgender men who have a cervix should be advised to undergo cervical cancer screening according to the guidelines described earlier. Transgender men who have not had mastectomy (or who have had a partial mastectomy) should be offered routine breast cancer screening. The evidence regarding breast cancer screening in transgender women is less clear but most guidelines recommend that screening mammograms be offered for those who have taken estrogen for 10 years or longer and otherwise meet the age criteria established for cisgender women. Transgender women should be counseled regarding prostate cancer screening in the same way that cisgender men should.[48]

SUMMARY

Despite the demonstrable benefits of early detection on morbidity, mortality in women, and health care system cost, cancer screening efforts have lagged the goals set out by Healthy People initiatives. Additionally, there remain large health disparities among minoritized communities. Closing these care gaps will require specific cancer screening program efforts on the part of clinicians and health systems to target under-screened populations. Lung cancer is both the cancer with the highest mortality rate in US women and the cancer with the lowest participation in screening programs. While tobacco use cessation is key to improving mortality from lung cancer, improving lung cancer screening rates in appropriate patients may be beneficial. A new multicancer early detection option, yet to be approved by the FDA, may soon be available. The technology detects novel DNA methylation patterns shared among multiple cancer subtypes and can detect cancer derived from multiple organ systems.[49,50] Further clinical trials are currently in process to further determine efficacy, utility, and safety. Looking toward the future, innovative technology as well as other strategies that reduce cultural, socio-economic, racial, and physical barriers to screening, may shift cancer screening toward a more equitable landscape.

CLINICS CARE POINTS

- Cervical cancer screening via HPV testing alone is often not available to clinicians and patients due to limitations in lab equipment.

- HPV self-collection has the potential to improve cervical cancer screening rates in those who avoid testing due to the need for a pelvic examination.

- It is estimated that 81% of the mortality benefit of breast cancer screening is maintained with every other year screening compared to annual screening, with about half of the false-positive results.[13]

- The best test for colon cancer screening is the one that the patient will complete.

- Only 5.8% of eligible individuals were screened for lung cancer in 2021.

DISCLOSURE

The authors have nothing to disclose.

REFERENCES

1. Roser M, Ritchie H. Cancer. 2015. Available at: https://ourworldindata.org/cancer. Accessed August 29, 2024.
2. Hahn RA, Chang MH, Parrish RG, et al. Trends in mortality among females in the United States, 1900-2010: progress and challenges. Prev Chronic Dis 2018;15: E30. Erratum in: Prev Chronic Dis. 2018;15:E76.
3. Heron M. Deaths: leading causes for 2019. Natl Vital Stat Rep 2021;70:1–114.
4. Knudsen AB, Trentham-Dietz A, Kim JJ, et al. Estimated US cancer deaths prevented with increased use of lung, colorectal, breast, and cervical cancer screening. JAMA Netw Open 2023;6:e2344698.
5. Sharma KP, Grosse SD, Maciosek MV, et al. Preventing breast, cervical, and colorectal cancer deaths: assessing the impact of increased screening. Prev Chronic Dis 2020;17:200039.
6. Bretthauer M, Wieszczy P, Løberg M, et al. Estimated lifetime gained with cancer screening tests: a meta-analysis of randomized clinical trials. JAMA Intern Med 2023;183:1196–203.
7. Stang A, Jöckel KH. The impact of cancer screening on all-cause mortality. Dtsch Arztebl Int 2018;115:481–6.
8. Healthy People 2030. Washington, DC: U.S. Department of health and human Services, office of disease prevention and health promotion. Available at: https://health.gov/healthypeople/objectives-and-data/browse-objectives/cancer. Accessed August 29, 2024.
9. U.S. Cancer Statistics Working Group. U.S. Cancer Statistics data visualizations tool, based on 2022 submission data (1999-2020). U.S. Department of Health and Human Services, Centers for Disease Control and Prevention and National Cancer Institute; 2023. Available at: https://www.cdc.gov/cancer/dataviz. Accessed August 29, 2024.
10. Duffy SW, Tabár L, Yen AM, et al. Mammography screening reduces rates of advanced and fatal breast cancers: results in 549,091 women. Cancer 2020; 126:2971–9.
11. Hussein H, Abbas E, Keshavarzi S, et al. Supplemental breast cancer screening in women with dense breasts and negative mammography: a systematic review and meta-analysis. Radiology 2023;306:e221785.
12. US Preventive Services Task Force, Nicholson WK, Silverstein M, Wong JB, et al. Screening for breast cancer: US preventive Services Task Force recommendation statement. JAMA 2024;331:1918–30.
13. Oeffinger KC, Fontham ET, Etzioni R, et al, American Cancer Society. Breast cancer screening for women at average risk: 2015 guideline update from the American Cancer Society. JAMA 2015;314:1599–614.
14. Committee on Practice Bulletins - Gynecology. Committee opinion no. 625: management of women with dense breasts diagnosed by mammography. Obstet Gynecol 2015;125:750–1. Erratum in: Obstet Gynecol. 2016;127:166.
15. Bevers TB, Niell BL, Baker JL, et al. NCCN guidelines® insights: breast cancer screening and diagnosis. J Natl Compr Cancer Netw 2023;21:900–9.
16. Weinstein SP, Slanetz PJ, Lewin AA, et al. ACR Appropriateness Criteria® supplemental breast cancer screening based on breast density. J Am Coll Radiol 2021; 18:S456–73.
17. Glechner A, Wagner G, Mitus JW, et al. Mammography in combination with breast ultrasonography versus mammography for breast cancer screening in women at average risk. Cochrane Database Syst Rev 2023;3:CD009632.

18. Cancer trends progress report national cancer institute, NIH, DHHS, Bethesda, MD. 2024. Available at: https://progressreport.cancer.gov. Accessed August 29, 2024.
19. Committee on Practice Bulletins - Gynecology. Practice bulletin number 179: breast cancer risk assessment and screening in average-risk women. Obstet Gynecol 2017;130:e1–16.
20. Monticciolo DL, Malak SF, Friedewald SM, et al. Breast cancer screening recommendations inclusive of all women at average risk: update from the ACR and Society of Breast Imaging. J Am Coll Radiol 2021;18:1280–8.
21. Pal Choudhury P, Brook MN, Hurson AN, et al. Comparative validation of the BOADICEA and Tyrer-Cuzick breast cancer risk models incorporating classical risk factors and polygenic risk in a population-based prospective cohort of women of European ancestry. Breast Cancer Res 2021;23:22.
22. Fuzzell LN, Perkins RB, Christy SM, et al. Cervical cancer screening in the United States: challenges and potential solutions for underscreened groups. Prev Med 2021;144:106400.
23. Lei J, Ploner A, Elfström KM, et al. HPV vaccination and the risk of invasive cervical cancer. N Engl J Med 2020;383:1340–8.
24. Siegel RL, Wagle NS, Cercek A, et al. Colorectal cancer statistics, 2023. CA Cancer J Clin 2023;73:233–54.
25. Melnikow J, Henderson JT, Burda BU, et al. Screening for cervical cancer with high-risk human papillomavirus testing: updated evidence report and systematic review for the US Preventive Services Task Force. JAMA 2018;320:687–705.
26. Fontham ETH, Wolf AMD, Church TR, et al. Cervical cancer screening for individuals at average risk: 2020 guideline update from the American Cancer Society. CA Cancer J Clin 2020;70:321–46.
27. Zaborowski AM. REACCT Collaborative. Colorectal cancer in the young: research in early age colorectal cancer trends (REACCT) collaborative. Cancers 2023;15:2979.
28. Lewandowska A, Rudzki G, Lewandowski T, et al. Risk factors for the diagnosis of colorectal cancer. Cancer Control 2022;29:10732748211056692.
29. Fedirko V, Tramacere I, Bagnardi V, et al. Alcohol drinking and colorectal cancer risk: an overall and dose-response meta-analysis of published studies. Ann Oncol 2011;22:1958–72.
30. Lin JS, Perdue LA, Henrikson NB, et al. Screening for colorectal cancer: updated evidence report and systematic review for the US Preventive Services Task Force. JAMA 2021;325:1978–98.
31. Wolf AMD, Fontham ETH, Church TR, et al. Colorectal cancer screening for average-risk adults: 2018 guideline update from the American Cancer Society. CA Cancer J Clin 2018;68:250–81.
32. Patel SG, May FP, Anderson JC, et al. Updates on age to start and stop colorectal cancer screening: recommendations from the U.S. Multi-Society Task Force on Colorectal Cancer. Gastroenterology 2022;162:285–99. Erratum in: Gastroenterology. 2022 Jul;163:339.
33. Shaukat A, Kahi CJ, Burke CA, et al. ACG clinical guidelines: colorectal cancer screening 2021. Am J Gastroenterol 2021;116:458–79.
34. Jain S, Maque J, Galoosian A, et al. Optimal strategies for colorectal cancer screening. Curr Treat Options Oncol 2022;23:474–93.
35. Chung DC, Gray DM 2nd, Singh H, et al. A cell-free DNA blood-based test for colorectal cancer screening. N Engl J Med 2024;390:973–83.

36. State of lung cancer: 2022 report. American lung association. Available at: https://www.lung.org/getmedia/647c433b-4cbc-4be6-9312-2fa9a449d489/solc-2022-print-report. Accessed August 29, 2024.

37. Jonas DE, Reuland DS, Reddy SM, et al. Screening for lung cancer with low-dose computed tomography: updated evidence report and systematic review for the US Preventive Services Task Force. JAMA 2021;325:971–87.

38. Wolf AMD, Oeffinger KC, Shih TY, et al. Screening for lung cancer: 2023 guideline update from the American Cancer Society. CA Cancer J Clin 2024;74:50–81.

39. Aberle DR, Adams AM, Berg CD, et al. National lung screening trial research team. Reduced lung-cancer mortality with low-dose computed tomographic screening. N Engl J Med 2011;365:395–409.

40. Sosa E, D'Souza G, Akhtar A, et al. Racial and socioeconomic disparities in lung cancer screening in the United States: a systematic review. CA Cancer J Clin 2021;71:299–314.

41. Barbeau EM, Wolin KY, Naumova EN, et al. Tobacco advertising in communities: associations with race and class. Prev Med 2005;40:16–22.

42. Gareen IF, Gutman R, Sicks J, et al. Significant incidental findings in the national lung screening trial. JAMA Intern Med 2023;183:677–84.

43. Grossman DC, Curry SJ, Owens DK, et al. Screening for ovarian cancer: US preventive Services Task Force recommendation atatement. JAMA 2018;319:588–94.

44. Committee Opinion No. 716. The role of the obstetrician-gynecologist in the early detection of epithelial ovarian cancer in women at average risk. Obstet Gynecol 2017;130:e146–9.

45. Sideris M, Menon U, Manchanda R. Screening and prevention of ovarian cancer. Med J Aust 2024;220:264–74.

46. Mei S, Chelmow D, Gecsi K, et al. Health disparities in ovarian cancer: report from the ovarian cancer evidence review conference. Obstet Gynecol 2023;142:196–210.

47. Karanth S, Fowler ME, Mao X, et al. Race, socioeconomic status, and health-care access disparities in ovarian cancer treatment and mortality: systematic review and meta-analysis. JNCI Cancer Spectr 2019;3:pkz084.

48. Leone AG, Trapani D, Schabath MB, et al. Cancer in transgender and gender-diverse persons: a review. JAMA Oncol 2023;9:556–63.

49. Schrag D, Beer TM, McDonnell CH 3rd, et al. Blood-based tests for multicancer early detection (PATHFINDER): a prospective cohort study. Lancet 2023;402:1251–60.

50. Klein EA, Richards D, Cohn A, et al. Clinical validation of a targeted methylation-based multi-cancer early detection test using an independent validation set. Ann Oncol 2021;32:1167–77.

Contraception Updates

Kelita Fox, MD[a],*, Rachel Lee, MD[a,b], Emilyn Anderi, MD, MS[a,b]

KEYWORDS

- Contraception • Contraception counseling • Family planning
- Hormonal contraception • Nonhormonal contraception

KEY POINTS

- Clinicians should be well informed of all contraceptive methods to ensure noncoercive, person-centered contraceptive counseling.
- The levonorgestrel 52 mg intrauterine device (IUD) has recently been Food and Drug Administration (FDA) approved for use up to 8 years.
- The norgestrel progestin-only pill is the first contraceptive pill available over the counter.
- A vaginal acidifying gel that is placed precoitally named Phexxi was FDA approved in 2020.

INTRODUCTION

Family planning, as defined by the World Health Organization, "allows people to attain their desired number of children, if any, and to determine the spacing of their pregnancies."[1] This article will focus on the use of contraception options in pregnancy prevention. However, it is important to acknowledge the plethora of indications for contraception outside of family planning. Hormonal contraception can be beneficial in treating conditions such as abnormal uterine bleeding, endometriosis, endometrial hyperplasia, adenomyosis, menopause, and gender dysphoria. The information presented in this article will provide an update on modern contraception in the United States.

In the past 20 years in North America, there has been increased acknowledgment of inequity and bias in reproductive health care spaces. Marginalized groups, including Black, indigenous and people of color, young, lower socioeconomic status (SES), disabled, and sexual and gender minority (SGM) individuals, bear the brunt of these inequities. Black and Latina women of lower SES are more likely to be counseled

a Department of Family Medicine Residency Program, Henry Ford Health, Detroit, MI, USA;
b Henry Ford Department of Family Medicine, One Ford Place, Detroit, MI 48202, USA
* Corresponding author. Department of Family Medicine, One Ford Place, 2E, Detroit, MI 48202.
E-mail address: kfox10@hfhs.org

Prim Care Clin Office Pract 52 (2025) 249–263
https://doi.org/10.1016/j.pop.2024.12.008   **primarycare.theclinics.com**
0095-4543/25/© 2025 Elsevier Inc. All rights reserved, including those for text and data mining, AI training, and similar technologies.

Abbreviations

DMPA	depot medroxyprogesterone acetate
EE	ethinyl estradiol
FDA	Food and Drug Administration
FABM	fertility awareness–based methods
IUD	intrauterine device
OTC	over the counter
PID	pelvic inflammatory disease
POP	progestin-only pill
RJ	reproductive justice
SES	socioeconomic status
SGM	sexual and gender minority
STI	sexually transmitted infection
UTIs	urinary tract infections
VTE	venous thromboembolism

about sterilization and contraception,[2] advised to restrict childbearing,[3] and be recommended to use long-acting reversible contraceptives for contraception.[4] A qualitative study found that young Black and Latina women receive implicit pressure to use contraception from providers which can negatively impact their willingness to engage with reproductive health care in the future.[5] Regardless of race and ethnicity, younger women are more likely to receive provider-driven contraceptive counseling.[6] Significant gaps exist in our knowledge of the contraceptive needs and experiences of SGM individuals who are assigned female at birth. One study showed that lesbian and bisexual cis-women are less likely to receive contraception counseling even though they may engage in sexual practices that could result in pregnancy.[7] The experiences of transmasculine individuals in regard to contraception counseling is even less studied, but the need is great. One study showed that 17% of transmasculine individuals had been pregnant and 60% used contraception.[8]

The Reproductive Justice (RJ) movement has helped to bring these inequities to the forefront. Sister Song, an early RJ organization, defines reproductive justice as "the human right to maintain personal bodily autonomy, have children, not have children, and parent the children we have in safe and sustainable communities."[9] Employing an RJ lens to reproductive health care includes honoring patient autonomy. This involves considering a patient's contraception priorities and preferences rather than promoting methods based on the provider's assumptions and beliefs. It empowers patients to have autonomy over their reproductive journey, which can sometimes include the choice not to use contraception. And lastly, it includes understanding the longstanding impact of systemic racism and eugenics, including forced sterilization of Black, Latina, poor, and disabled individuals, throughout the past century in North America. While much of the data cited in this article is US-based, discrimination based on race, gender, ethnicity, sexual orientation, ability, and age is not unique to the United States and exists across North America.

NEW CONTRACEPTIVE METHODS
Drospirenone Progestin-Only Pill

Slynd is a progestin-only pill (POP) that was Food and Drug Administration (FDA) approved for use in 2019.[10] Previously, the only POP available was the norethindrone POP (**Table 1**). Norethindrone POPs are packaged in a continuous use form, without a hormone-free interval. Slynd includes a 4-day hormone-free interval.[11] This interval allows time for withdrawal bleeding and can improve the often-bothersome bleeding

Table 1
Oral contraceptive pill options

	Hormone Type/Strength	Frequency/Duration of Use	Contraindications
Norethindrone POP	0.35 mg norethindrone	Once daily continuous, no hormone-free interval	Current breast cancer[16]
Norgestrel POP	0.075 mg of norgestrel	Once daily continuous, no hormone-free interval	
Drospirenone POP	4 mg drospirenone	Once daily hormonal pills × 24, nonhormonal pills × 4 d	Current breast cancer Chronic kidney disease with known hyperkalemia[16]
Combined oral contraceptive pills	20–50 mcg of ethinyl estradiol Varying doses of progestins	Once daily hormonal pills followed by nonhormonal pills during time of withdrawal bleeding	Chronic kidney disease Current breast cancer Severe hypertension Vascular disease Complicated valvular heart disease Severe cardiomyopathy <3 wk postpartum Systemic lupus erythematosus with positive or unknown antiphospholipid antibodies Migraines with aura High risk for venous thromboembolism (VTE) Smoking 15 or more cigarettes per day + age 35 y or older[16]

profile users experience with other progestin-only pills. Drospirenone is a fourth-generation progestin which has antiandrogenic properties and a longer half-life than norethindrone. The dose contained in Slynd is a relatively higher dose of progestin compared to other combined oral contraceptives or POPs.[12] Users may experience less irregular bleeding and better efficacy compared to norethindrone-containing POPs. Where norethindrone POPs have a 3-hour missed pill interval, drospirenone POPs remain effective longer, with some studies suggesting up to 24 hours of continued protection after a missed pill.[12,13]

Mechanism of action: ovulation suppression, cervical mucus thickening, and endometrial thinning.

Trouble shooting: If one pill is missed, take the next pill as soon as possible. Back up method is not indicated. If 2 or more pills are missed, take the next pill as soon as possible. Use back up method for the next 7 days.

Norgestrel, Progestin-Only Pill

On July 13, 2023, the FDA approved the first over-the-counter (OTC) hormonal contraceptive method, a norgestrel-containing progestin-only pill, brand name Opill.[14] This POP contains 0.075 mg of norgestrel, a second-generation progestin. The short half-life of norgestrel requires daily administration at almost exactly the same time. In the United States, this has been a groundbreaking change to expand access to contraception especially in low-resource areas as individuals do not have to present personal identification or insurance to purchase the pill. Despite the improved access, cost remains a potential barrier to use. Without a prescription, the norgestrel pill costs $49.99 for a 3-month supply and $89.99 for a 6-month supply. Some insurance plans fully cover the cost of the OTC POP even without a prescription and some may allow use of flexible spending account funds to purchase the POPs.[15]

Mechanism of action: Ovulation suppression, cervical mucus thickening, and endometrial thinning.

Troubleshooting: If a missed pill is less than 3 hours late, take the pill as soon as possible. Back up is not needed. If the pill is more than 3 hours late, take it as soon as remembered and continue the remainder of the pills at their regularly scheduled time. Use a backup method for 2 days (48 hours). The norgestrel pill will start working again after 2 days of continuous, on-time use.[15]

Combined Contraceptive Rings: Annovera and NuvaRing

A new combined hormonal vaginal contraceptive ring was approved for use by the FDA in 2018.[17] The segesterone acetate and ethinyl estradiol vaginal system, Annovera, is 97.5% effective in preventing pregnancy,[18] similar in efficacy and mechanism of action as the NuvaRing but reusable up to 1 year. While NuvaRing requires placement of a new vaginal ring each month and multiple prescriptions or refills during a year of use, Annovera users require only 1 visit to the pharmacy for each year of use. Similar to the NuvaRing, Annovera should be used on a 28-day cycle with intravaginal placement for 3 weeks, followed by removal for 1 week. While not in use, Annovera ring should be washed with cold to lukewarm temperature water and will tolerate storage temperatures at 30°F or less. Hormonally, Annovera contains 17.4 mg of ethinyl estradiol (EE) and 103 mg of the progestin segesterone acetate. The average daily release of hormones is 13 mcg/day of EE and 150 mcg/day of segesterone acetate.[19] Compared to Annovera, the NuvaRing intravaginal system contains 2.7 mg of EE and 11.7 mg of a different progestin, etonogestrel. The daily release rates are 15 mcg/d and 120 mcg/d, respectively.[20] Extended cycling has not yet been studied in Annovera users. However, similar to other combined hormonal methods, it would be reasonable to discuss the benefits of extended cycling with a shared decision-making approach. Unscheduled bleeding was seen in 13% to 22% of Annovera users per cycle during 1 year of use.[21] Whereas 7.2% to 11.7% of NuvaRing users may have unscheduled bleeding.[20]

Mechanism of action: Ovulation suppression.

Contraindications: Severe hypertension, vascular disease, complicated valvular heart disease, severe cardiomyopathy, end-stage renal disease, nephrotic syndrome, less than 3 weeks postpartum, systemic lupus erythematosus with positive antiphospholipid antibodies, migraines with aura, current breast cancer, and those at high risk for venous thromboembolism (VTE).[16]

Troubleshooting: Avoid removal of the vaginal ring for more than 2 hours during the 21-day period of active use.[13]

Contraceptive Patches

	Hormone Dose per day	Size	Food and Drug Administration Approved	Efficacy	Special Considerations
Twirla	30 mcg of ethinyl estradiol and 120 mcg of levonorgestrel	28 cm²	2020	95%[22,23]	Higher risk of pregnancy in patients with body mass index (BMI) >30 kg/m².[22]
Zafemy	35 mcg ethinyl estradiol, 150 mcg norelgestromin	12.5 cm²	2021	99%[24]	FDA packaging lists concern for higher VTE risk in patients with BMI >30 kg/m²,[2,25,26]; however, this is not a true contraindication per Centers for Disease Control and Prevention Medical Eligibility Criteria[21] and can be prescribed regardless of BMI.
Xulane	35 mcg ethinyl estradiol, 150 mcg norelgestromin	14 cm²	2014	99%[24]	

Mechanism of action: ovulation suppression

Costs are similar

Instructions: Place a new patch weekly × 3 wk, no patch × 1 wk.

Troubleshooting: If <24 h without the patch, replace as soon as possible, back up method is not needed. If 24 h or greater without the patch, use a backup method for 7 d.

Vaginal Acidifying Gel

Vaginal pH regulating gel (commercially known as Phexxi) is an on-demand vaginal gel that contains lactic acid, citric acid, and potassium bitartrate. This formulation maintains the vagina at a pH of 3.5 to 4.5, despite the presence of alkaline semen, and immobilizes sperm from ascending into the upper reproductive tract.[27] Recently approved in 2020, there are limited data on the efficacy of the product; however, initial clinical trials reported the 7-cycle typical use cumulative pregnancy rate of 13%.[27,28] Vaginal acidifying gel requires a prescription which will provide 1 box of 12 prefilled applicators. If not covered by insurance, the cost is about $285 per box.[29] Each dose is inserted into the vagina up to an hour before coitus. If more than 1 act of vaginal intercourse occurs, additional doses must be applied. This gel can be used alongside other barrier methods of contraception; however, it is not recommended to be used with a hormonal vaginal ring.[27] Some reported complications include vulvovaginal burning, itching, urinary tract infections (UTIs), bacterial vaginosis, and candidiasis.[27,28]

UPDATES IN DURATION OF USE
Progestin Intrauterine Devices

In North America, there are 4 different progestin intrauterine devices (IUDs) available. In the United States, this includes Mirena, Liletta, Kyleena, and Skyla. The Mirena IUD has been available since 2000 when it was first FDA approved for 5 years of use. Most recently in 2022 after a phase 3 trial showed Mirena remains up to 99% effective at preventing pregnancy after 6 to 8 years, it was approved by the FDA for 8 years of use. FDA approval of Liletta was updated and approved for use up to 8 years. If using the levonorgestrel 52 mg IUD for treatment of heavy menstrual bleeding, it is FDA approved for 5 years[30,31] **(Table 2)**.[32]

Mechanism of action: Like other exogenous progestin methods, progestin IUDs help prevent pregnancy through a combination of endometrial thinning and thickening of cervical mucus. Intermittent suppression of ovulation may occur, but most patients will have ovulatory cycles with a progestin IUD.[31,33]

Contraindications: Do not initiate or place a progestin IUD in a patient with known cervical or uterine cancer.

- Gestational trophoblastic disease and intrauterine involvement,
- Active cervicitis or pelvic inflammatory disease (PID),
- Current pregnancy.[16]

UPDATES TO THE ROUTE OF ADMINISTRATION
SubQ Depo Provera

Until 2004, when the FDA approved subcutaneous depot medroxyprogesterone acetate (DMPA-SC), DMPA was only available in an intramuscular formulation (DMPA-IM). There has been an increase in clinicians offering DMPA-SC during the coronavirus disease 2019 pandemic[35] which allowed DMPA users to self-administer at home. DMPA-SC comes in a disposable package containing a prefilled syringe and needle. It contains 104 mg of progestin compared to 150 mg in DMPA-IM, Step by step instructions are available online on the Pfizer website.[36] Self-administered DMPA-SC may lead to higher continuation rates at 12 months of use compared to DMPA-IM, without an increase in pregnancy rates or serious adverse events.[37]

Mechanism of action: ovulation suppression, cervical mucus thickening, endometrial thinning.

Frequency/Duration of use: 1 injection every 12 to 13 weeks.

Contraindications: Current breast cancer[16]

Troubleshooting: Injection site reactions might be higher with self-administration of DMPA-SC, but this difference did not persist with subsequent injections.[38]

EMERGENCY CONTRACEPTION UPDATES

Table 3 summarizes updates on available emergency contraception methods. Increasing evidence shows that the 52 mg levonorgestrel IUD can be used for emergency contraception with efficacy similar to that of the copper IUD.[39,40]

Table 2
Hormonal long-acting reversible contraceptives methods

	FDA Approved Duration of Use	Insertion Tube Size	Hormone type/Strength	Dose/d
Intrauterine device				
Mirena	8 y	4.4 mm	52 mg Levonorgestrel	21 mcg/d
Liletta	8 y	4.8 mm	52 mg Levonorgestrel	20 mcg/d
Kyleena	5 y	3.8 mm	19.5 mg Levonorgestrel	17.5 mcg/d
Skyla	3 y	3.8 mm	13.5 mg Levonorgestrel	14 mcg/d
Contraceptive Implant				
Nexplanon	3 y	2 mm × 4 cm	68 mg etonogestrel	70 mcg/d, slowly declines to 25 mcg/d[34]

Table 3
Emergency contraception options

EC Method	Timing of Use	Pregnancy Risk/Efficacy	Special Considerations
Copper IUD	5 d postcoital	0%–0.1%[39,40]	Method can be continued for long-term contraception.
Levonorgestrel 52 mg IUD	5 d postcoital	0.4%[39,40]	
Ulipristal 30 mg, single dose	5 d postcoital	0.9%–2.1%[40]	Lower efficacy if BMI >30[41] Requires a prescription
Levonorgestrel 1.5 mg single dose	3 d postcoital	0.6%–3.1%[40]	Lower efficacy if BMI >25[41] Available without a prescription.

NONHORMONAL

There are many reasons a patient may choose a nonhormonal source of contraception, including but not limited to personal choice, financial restrictions, or a medical contraindication to exogenous hormones.

Copper Intrauterine Device

The copper IUD is one of the most highly effective nonhormonal long-acting reversible contraception methods.[42,43] The percentage of users who experience pregnancy in the first year is 0.6% with "perfect use" and 0.8% with "typical use."

Mechanism of Action: Spermicidal as the copper ions adversely affect sperm viability and motility.[44] Local inflammatory response within the endometrial cavity prevents fertilization.[42]

Frequency/Duration of use: FDA approved for 10 years, data support use for up to 12 years.[42,45]

Contraindications: Uterine cavity abnormalities (bicornate uterus, leiomyomas that distort the endometrial cavity), acute PID, postpartum/postabortive endometritis within 3 months, Wilson's disease, or genital bleeding of unknown origin.[42,45] While it was previously thought to increase the risk of PID if a sexually transmitted infection (STI) was present, the absolute risk remains low (less than 5%) in patients with existing gonorrhea or chlamydial infection.[46]

Menstrual cycle changes: Increased dysmenorrhea and volume of bleeding in the first 3 to 6 months after insertion.[45]

Trouble shooting: Limited studies show nonsteroidal antiinflammatory drugs, antifibrinolytics, and vitamin B1 may reduce heavy menstrual bleeding and pain associated with use of the copper IUD.[47,48]

Barrier Methods

Barrier methods such as diaphragm, cervical cap, and condoms prevent pregnancy by blocking sperm from entering the upper reproductive tract. The percentage of users who experience pregnancy in the first year is around 13%, but can range to upwards of 29%.[46,49,50]

Diaphragms

Diaphragms require a prescription, and a physician will determine the appropriate size for a given patient. The diaphragm should sit comfortably with the posterior rim in the posterior vaginal fornix and the anterior rim sitting behind the pubic bone. They are inserted before coitus and removed 6 to 24 hours after. Contraindications include those with an allergy to the material, or those with significant pelvic organ prolapse. Some reported complications include increased risk of UTIs and toxic shock syndrome.[49] **Table 4** shows the available diaphragms in the United States.[51–53]

Cervical cap

The FemCap device is the only silicone cervical cap available in the United States. Like the diaphragm, a prescription is required and evaluation by a clinician for sizing (available in 22 mm, 26 mm, and 30 mm sizes). It is intended to be used with spermicide and washed between uses. They are inserted before coitus and removed 6 to 48 hours after.[49] Some reported complications include increased risk of urinary tract infections, vaginal candidiasis, and blood in the device.[54]

Table 4
Diaphragm types

Brand Name	Available Sizes	Spring Type	Material
Caya	Single size.	Contoured	Silicone
Milex	60 mm, 65 mm, 70 mm, 75 mm, 80 mm, 85 mm, 90 mm, and 95 mm	Arcing (easier to insert, best for decreased pelvic tone) Omniflex (best for average pelvic muscle tone)	Silicone

Condoms

There are 2 types of condoms, internal and external. Both help prevent transmission of STIs. Internal condoms consist of a polyurethane or nitrile ring that is inserted into the vagina and covers the cervix, with the other end of the ring open and extending outside the vagina. They are available OTC and do not require a physician examination.[49]

External condoms can be made of latex or nonlatex materials like polyisoprene. They are placed over an erect penis. Users should be mindful of handling techniques to avoid ripping the material, and if lubricants are needed, the use of a water-based lubricant is preferred as oil-based lubricants can increase the risk of the material breaking.[49]

Spermicide

Spermicide is a chemical agent that immobilizes sperm from ascending into the upper reproductive tract. Spermicidal preparations are formulated using Noxonyl-9 and can be used as a gel, foam, or suppository. The percentage of users who experience pregnancy in the first year is around 18% for "perfect use" and 20% with "typical use."[50] Spermicide must be inserted at least 10 minutes prior to coitus, and no longer than an hour before. Some reported complications include vaginal or penile irritation, transmission of STIs, and a small risk of bacterial vaginosis.[55]

Fertility Awareness–Based Methods

Fertility awareness–based methods (FABMs) of family planning involve monitoring signs and symptoms of fertility throughout the menstrual cycle to identify the days of the cycle when pregnancy is most likely if unprotected intercourse occurs. The physiologic basis behind these methods relies on the knowledge that ovulation occurs on a single day within each cycle, the ovum released remains viable for approximately 24 to 48 hours, and sperm present in the vaginal canal prior to ovulation can survive for up to 5 days.[56] Efficacy studies for the various FABM methods have found a range for percentage of users who experience pregnancy in the first year to be from 0.4% to 12.1% with "perfect use" and from 1.8% to 33.6% with "typical use."[57]

FABMs can generally be classified into the following categories[57]:

- Calendar-based methods that track menstrual cycle dates,
- Mucus-based methods that track changes in cervical mucus,
- Basal body temperature methods that track changes in the basal body temperature in relation to calendar days,
- Symptothermal methods which combine the tracking of cervical mucus and basal body temperature,
- Urine hormone-based methods that track metabolites of estradiol and luteinizing hormone in the urine.

Circumstances and conditions that make FABMs difficult:

- Long or irregular menstrual cycles;
- Recent childbirth or current breastfeeding;
- Being on medications that affect cervical mucus (vaginal creams or antihistamines);
- Irregular work, sleep, or travel patterns.

Withdrawal

The withdrawal method, or coitus interruptus, involves removal of the penis from the vaginal canal prior to ejaculation of sperm. First year pregnancy rates are around 4% for "perfect use" and 20% with "typical use."[58]

Tubal Ligation

For individuals who are certain they no longer desire future pregnancies, permanent sterilization via tubal ligation is an option. This method requires surgical intervention to perform a salpingectomy with the removal of fallopian tubes. The percentage of users who experience pregnancy in the first year after sterilization is 0.5%.[58] If there is concern that an individual may be pregnant after sterilization, the risk of an ectopic pregnancy is high, and prompt evaluation is necessary.

SUMMARY

Over the past decade, access to contraception in the United States has markedly increased with the addition of new contraceptive methods and the passage of the Affordable Care Act, which guarantees access to FDA-approved contraception to nearly all individuals of child-bearing potential at no out-of-pocket cost. However, people who are uninsured do not benefit from this provision. In the past year, barriers to contraception have been further reduced by the FDA approval of the norgestrel, progesterone-only contraception pills which can be purchased OTC at pharmacies without insurance. This is following in the footsteps of Mexico, where multiple types of hormonal oral contraceptive pills are available without prescription at pharmacies. It is essential to employ a reproductive justice lens when counseling patients about their contraception options. North American patients have a wide variety of both hormonal and nonhormonal contraception options.

CLINICS CARE POINTS

- The drospirenone-only progestin only pills may offer better bleeding profile and higher efficacy compared to the norethindrone POP.
- The norgestrel progestin-only pill is available without a prescription and may cost around $49.99 for a 3-month supply.
- The segesterone acetate and ethinyl estradiol vaginal system, Annovera is available as a reusable, yearly vaginal ring and may reduce barriers to use by not needing refills.
- A newly approved, nonhormonal, nonspermicidal, vaginal acidifying gel, available with a prescription. It can be used on-demand up to 1 hour before coitus.
- The levonorgestrel 52 mg intrauterine device is FDA approved for use up to 8 years.
- The copper IUD, while FDA approved for 10 years, has strong evidence to support use for up to 12 years.
- DMPA is now available as a subcutaneous formulation. Data support similar efficacy to DMPA-IM and higher adherence when available to be self-administered at home.

DISCLOSURE

The authors have nothing to disclose.

REFERENCES

1. Contraception (who.int). Available at: https://www.who.int/health-topics/contraception#tab=tab_1. Accessed June 1, 2024.
2. Borrero S, Schwarz EB, Creinin M, et al. The impact of race and ethnicity on receipt of family planning services in the United States. J Womens Health (Larchmt) 2009;18(1):91–6.

3. Downing RA, LaVeist TA, Bullock HE. Intersections of ethnicity and social class in provider advice regarding reproductive health. Am J Publ Health 2007;97(10):1803–7.
4. Dehlendorf C, Ruskin R, Grumbach K, et al. Recommendations for intrauterine contraception: a randomized trial of the effects of patients' race/ethnicity and socioeconomic status. Am J Obstet Gynecol 2010;03(4):319.e1–8.
5. Gomez AM, Wapman M. Under (implicit) pressure: young Black and Latina women's perceptions of contraceptive care. Contraception 2017;96(4):221–6.
6. Dehlendorf C, Kimport K, Levy K, et al. A qualitative analysis of approaches to contraceptive counseling. Perspect Sex Reprod Health 2014;46(4):233–40.
7. Everett BG, Higgins JA, Haider S, et al. Do sexual minorities receive appropriate sexual and reproductive health care and counseling? J Womens Health (Larchmt). 2019;28(1):53–62.
8. Light A, Wang LF, Zeymo A, et al. Family planning and contraception use in transgender men. Contraception 2018;98(4):266–9. Epub 2018 Jun 23.
9. Reproductive justice. Available at: https://www.sistersong.net/reproductive-justice. Accessed June 1, 2024.
10. Exeltis USA Inc. Slynd (drospirenone pills) [package insert]. U.S. Food and Drug Administration website. 2019. Available at: https://www.accessdata.fda.gov/drugsatfda_docs/label/2019/211367s000lbl.pdf. Accessed June 1, 2024.
11. Kimble T, Burke AE, Barnhart KT, et al. A 1-year prospective, open-label, single-arm, multicenter, phase 3 trial of the contraceptive efficacy and safety of the oral progestin-only pill drospirenone 4 mg using a 24/4-day regimen. Contracept X 2020;2:100020.
12. Palacios S, Regidor PA, Colli E, et al. Oestrogen-free oral contraception with a 4 mg drospirenone-only pill: new data and a review of the literature. Eur J Contracept Reprod Health Care 2020;25(3):221–7.
13. Baker CC, Chen MJ. New contraception update - Annovera, Phexxi, Slynd, and twirla. Curr Obstet Gynecol Rep 2022;11(1):21–7.
14. U.S. Food and Drug Administration. FDA approves first nonprescription daily oral contraceptive. 2023. Available at: https://www.fda.gov/news-events/press-announcements/fda-approves-first-nonprescription-daily-oral-contraceptive. Accessed June 1, 2024.
15. Opill manufacturers website. 2024. Available at: https://opill.com/products/opill. Accessed June 1, 2024.
16. Nguyen AT, Curtis KM, Tepper NK, et al. U.S. Medical eligibility criteria for contraceptive use, 2024. MMWR Recomm Rep (Morb Mortal Wkly Rep) 2024;73(RR-4):1–126.
17. FDA News. FDA approves new vaginal ring for one year of birth control. 2018. Available at: https://www.fda.gov/news-events/press-announcements/fda-approves-new-vaginal-ring-one-year-birth-control. Accessed June 1, 2024.
18. Archer DF, Merkatz RB, Bahamondes L, et al. Efficacy of the 1-year (13-cycle) segesterone acetate and ethinylestradiol contraceptive vaginal system: results of two multicentre, open-label, single-arm, phase 3 trials. Lancet Glob Health 2019;7(8):e1054–64.
19. Pharma M. Annovera (segesterone acetate and ethinyl estradiol vaginal system) [package insert]. U.S. Food and Drug Administration website. 2020. Available at: https://www.annovera.com/pi.pdf. Accessed June 1, 2024.
20. Organon USA. NuvaRing (etonogestrel/ethinyl estradiol vaginal ring) [package insert] U.S. Food and Drug Administration website. 2024. Available at: https://www.accessdata.fda.gov/drugsatfda_docs/label/2013/021187s022lbl.pdf. Accessed June 15, 2024.

21. Vieira CS, Fraser IS, Plagianos MG, et al. Bleeding profile associated with 1-year use of the segesterone acetate/ethinyl estradiol contraceptive vaginal system: pooled analysis from phase 3 trials. Contraception 2019;100:438–44. https://doi.org/10.1016/j.contraception.2019.07.145.

22. Nelson AL, Kaunitz AM, Kroll R, et al. Efficacy, safety, and tolerability of a levonorgestrel/ethinyl estradiol transdermal delivery system: phase 3 clinical trial results. Contraception 2021;103(3):137–43.

23. Trussell J, Aiken ARA, Micks E, et al. Efficacy, safety, and personal considerations. In: Hatcher RA, Nelson AL, Trussell J, et al, editors. Contraceptive technology. 21st ed. New York, NY: Ayer Company Publishers; 2018. p. 95–128.

24. Smallwood GH, Meador ML, Lenihan JP, et al, ORTHO EVRA/EVRA 002 Study Group. Efficacy and safety of a transdermal contraceptive system. Obstet Gynecol 2001;98(5 Pt 1):799–805.

25. Xulane- norelgestromin and ethinyl estradiol patch. US Food and Drug Administration (FDA) approved product information. US National Library of Medicine. 2020. Available at: https://dailymed.nlm.nih.gov/dailymed/fda/fdaDrugXsl.cfm?setid=f7848550-086a-43d8-8ae5-047f4b9e4382&type=display#ID_8a7fd083-8861-4485-a5fd-8bbc77f8cf61. Accessed June 15, 2024.

26. Zafemy- Norelgestromin and ethinyl estradiol patch. DailyMed. 2022. Available at: https://dailymed.nlm.nih.gov/dailymed/drugInfo.cfm?setid=5ee34c07-65af-42b8-a98f-e299ff90a8a1. Accessed June 16, 2024.

27. Thomas MA, Chappell BT, Maximos B, et al. A novel vaginal pH regulator: results from the phase 3 AMPOWER contraception clinical trial. Contracept X 2020;2: 100031.

28. Evofem biosciences. Phexxi [package insert] U.S. Food and Drug Administration website. 2020. Available at: https://www.accessdata.fda.gov/drugsatfda_docs/label/2020/208352s000lbl.pdf. Accessed June 17, 2024.

29. Steinberg J, Lynch SE. Lactic acid, citric acid, and potassium bitartrate (Phexxi) vaginal gel for contraception. Am Fam Physician 2021;103(10):628–9.

30. FDA News. FDA expands approval of Mirena IUD device. 2022. Available at: https://www.fdanews.com/articles/209140-fda-expands-approval-of-mirena-iud-device. Accessed June 15, 2024.

31. AbbVie and Medicines360; Liletta [package insert]. 2023. Available at: https://www.accessdata.fda.gov/drugsatfda_docs/label/2023/206229s013lbledt.pdf. Accessed June 15, 2024.

32. Paradise SL, Landis CA, Klein DA. Evidence-based contraception: common questions and answers. Am Fam Physician 2022;106(3):251–9.

33. Bayer HealthCare pharmaceuticals. [Package insert]. 2023. Available at: https://www.accessdata.fda.gov/drugsatfda_docs/label/2022/021225s043lbl.pdf. Accessed June 15, 2024.

34. Merck. Nexplanon [package insert] U.S. Food and drug administration website. 2015. Available at: https://www.accessdata.fda.gov/drugsatfda_docs/label/2019/021529s018lbl.pdf. Accessed June 1, 2024.

35. Comfort AB, Alvarez A, Goodman S, et al. Provision of DMPA-SC for self-administration in different practice settings during the COVID-19 pandemic: data from providers across the United States. Contraception 2024;131:110360.

36. Pfizer. SubQ depo [package insert]. 2020. Available at: https://labeling.pfizer.com/ShowLabeling.aspx?id=549. Accessed June 17, 2024.

37. Kennedy CE, Yeh PT, Gaffield ML, et al. Self-administration of injectable contraception: a systematic review and meta-analysis. BMJ Glob Health 2019;4(2): e001350.

38. Cover J, Ba M, Drake JK, et al. Continuation of self-injected versus provider-administered contraception in Senegal: a nonrandomized, prospective cohort study. Contraception 2019;99(2):137–41.

39. Turok DK, Gero A, Simmons RG, et al. Levonorgestrel vs. Copper intrauterine devices for emergency contraception. N Engl J Med 2021;384:335.

40. Cleland K, Raymond EG, Westley E, et al. Emergency contraception review: evidence-based recommendations for clinicians. Clin Obstet Gynecol 2014; 57(4):741–50.

41. Glasier A, Cameron ST, Blithe D, et al. Can we identify women at risk of pregnancy despite using emergency contraception? Data from randomized trials of ulipristal acetate and levonorgestrel. Contraception 2011;84(4):363–7.

42. Baker C, Creinin M. Long-acting reversible contraception. Obstet Gynecol 2022; 140(5):883–97.

43. Winner B, Peipert JF, Zhao Q, et al. Effectiveness of long-acting reversible contraception. N Engl J Med 2012;366(21):1998–2007.

44. Ortiz ME, Croxatto HB. Copper-T intrauterine device and levonorgestrel intrauterine system: biological bases of their mechanism of action. Contraception 2007; 75(6):S16–30, suppl.

45. ParaGard T380A. Intrauterine copper contraceptive efficacy-labeling change with clinical data; Food and Drug Administration Web site. 2005. Available at: https://www.accessdata.fda.gov/drugsatfda_docs/label/2005/018680s060lbl. pdf. Accessed June 16, 2024.

46. Teal S, Edelman A. Contraception selection, effectiveness, and adverse effects: a review. JAMA 2021;326(24):2507–18.

47. Christelle K, Norhayati MN, Jaafar SH. Interventions to prevent or treat heavy menstrual bleeding or pain associated with intrauterine-device use. Cochrane Database Syst Rev 2022;8(8):CD006034.

48. Godfrey EM, Folger SG, Jeng G, et al. Treatment of bleeding irregularities in women with copper-containing IUDs: a systematic review. Contraception 2013; 87(5):549–66.

49. Tracy E. Contraception. Obstetrics and Gynecology Clinics 2017;44(2):143–58.

50. CDC contraception. Available at: https://www.cdc.gov/reproductive-health/contraception/index.html. Accessed June 17, 2024.

51. Schwartz Jill, Weiner Debra, Lai Jaim, et al. Contraceptive efficacy, safety, fit, and acceptability of a single-size diaphragm developed with end-user input. Obstet Gynecol 2015;125(4):895–903.

52. Milex diaphragm. Available at: https://www.coopersurgical.com/product/milex-omniflex-style-diaphragm/. Accessed July 20, 2024.

53. Allen RE. Diaphragm fitting. Am Fam Physician 2004;69(1):97–100.

54. FemCap [package insert. U.S. Food and drug administration web site. Available at: https://www.accessdata.fda.gov/cdrh_docs/pdf2/P020041b.pdf. Accessed June 16, 2024.

55. Schreiber CA, Meyn LA, Creinin MD, et al. Effects of long-term use of nonoxynol-9 on vaginal flora. Obstet Gynecol 2006;107(1):136–43.

56. Simmons R, Jennings V. Fertility awareness-based methods of family planning. Best Pract Res Clin Obstet Gynaecol 2020;66:68–82.

57. Urrutia RP, Polis CB. Fertility based methods for pregnancy prevention. BMJ 2019;366:l4245.

58. Woodhams EJ, Gilliam M. Contraception. Ann Intern Med 2019;170(3):ITC18–32.

Management of Menopause Symptoms

Jonathan Snyder, MPAS[a,1], Coral Matus, MD[b,c,2], Emily Landis, MSPAS[a,1], Robin Barry, PhD[c], Linda Speer, MD[c,*]

KEYWORDS

- Menopause • Treatment • Vasomotor symptoms
- Genitourinary syndrome of menopause

KEY POINTS

- Menopausal hormone therapy remains the most effective treatment for patients with vasomotor symptoms of menopause (VSM) without contraindications to hormonal therapy.
- Topical estrogen is first-line treatment for isolated genitourinary syndrome of menopause.
- Fezolinetant is the first in a new class of nonhormonal medications for treatment of VSM.
- Selectoive serotonin reuptake inhibitors (SSRIs), serotonin-norepinephrine reuptake inhibitors (SNRIs), gabapentin, and nonmedication treatments may also be effective for the treatment of VSM.

INTRODUCTION

Up to 75% of women experience vasomotor symptoms, mood changes, sleep disturbances, genitourinary symptoms, and hair loss associated with menopause leading to decreased quality of life, lost production at work, and increased health care visits.[1] The natural onset of menopause typically occurs between the ages of 48 and 52 in developed countries,[1] and women often live 30 years or more postmenopause.[2] Vasomotor symptoms tend to peak in the first year after the last menstrual period, and last 7 years on average. Elevated body mass index (BMI) and tobacco use are factors associated with menopausal symptoms.[3] Barriers to treatment may include insufficient knowledge of treatment options, patient embarrassment, or lingering anxiety about menopausal hormone therapy (MHT) due to risks found in the Women's Health Initiative (WHI).[4] Further analysis has shown that the initially reported risks of MHT were not necessarily accurate and treatment indications have changed over time.[5,6]

[a] Division of the Department of Family Medicine, University of Toledo, Toledo, OH 43514, USA;
[b] Department of Medical Education, University of Toledo, Toledo, OH 43514, USA;
[c] Department of Family Medicine, University of Toledo, Toledo, OH 43514, USA
[1] Present address: 3000 Arlington Avenue MS 1027, Toledo, OH 43614.
[2] Present address: 3000 Arlington Avenue MS 1050, Toledo, OH 43614.
* Corresponding author. 3000 Arlington Avenue MS 1170, Toledo, OH 43614.
E-mail address: linda.speer@utoledo.edu

Prim Care Clin Office Pract 52 (2025) 265–276
https://doi.org/10.1016/j.pop.2025.01.001
0095-4543/25/© 2025 Elsevier Inc. All rights reserved, including those for text and data mining, AI training, and similar technologies.
primarycare.theclinics.com

Abbreviations	
CBT	cognitive behavioral therapy
DHEA	dehydroepiandrosterone
FPHL	female pattern hair loss
GSM	genitourinary syndrome of menopause
KNB	kisspeptin-neurokinin B
MHT	menopausal hormone therapy
NK3Ra	neurokinin receptor antagonists
UTI	urinary tract infection
VSM	vasomotor symptoms of menopause
WHI	Women's Health Initiative

Nonhormonal pharmacologic treatments and complementary therapies are also options to treat symptoms related to menopause, and topical options are available for isolated genitourinary syndrome of menopause (GSM).

MENOPAUSAL HORMONE THERAPY

Hormone therapy continues to be the most effective treatment for vasomotor symptoms of menopause (VSM) including hot flashes, night sweats, and palpitations. Estrogen alone and combination estrogen-progestogen regimens effectively reduce the severity and intensity of vasomotor symptoms.[7–12] Estrogen-only regimens are appropriate for patients without a uterus, but estrogen combined with a progestogen or bazedoxifene must be used in those with a uterus to prevent endometrial hyperplasia or cancer.[13] Bazedoxifene is a selective estrogen receptor modulator that prevents endometrial hyperplasia, maintains the benefits of estrogen, and decreases the potential side effects of breast pain and vaginal bleeding from progestogens.[14–18] Multiple formulations of systemic estrogen with similar efficacy are available (**Table 1**).[11,22] The transdermal patch is the least likely to be discontinued.[11] **Table 2** shows common effects of MHT. Progestogen only regimens can be effective for treating VSM but are not Food and Drug Administration (FDA) approved, and no long-term studies have been conducted on safety.[19,23,28,29] Compounded bioidenticals are not recommended due to lack of safety and efficacy data.[22]

Guidelines recommend making individualized decisions for MHT to achieve maximum benefit with minimal risk.[22,30,31] Patients younger than 60 and within 10 years of menopause have the most favorable benefit-risk ratio, and MHT should be considered in these patients if they do not have contraindications like history of myocardial infarction, stroke, venous thromboembolism (VTE), or estrogen-dependent cancers (ie, breast).[5,22,30] Patients over 60 years old and more than 10 years past the onset of menopause have a less favorable benefit-risk ratio, but it is still reasonable to consider MHT if benefits outweigh risks.[22,30] To minimize adverse events, all patients should receive the lowest effective dose of MHT for the shortest amount of time needed with annual evaluation.[30] There are no specific guidelines on when to discontinue MHT, so decisions must be individualized. Tapering the dose has no proven benefit in mitigating symptom return.[22]

MHT is not FDA approved for treatment of depressive symptoms but data are mixed.[32] Studies have also shown improvement in insomnia.[10,33,34]

NONHORMONAL PHARMACOLOGIC TREATMENTS FOR VSM

SSRIs Paroxetine, escitalopram, citalopram, and SNRIs venlafaxine, and desvenlafaxine have all been shown to reduce VSM with a range in the reduction for VSM

Table 1
Sample systemic medication regimens

Hormone Therapy	Dosing	Use Recommendations
Conjugated equine estrogen oral	0.3–1.25 mg/d	Avoid in hypertriglyceridemia, active gallbladder disease, known thrombophilia and history of VTE[5,8,19–21]
Esterified estrogens oral	0.3–1.25 mg/d	
Ethinyl estradiol oral	0.5–2 mg/d	
Ethinyl estradiol topical gel	0.25–1.25 g/d	Preferred in migraine headache with aura and may mitigate VTE risk[8,21]
Ethinyl estradiol topical spray	1–3 sprays/d	
Ethinyl estradiol transdermal patch	0.025–0.1 mg/d once weekly	
Ethinyl estradiol vaginal ring	0.05–0.1 mg/d intravaginally q3 months	
Ethinyl estradiol cypionate intramuscularly	1–5 mg q 3–4 wk	Not generally used
Ethinyl estradiol valerate IM	10–20 mg q4 weeks	
Progesterone oral	200 mg daily 12 d each mo	
Conjugated estrogen/ bazedoxifene oral	0.45 mg/20 mg daily	

Abbreviation: VTE, venous thromboembolism.

frequency of 25% to 69%.[35] Paroxetine was the first nonhormonal treatment of VSM to be FDA approved. Paroxetine and venlafaxine both reduce VSM frequency by about 50%, and the latter is more often used.[36] Duloxetine has been shown effective in smaller studies.[37,38] Research has indicated that 10 to 20 mg escitalopram and 75 mg venlafaxine are equivalent to 0.5 mg oral 17β-estradiol.[7]

Gabapentin 900 mg daily improves VSM, and higher doses are more effective.[39] Side effects of drowsiness, dizziness, headache, and disorientation are more common at higher doses. A meta-analysis showed gabapentin was associated with significant reductions versus placebo for VSM frequency, duration, and composite score.[40] One study found that pregabalin at doses of 75 or 150 mg twice daily reduced VSM by about 60% compared with 35% for placebo.[41]

Table 2
Effects of menopausal hormone therapy

Increasing age and duration of use increase risk for adverse effects[20,23]	
Common side effects	Breast tenderness, nausea, bloating, headaches, abnormal uterine bleeding
Gallbladder disease	Increased incidence[20]
Venous thromboembolism (VTE)	Increased risk, highest with estrogen-progesterone[5,8,20,21] Mitigated with transdermal estrogen[8,21]
Breast cancer	Inconsistent findings with possible decreased or slightly increased incidence with estrogen only[4,20,24–27] Slight increase with combined therapy[5,20,24]
Endometrial cancer	Increased risk with estrogen only[23] Decreased incidence with combined therapy[23]
Coronary heart disease	Increased risk with combined therapy[23,27]
Stroke	Increased risk with oral MHT, MHT use > 5 y[21] Decreased risk with nonoral MHT[21]

Fezolinetant represents a new class of drugs called neurokinin receptor antagonists (NK3Ra). The mechanism of action is via a group of neurons in the hypothalamus, kisspeptin-neurokinin B (KNB) neurons. Menopausal decrease in estrogen levels leads to hyperstimulation of KNB neuron production of kisspeptin, which in turn stimulates the thermoregulatory center to increase sensitivity to external cues and triggers more frequent heat dissipation responses, such as VSM. Antagonist blockade of NK3 receptors alleviates thermoregulatory disturbances related to the female low estrogen state.

Fezolinetant is the second nonhormonal medication approved by the FDA to treat menopausal vasomotor symptoms. Although significantly more effective than other nonhormonal medications,[9] the cost of approximately $540/mo may limit use. Approval trials had durations of up to 1 year, so postmarketing surveillance is required to evaluate longer-term use.

A meta-analysis comparing fezolinetant to placebo among postmenopausal participants with moderate to severe VSM showed a pooled odds ratio for reduction of symptoms by at least 50% versus placebo of 2.78 (95% confidence interval: 1.81–4.27) with 70% decreased odds of sleep problems. There was about a 1% incidence above placebo of elevated alanine transaminase.[42]

Another meta-analysis compared the results of venlafaxine or desvenlafaxine placebo-controlled trials to NK3Ra placebo-controlled trials for VSM frequency and severity, and night-time awakenings/night sweats. NK3Ra treatment resulted in reduction in frequency from baseline to week 12 by 62% to 93% (placebo 28%–55%) compared with 48% to 67% for SNRIs (placebo 25%–51%) and were better tolerated regarding nausea, dry mouth, insomnia, dizziness, and constipation.[43]

Other nonhormonal pharmacologic treatments for VSM include clonidine and oxybutynin. Clonidine is more effective than placebo, but less effective than other options and limited by anticholinergic effects. Oxybutynin is somewhat effective but associated with cognitive decline in older persons.[44] See **Table 3** for a summary of nonhormonal pharmacologic treatments.

NONPHARMACOLOGICAL TREATMENTS FOR MENOPAUSAL SYMPTOMS

The 2023 North American Menopause Society position statement recommended the use of cognitive behavioral therapy (CBT), clinical hypnosis, weight loss, and stellate ganglion blocks as scientifically supported modalities for management.[31]

As elevated (BMI) and tobacco use are risk factors for VSM, weight reduction, and smoking cessation are encouraged.[3] Dietary guidelines include a whole food, plant-based diet with an emphasis on protein intake of at least 0.8 g/kg of body weight/day.[45,46] Strength training is encouraged to mitigate metabolic changes associated with menopause, help prevent osteoporosis, and decrease VSM.[47]

CBT utilizes psychotherapeutic behavior modifications to change negative patterns associated with VSM of menopause.[3,48] Sessions focus on developing deep awareness of one's mind and body with meditation, breathing techniques, and yoga.[49] CBT decreases the frequency and severity of VSM, anxiety, and sleep problems.[50–52] CBT provided in individual sessions, group sessions, virtual sessions, and self-guided online modules is efficacious and cost-effective.[53,54]

Clinical hypnosis has shown similar efficacy to CBT for short-term reduction of VSM and associated sleep disturbances.[52] Sleep quality significantly improved in groups that had either phone or in-person delivery of hypnosis.[55]

Stellate ganglion blocks can be effective for VSM.[31] These blocks are performed at the anterolateral aspect of the right C6 vertebra under fluoroscopy and may alleviate

Table 3
Nonhormonal pharmacologic treatments of vasomotor symptoms of menopause

Medication	Dosing	Notes
Paroxetine	7.5 mg IR capsule nightly	FDA approved. SSRI/SNRIs may increase rate of fragility fractures[31]
Escitalopram	10–20 mg daily	Start at 10 mg daily and increase after 4 wk if symptoms are not adequately controlled, SSRI/SNRIs may increase rate of fragility fractures[31]
Citalopram	10–20 mg daily	Off-label use, SSRI/SNRIs may increase rate of fragility fractures[31]
Venlafaxine	37.5–75 mg daily	Off-label use, SSRI/SNRIs may increase rate of fragility fractures[31]
Desvenlafaxine	50–100 mg daily	Off-label use, SSRI/SNRIs may increase rate of fragility fractures[31]
Gabapentin	900 mg	Off-label use, start 100–300 mg nightly and increase gradually over 3–12 d based on response and tolerability[39,40]
Pregabalin	75–150 mg twice daily	Off-label use, start 50 mg nightly and increase weekly based on response and tolerability, may cause weight gain[41]
Fezolinetant	45 mg daily	FDA approved Cost may be prohibitive. Associated with abdominal pain, diarrhea, and increased risk of hepatic transaminase elevation. Liver function tests should be obtained prior to initiation and at 3, 6, and 9 mo[42]
Clonidine	0.05 mg twice daily	Anticholinergic effects, may titrate up based on response and tolerability to a dosage range of 0.1–1 mg/d in divided doses[31,44]

symptoms for up to 12 weeks but is reserved for patients with severe or refractory VSM due to limited availability and higher risk.[3]

While not recommended by North American Menopause Society (NAMS), phytoestrogen ("plant" estrogen) use is a popular form of alternative therapy for VSM. All classes of phytoestrogens have varying efficacy. Supplementation is effective in some patients; however, the lack of regulation of supplements introduces challenges to therapy. Genistein, the most prevalent isoflavone in soy, can stimulate breast cancer growth and may interfere with the antitumor activity of tamoxifen and should not be utilized in this population.[31,56]

GENITOURINARY SYNDROME OF MENOPAUSE

GSM is a prevalent condition affecting up to 90% of postmenopausal women. Symptoms include vaginal burning, itching, dryness, and pain (including dyspareunia), and recurrent urinary tract infections (UTIs). These symptoms can significantly impair quality of life and sexual function.[57]

The pathophysiology of GSM involves thinning, dryness, and inflammation of vaginal tissue due to decreased estrogen stimulation resulting in a reduced number of epithelial cells, degeneration of collagen and elastin fibers in connective tissue, and an overall increase in mucosal fragility which impacts sexual and urinary function.[58]

Diagnosis of GSM is based on patient history, physical examination, and vaginal pH measurement. Visual inspection for signs of keratinization and loss of rugae can be helpful.

Treatment options for GSM include lifestyle modifications, vaginal moisturizers/lubricants, estrogen, dehydroepiandrosterone (DHEA), and ospemifene. Lifestyle modifications that can mitigate symptoms include smoking cessation, regular sexual activity, which helps to maintain vaginal elasticity and lubricative response to sexual arousal, and pelvic floor exercises. Vaginal moisturizers and lubricants offer relief from coital discomfort without reversing atrophic changes.

Estrogen therapy in the form of topical creams, suppositories, or rings, effectively decreases GSM symptoms, reducing the incidence of incontinence and recurrent UTIs in postmenopausal women.[59] Systemic estrogen can be considered for more severe symptoms. In one study, vaginal estrogen improved incontinence symptoms (relative risk [RR]: 0.74; CI: 0.64–0.86) while systemic estrogen alone worsened incontinence (RR: 1.32).[60] In a small study, vaginal estrogen reduced the frequency of recurrent UTIs in postmenopausal women,[61] while the serum estrogen levels remained within postmenopausal range in another study of women treated with low-dose vaginal estrogen therapy.[62] Vaginal estrogen therapy should be used at the lowest effective dose and frequency and avoided in cases of undiagnosed vaginal or uterine bleeding.

DHEA, an intermediate in androgen and estrogen biosynthesis, is a newer treatment option. A low-dose DHEA vaginal insert is approved in the United States for treatment of moderate to severe dyspareunia in menopausal women. It has been shown to have no significant impact on endometrial cytology. The most common side effect of this treatment is vaginal discharge.[63]

Ospemifene is an estrogen agonist/antagonist indicated for treatment of vaginal dryness and moderate to severe dyspareunia. A 52-week study showed sustained improvement without any cases of venous thromboembolism, endometrial hyperplasia, or cancer. The most common side effect was vasomotor symptoms.[64] Ospemifene reduced recurrent UTIs in a 6-month retrospective observational study.[65] It should not be recommended for patients with known or suspected breast cancer. Treatment options are summarized in **Table 4**.

There is insufficient data to recommend vaginal testosterone, including combinations of estradiol and compounded vaginal testosterone cream.[66]

Unlike VSM, genitourinary symptoms typically worsen over time. As women are often reluctant to voice concerns over these symptoms, it is essential to provide ongoing education about typical symptoms of GSM as well as potential treatments for this condition.

Table 4 Treatments of genitourinary syndrome of menopause		
Medication	**Targeted Symptoms**	**Notes**
Topical estrogen	Incontinence and UTIs[59–61]	Use lowest dose possible, avoid in undiagnosed vaginal or uterine bleeding[22]
DHEA	Moderate to severe dyspareunia[63]	
Ospemifene	Vaginal dryness and moderate to severe dyspareunia, may reduce recurrent UTIs[64,65]	Should not be used in patients with known or suspected breast cancer[64]

HAIR LOSS

Female pattern hair loss (FPHL) affects about 50% of menopausal women. Topical minoxidil and topical or oral finasteride may be effective.[67–69] Current guidelines recommend topical minoxidil as first-line treatment for FPHL while some studies have shown that oral finasteride is more effective.[70,71]

CASE

Brenda, a 54-year-old female, presents to her primary care physician with 10 months of daily hot flashes, night sweats, and insomnia. She has a past medical history of hypertension and depression, well controlled on 10 mg of lisinopril and 150 mg of venlafaxine XR. Hot flashes occur several times a day and affect her personal and professional life. Brenda's last menstrual cycle was 15 months ago. Brenda has not had a hysterectomy. She denies any family history of breast or gynecologic cancer. She is a nonsmoker. Her current BMI is 29 without regular exercise. She endorses experiencing vaginal dryness and dyspareunia for several months with no urinary symptoms. She is interested in medication options to relieve her symptoms. She read on social media that hormone therapy is not safe due to risks of breast cancer and blood clots. What is your advice for Brenda?

As Brenda is younger than 60 and less than 5 years from menopause onset with no contraindications, MHT is the recommended first-line treatment for her vasomotor and genitourinary symptoms. You advise Brenda that transdermal estrogen in combination with progesterone is a safe, effective option which is low risk for developing breast cancer or blood clots.

Despite assurances, Brenda refuses MHT. She declines gabapentin due to the side effects of drowsiness and dizziness. She is interested in fezolinetant and states that she has great insurance, so she is not worried about the high cost. You advise Brenda this will not help with her genitourinary symptoms. She is still hesitant to use even topical hormones and states she will try vaginal moisturizers and lubricants and consider other options in the future. You recommend that she start exercising regularly to help maintain bone mineral density and to lose weight which may improve her vasomotor symptoms.

CLINICS CARE POINTS

- Menopausal hormone therapy (MHT) with estrogen only or estrogen plus progestogen therapy at the lowest effective dose for the shortest amount of time with regular monitoring should be considered first-line treatment for vasomotor symtomptoms of menopause (VSM) in patients under 60 and less than 10 years from start of menopause without contraindications and may be considered for patients with VSM over 60 or more than 10 years from start of menopause with individualized decisions made considering the risks versus benefits. Transdermal estrogen has the greatest adherence and lowest risk factor profile.

- selective serotonin reuptake inhibitors (SSRIs), serotonin-norpepnephrine inhibitors (SNRIs), gabapentin, and fezolinetant are effective nonhormonal options for treatment of VSM of menopause.

- Improving lifestyle factors such as weight loss and tobacco cessation help manage VSM and are encouraged in all women. Cognitive behavioral therapy is recommended for VSM management in those who are not good candidates for pharmacologic treatments.

- Nonhormonal lubricants, including long-acting vaginal moisturizers, are first-line therapies for women with genitourinary syndrome of menopause (GSM).

- Low-dose vaginal estrogen therapy is safe and effective for women with moderate to severe GSM symptoms that do not respond to nonhormonal options.
- Topical minoxidil or oral/topical finasteride may be effective to help with hair loss due to menopause.

DISCLOSURE

The authors have nothing to disclose.

REFERENCES

1. Whiteley J, daCosta DiBonaventura M, Wagner J-S, et al. The impact of menopausal symptoms on quality of life, productivity, and economic outcomes. J Wom Health 2013;22(11):983–90.
2. GBD 2017 Mortality Collaborators. Global, regional, and national age-sex-specific mortality and life expectancy, 1950-2017: a systematic analysis for the Global Burden of Disease Study 2017. Lancet 2018;392(10159):1684–735 [published correction appears in Lancet 2019;393(10190):e44. doi: 10.1016/S0140-6736(19)31046-3].
3. Davis SR, Taylor S, Hemachandra C, et al. The 2023 practitioner's toolkit for managing menopause. Climacteric 2023;26(6):517–36.
4. Crawford SL, Crandall CJ, Derby CA, et al. Menopausal hormone therapy trends before versus after 2002: impact of the women's health initiative study results. Menopause 2018;26(6):588–97. PMID: 30586004; PMCID: PMC6538484.
5. Prentice RL, Aragaki AK, Chlebowski RT, et al. Randomized trial evaluation of the benefits and risks of menopausal hormone therapy among women 50-59 Years of age. Am J Epidemiol 2021;190(3):365–75. PMID: 33025002; PMCID: PMC8086238.
6. Cho L, Kaunitz AM, Faubion SS, et al. Rethinking menopausal hormone therapy: for whom, what, when, and how long? Circulation 2023;147(7):597–610.
7. Joffe H, Guthrie KA, LaCroix AZ, et al. Low-dose estradiol and the serotonin-norepinephrine reuptake inhibitor venlafaxine for vasomotor symptoms: a randomized clinical trial. JAMA Intern Med 2014;174(7):1058–66. PMID: 24861828; PMCID: PMC4179877.
8. Marko KI, Simon JA. Clinical trials in menopause. Menopause 2018;25(2):217–30. PMID: 28953214.
9. Morga A, Ajmera M, Gao E, et al. Systematic review and network meta-analysis comparing the efficacy of fezolinetant with hormone and nonhormone therapies for treatment of vasomotor symptoms due to menopause. Menopause 2024; 31(1):68–76.
10. Santoro N, Allshouse A, Neal-Perry G, et al. Longitudinal changes in menopausal symptoms comparing women randomized to low-dose oral conjugated estrogens or transdermal estradiol plus micronized progesterone versus placebo: the Kronos Early Estrogen Prevention Study. Menopause 2017;24(3):238–46. PMID: 27779568; PMCID: PMC5323337.
11. Sarri G, Pedder H, Dias S, et al. Vasomotor symptoms resulting from natural menopause: a systematic review and network meta-analysis of treatment effects from the National Institute for Health and Care Excellence guideline on menopause. BJOG 2017;124:1514–23.

12. Simon JA, Kaunitz AM, Kroll R, et al. Oral 17β-estradiol/progesterone (TX-001HR) and quality of life in postmenopausal women with vasomotor symptoms. Menopause 2019;26(5):506–12. PMID: 30489424; PMCID: PMC6493699.

13. Sjögren LL, Mørch LS, Løkkegaard E. Hormone replacement therapy and the risk of endometrial cancer: a systematic review. Maturitas 2016;91:25–35. Epub 2016 Jun 1. PMID: 27451318.

14. Lobo RA, Pinkerton JV, Gass MLS, et al. Evaluation of bazedoxifene/conjugated estrogens for the treatment of menopausal symptoms and effects on metabolic parameters and overall safety profile. Fertil Steril 2009;92(3):1025–38. Epub 2009 Jul 26. PMID: 19635615.

15. Mirkin S, Komm B, Pickar JH. Conjugated estrogen/bazedoxifene tablets for the treatment of moderate-to-severe vasomotor symptoms associated with menopause. Womens Health (Lond) 2014;10(2):135–46. PMID: 24601804.

16. Pinkerton JV, Harvey JA, Pan K, et al. Breast effects of bazedoxifene-conjugated estrogens: a randomized controlled trial. Obstet Gynecol 2013;121(5):959–68. PMID: 23635731.

17. Pinkerton JV, Utian WH, Constantine GD, et al. Relief of vasomotor symptoms with the tissue-selective estrogen complex containing bazedoxifene/conjugated estrogens: a randomized, controlled trial. Menopause 2009;16(6):1116–24. Erratum in: Menopause. 2015 Feb;22(2):245. PMID: 19546826.

18. Utian W, Yu H, Bobula J, et al. Bazedoxifene/conjugated estrogens and quality of life in postmenopausal women. Maturitas 2009;63(4):329–35. Epub 2009 Jul 31. PMID: 19647382.

19. Goodwin JW, Green SJ, Moinpour CM, et al. Phase III randomized placebo-controlled trial of two doses of megestrol acetate as treatment for menopausal symptoms in women with breast cancer: southwest Oncology Group Study 9626. J Clin Oncol 2008;26:1650–6.

20. Marjoribanks J, Farquhar C, Roberts H, et al. Long-term hormone therapy for perimenopausal and postmenopausal women. Cochrane Database Syst Rev 2017;1(1):CD004143. PMID: 28093732; PMCID: PMC6465148.

21. Rovinski D, Ramos RB, Fighera TM, et al. Risk of venous thromboembolism events in postmenopausal women using oral versus non-oral hormone therapy: a systematic review and meta-analysis. Thromb Res 2018;168:83–95. Epub 2018 Jun 19. PMID: 29936403.

22. "The 2022 hormone therapy position statement of the North American menopause society" advisory panel. The 2022 hormone therapy position statement of the North American menopause society. Menopause 2022;29(7):767–94.

23. Hitchcock CL, Prior JC. Oral micronized progesterone for vasomotor symptoms—a placebo-controlled randomized trial in healthy postmenopausal women. Menopause 2012;19:886–93.

24. Manson JE, Chlebowski RT, Stefanick ML, et al. Menopausal hormone therapy and health outcomes during the intervention and extended poststopping phases of the Women's Health Initiative randomized trials. JAMA 2013;310:1353–68.

25. Chlebowski RT, Aragaki AK. The Women's Health Initiative randomized trials of menopausal hormone therapy and breast cancer: findings in context. Menopause 2023;30(4):454–61. Epub 2023 Jan 22. PMID: 36727752.

26. Collaborative Group on Hormonal Factors in Breast Cancer. Type and timing of menopausal hormone therapy and breast cancer risk: individual participant meta-analysis of the worldwide epidemiological evidence. Lancet 2019;394(10204):1159–68. Epub 2019 Aug 29. PMID: 31474332; PMCID: PMC6891893.

27. Kim JE, Chang JH, Jeong MJ, et al. A systematic review and meta-analysis of effects of menopausal hormone therapy on cardiovascular diseases. Sci Rep 2020; 10(1):20631. PMID: 33244065; PMCID: PMC7691511.

28. Prior JC, Nielsen JD, Hitchcock CL, et al. Medroxyprogesterone and conjugated oestrogen are equivalent for hot flushes: a 1-year randomized double-blind trial following premenopausal ovariectomy. Clin Sci (Lond) 2007;112:517–25.

29. Schiff I, Tulchinsky D, Cramer D, et al. Oral medroxyprogesterone in the treatment of postmenopausal symptoms. JAMA 1980;244:1443–5.

30. ACOG Practice Bulletin No. 141: management of menopausal symptoms. Obstet Gynecol 2014;123(1):202–16 [published correction appears in Obstet Gynecol 2016;127(1):166. doi:10.1097/AOG.0000000000001230] [published correction appears in Obstet Gynecol 2018;131(3):604. doi:10.1097/AOG.0000000000002513].

31. "The 2023 nonhormone therapy position statement of the North American menopause society" advisory panel. The 2023 nonhormone therapy position statement of the North American menopause society. Menopause 2023;30(6):573–90.

32. Maki PM, Kornstein SG, Joffe H, et al. Guidelines for the evaluation and treatment of perimenopausal depression: summary and recommendations. J Womens Health (Larchmt) 2019;28(2):117–34. Epub 2018 Sep 5. PMID: 30182804.

33. Cintron D, Lahr BD, Bailey KR, et al. Effects of oral versus transdermal menopausal hormone treatments on self-reported sleep domains and their association with vasomotor symptoms in recently menopausal women enrolled in the Kronos Early Estrogen Prevention Study (KEEPS). Menopause 2018;25(2):145–53. PMID: 28832429; PMCID: PMC5771895.

34. Geiger PJ, Eisenlohr-Moul T, Gordon JL, et al. Effects of perimenopausal transdermal estradiol on self-reported sleep, independent of its effect on vasomotor symptom bother and depressive symptoms. Menopause 2019;26(11):1318–23. PMID: 31688579; PMCID: PMC8294069.

35. Shufelt CL, Brown V, Carpenter JS, et al, for the North American Menopause Society. The 2023 nonhormone therapy position statement of the North American Menopause Society. Menopause 2023;30:573–90.

36. Crandall CJ, Mehta JM, Manson JE. Management of menopausal symptoms. JAMA 2023;329:405–20.

37. Biglia N, Bounous VE, Susini T, et al. Duloxetine and escitalopram for hot flushes: efficacy and compliance in cancer survivors. Eur J Cancer Care 2018;27. https://doi.org/10.1111/ecc.1284.

38. Freeman MP, Hirschberg AM, Wnag B, et al. Duloxetine for major depressive disorder and daytime and nighttime hot flashes associated with the menopause transition. Maturitas 2013;75:170–4.

39. Reddy SY, Warner H, Guttuso T, et al. Gabapentin, estrogen, and placebo for treatment of hot flushes: a randomized controlled trial. Obstet Gynecol 2006; 108:41–8.

40. Yoon SH, Li JY, Lee C, et al. Gabapentin for the treatment of hot flushes in menopause: a meta-analysis. Menopause 2020;27:485–93.

41. Loprinzi CL, Qin R, Balcueva EP, et al. Phase III, randomized, placebo-controlled evaluation of pregabalin for alleviating hot flashes. J Clin Oncol 2010;28:641–7.

42. Bonga KN, Mishra A, Maiti R, et al. Efficacy and safety of fezolinetant for the treatment of menopause-related vasomotor symptoms: a meta-analysis. Obstet Gynecol 2023;143:393–420.

43. Menown SJ, Tello J. Neurokinin3 receptor antagonists compared with serotonin norepinephrine reuptake inhibitors for non-hormonal treatment of menopausal hot flushes: a systematic qualitative review. Adv Ther 2021;38:5025–45.

44. Duong V, Iwamoto A, Pnnycuff J, et al. A systematic review of neurocognitive dysfunction with overactive bladder medications. Int Urogynecol J 2012;32:2693–702.
45. Barnard ND, Kahleova H, Holtz DN, et al. The Women's Study for the Alleviation of Vasomotor Symptoms (WAVS): a randomized, controlled trial of a plant-based diet and whole soybeans for postmenopausal women. Menopause 2021;28(10):1150–6.
46. McCarthy D, Berg A. Weight loss strategies, and the risk of skeletal muscle mass loss. Nutrients 2021;13(7):2473.
47. Capel-Alcaraz AM, García-López H, Castro-Sánchez AM, et al. The efficacy of strength exercises for reducing the symptoms of menopause: a systematic review. J Clin Med 2023;12(2):548.
48. American Psychological Association. What is cognitive behavioral therapy?. Available at: https://www.apa.org/ptsd-guideline/patients-and-families/cognitive-behavioral.pdf.
49. Hunter MS. Cognitive behavioral therapy for menopausal symptoms. Climacteric 2021;24(1):51–6.
50. Al Wattar BH, Talaulikar V. Non-oestrogen-based and complementary therapies for menopause. Best Pract Res Clin Endocrinol Metab 2024;38(1):101819.
51. John JB, Chellaiyan DVG, Gupta S, et al. How effective the mindfulness-based cognitive behavioral therapy on quality of life in women with menopause. J Midlife Health 2022;13(2):169–74.
52. Chang JG, Lewis MN, Wertz MC. Managing menopausal symptoms: common questions and answers. Am Fam Physician 2023;108(1):28–39.
53. Atema V, van Leeuwen M, Oldenburg HSA, et al. An Internet-based cognitive behavioral therapy for treatment-induced menopausal symptoms in breast cancer survivors: results of a pilot study. Menopause 2017;24(7):762–7.
54. Verbeek JGE, Atema V, Mewes JC, et al. Cost-utility, cost-effectiveness, and budget impact of Internet-based cognitive behavioral therapy for breast cancer survivors with treatment-induced menopausal symptoms. Breast Cancer Res Treat 2019;178(3):573–85.
55. Elkins G, Otte J, Carpenter JS, et al. Hypnosis intervention for sleep disturbance: determination of optimal dose and method of delivery for postmenopausal women. Int J Clin Exp Hypn 2021;69(3):323–45.
56. Drewe J, Bucher KA, Zahner C. A systematic review of non-hormonal treatments of vasomotor symptoms in climacteric and cancer patients. SpringerPlus 2015;4:65.
57. Kingsberg SA, Krychman M, Graham S, et al. The Women's EMPOWER Survey: identifying women's perceptions on vulvar and vaginal atrophy and its treatment. J Sex Med 2017;14(3):413–24. Epub 2017 Feb 12. PMID: 28202320.
58. Pérez-López FR, Vieira-Baptista P, Phillips N, et al. Clinical manifestations and evaluation of postmenopausal vulvovaginal atrophy. Gynecol Endocrinol 2021;37(8):740–5. Epub 2021 May 26. PMID: 34036849.
59. Robinson D, Cardozo LD. The role of estrogens in female lower urinary tract dysfunction. Urology 2003;62(4 Suppl 1):45–51. PMID: 14550837.
60. Cody JD, Jacobs ML, Richardson K, et al. Oestrogen therapy for urinary incontinence in post-menopausal women. Cochrane Database Syst Rev 2012;10:CD001405.
61. Ferrante KL, Wasenda EJ, Jung CE, et al. Vaginal estrogen for the prevention of recurrent urinary tract infection in postmenopausal women: a randomized clinical trial. Female Pelvic Med Reconstr Surg 2021;27(2):112–7. PMID: 31232721.

62. Lee JS, Ettinger B, Stanczyk FZ, et al. Comparison of methods to measure low serum estradiol levels in postmenopausal women. J Clin Endocrinol Metab 2006;91(10):3791–7. Epub 2006 Aug 1. PMID: 16882749.
63. Portman DJ, Labrie F, Archer DF, et al, other participating members of VVA Prasterone Group. Lack of effect of intravaginal dehydroepiandrosterone (DHEA, prasterone) on the endometrium in postmenopausal women. Menopause 2015; 22(12):1289–95. PMID: 25968836.
64. Simon JA, Lin VH, Radovich C, et al. The Ospemifene Study Group. One-year long-term safety extension study of ospemifene for the treatment of vulvar and vaginal atrophy in postmenopausal women with a uterus. Menopause 2013; 20(4):418–27.
65. Schiavi MC, Di Pinto A, Sciuga V, et al. Prevention of recurrent lower urinary tract infections in postmenopausal women with genitourinary syndrome: outcome after 6 months of treatment with ospemifene. Gynecol Endocrinol 2018;34(2):140–3. Epub 2017 Aug 30. PMID: 28853624.
66. Simon JA, Goldstein I, Kim Noel N, et al. The role of androgens in the treatment of genitourinary syndrome of menopause (GSM): international Society for the Study of Women's Sexual Health (ISSWSH) expert consensus panel review. Menopause 2018;25(7):837–47.
67. Hu AC, Chapman LW, Mesinkovska NA. The efficacy and use of finasteride in women: a systematic review. Int J Dermatol 2019;58(7):759–76. Epub 2019 Jan 3. PMID: 30604525.
68. Nobari NN, Roohaninasab M, Sadeghzadeh-Bazargan A, et al. A systematic review of clinical trials using single or combination therapy of oral or topical finasteride for women in reproductive age and postmenopausal women with hormonal and nonhormonal androgenetic alopecia. Adv Clin Exp Med 2023;32(7):813–23. PMID: 36897103.
69. van Zuuren EJ, Fedorowicz Z, Schoones J. Interventions for female pattern hair loss. Cochrane Database Syst Rev 2016;2016(5):CD007628. PMID: 27225981; PMCID: PMC6457957.
70. Carmina E, Azziz R, Bergfeld W, et al. Female pattern hair loss and androgen excess: a report from the multidisciplinary androgen excess and PCOS committee. J Clin Endocrinol Metab 2019;104(7):2875–91. PMID: 30785992.
71. Gupta AK, Wang T, Bamimore MA, et al. The relative effect of monotherapy with 5-alpha reductase inhibitors and minoxidil for female pattern hair loss: a network meta-analysis study. J Cosmet Dermatol 2024;23(1):154–60. Epub 2023 Jun 29. PMID: 37386777.

Abortion in Primary Care

Libby Wetterer, MD[a], Hannah Rosenfield, MD[b],
Hilary Gortler, MD, MS[c], Martha Simmons, MD[c],*

KEYWORDS

- Abortion • Reproductive Justice • Medication abortion • Mifepristone • Misoprostol
- Procedural abortion

KEY POINTS

- Medication and procedural abortion care is within the scope of most primary care clinicians including advanced practice clinicans; primary care integration increases access and promotes Reproductive Justice.
- Medication abortion via telemedicine, using a no-touch protocol, is safe and effective for most patients.
- Primary care clinicians should understand common follow-up concerns for patients undergoing clinician-led and self-managed abortion.
- Procedural abortion care should be trauma-informed and include options for pain control.
- Medication and procedural abortion are the same as evidenced-based treatment for early pregnancy loss.

INTRODUCTION

In the United States, 1 in 4 women[a] will have 1 or more abortions by age 45[1,2] and one-fifth of pregnancies end in abortion.[3] Most abortions occur in the first trimester.[2] First-trimester medication and procedural abortions are safe, effective, and within the scope of the primary care clinician, yet only 1% of abortions occur outside of a specialty clinic such as a primary care office.[4–6] Expanding abortion provision beyond obstetrics and gynecology to other specialties and advanced practice clinicians is fundamental to safeguarding and improving access, especially in rural communities.[7] Primary care integration promotes continuity of care, reduces the need for extra appointments, fees, and travel, reduces the odds of interactions with protestors, and

[a] Department of Family Medicine and Community Health, University of Pennsylvania, 51 N 39th Street, Philadelphia, PA 19104, USA; [b] Departments of OBGYN & Family Medicine, Western Michigan School of Medicine, Kalamazoo, MI 49006, USA; [c] Division of Family Medicine, Jefferson Einstein Philadelphia Hospital, Philadelphia, PA 19141, USA
* Corresponding author. 5201 Old York Road, Suite 311, Philadelphia, PA 19141.
E-mail address: MarthaASimmons@gmail.com

[a] Not only cis women have abortions, though most data collection is from this population. For this article, the authors will use gender-neutral language to include all people with the capacity for pregnancy except when referring to respective studied populations.

Prim Care Clin Office Pract 52 (2025) 277–290
https://doi.org/10.1016/j.pop.2025.01.002
0095-4543/25/© 2025 Elsevier Inc. All rights reserved, including those for text and data mining, AI training, and similar technologies.

Abbreviations	
hCG	human chorionic gonadotropin
IUD	intrauterine device
LMP	last menstrual period
MAB	medication abortion
NSAIDs	nonsteroidal anti-inflammatory drugs
PAB	procedural abortion
PCB	paracervical block
RJ	Reproductive Justice

allows patients to receive their abortion care in a place they know. It also reduces the burden on specialty abortion clinics and allows for increased access for those who need to travel or have abortions beyond the first trimester.

Assuring access to abortion care is rooted in Reproductive Justice (RJ). RJ is built from a Human Rights framework and combines reproductive rights and social justice. While the ideology has existed and been practiced within many communities for generations, the term was formalized by a group of Black women in 1994.[8] It posits that everyone has the right to bodily autonomy, and to have children, not have children, and parent in safe and sustainable communities. States with the least supportive parenting resources and the highest maternal mortality rates are also the states with the most restrictive abortion policies.[9–11] Twentieth-century public health messaging around abortion rights is centered around "choice." We cannot achieve RJ without shifting the narrative to access.

Excellent and equitable primary care for people with the capacity for pregnancy includes not only contraception, fertility, and perinatal services but also the ability to manage a miscarriage and provide early abortion care. This article aims to serve as an overview and jumping-off point for clinicians initiating or expanding their primary care-based abortion services.

OPTIONS COUNSELING

Some patients may present with a positive home pregnancy test while others have a test included in routine care. Clinicians should avoid assumptions and foster a trauma-informed space by providing silence, asking open-ended questions, and using neutral language. For example, "your pregnancy test is positive which means you are pregnant, how do you feel about that?" Every patient should be provided with the option of abortion or continuing the pregnancy with the option to parent or make an adoption plan. While some may chose adoption, it is not an alterative to abortion.

Terms and phrases such as "termination," "putting up for adoption," and "keeping the baby" should be avoided.

Options counseling may include assistance in deciding what type of abortion the patient would like. **Table 1** delineates key differences between medication and procedural abortion.

PREGNANCY DATING

There are multiple modalities for determining gestational age. Ultrasound, while commonly used, is not a requirement for medication or procedural abortion.

Use of last menstrual period (LMP) is an accurate means of establishing dating.[12] Obtaining a patient's history including irregular periods, hormone use, risk factors for ectopic pregnancy, and symptoms of ectopic pregnancy can help determine if

Table 1	
Key differences between medication and procedural abortion	
Medical Abortion (<77–84 d)	**Procedural Abortion**
• Less medicalized	• Shorter time overall
• Avoids a procedure	• Option for anesthesia in some locations
• May feel more "natural"	• Less at home bleeding
• Easier to disguise as having a miscarriage	• Can get intrauterine device (IUD) on day
• Option for no touch/telehealth	of procedure
• No pelvic examination needed	• No need for follow-up
• Follow-up sometimes needed	• Preferred option >77–84 d
• Completion rate 93%–99%	• Completion rate >99%
(depending on gestational age and regimen)	

the LMP is accurate or if further evaluation is indicated. If an ultrasound is needed, a patient can be referred if it is unavailable in the office.

Use of LMP for dating expands access to abortion care when ultrasound is not readily available. Patients report high confidence in protocols that allow for no or minimal testing.[13]

Pregnancy of Unknown Location

Patients often seek abortion care early in pregnancy. For patients with a positive pregnancy test and no pregnancy visualized on ultrasound, the differential includes a false positive test, early intrauterine pregnancy, early pregnancy loss, or ectopic pregnancy. For patients at low risk of ectopic pregnancy, medication and procedural abortion can be initiated while determining the location of the pregnancy.[14]

Medication abortion (MAB) protocols for pregnancy of unknown location utilize beta human chorionic gonadotropin (hCG) trending.[15] Expect a 50% decrease at 48 hours from misoprostol use. In most cases, trending to zero is not indicated. Patients should be given ectopic precautions while awaiting results. Procedural abortion (PAB) expedites care by allowing for direct visualization of products of conception (POCs). If no POCs are visualized, or decrease is <50%, referral should be made for suspected ectopic.

Serum hCG trending can also be used when patients prefer to identify pregnancy location prior to initiating care.

LABORATORY EVALUATION

There is no required laboratory testing before first-trimester medical or procedural abortion. Many restrictive states require certain tests, so it is important to review your local laws.

Routine testing of hemoglobin for first-trimester abortion has not been shown to improve clinical outcomes.[16] However, clinicians should screen patients for symptoms of anemia and/or increased risk of postabortion hemorrhage and check hemoglobin/hematocrit as indicated.

Extensive data demonstrate that Rh testing and administration of Rh immunoglobulin (RhIg) to Rh-negative patients before abortion or miscarriage up to 12 weeks is not necessary.[17–20]

MEDICATION ABORTION

MAB, also known as medical abortion or abortion with pills, is the most common form of abortion care in the United States.[21] The Food and Drug Adminsitration (FDA)-

approved regimen consists of mifepristone taken orally, followed by misoprostol which can be administered sublingually, buccally, or vaginally. MAB is safe via telemedicine using a no-test protocol as described earlier. The use of abortion pills is FDA approved up to 70 days gestation. Clinical practice guidelines support use through 77 days and World Health Organization guidelines supports MAB through 84 days.[22] The recommended evidence-based regimens are summarized in **Table 2**. Of note, simultaneous use of mifepristone and vaginal misoprostol has also been shown to be noninferior to 24-hour interval dosing up to 63 days gestation.[23] Vaginal dosing helps to reduce side effects.[24] Side effects of misoprostol can include low-grade fever, chills, sore throat, nausea, vomiting, and diarrhea.

Eligibility

There are few absolute contraindications to medical abortion with mifepristone and misoprostol which are summarized in **Table 3**. Breastfeeding, inhaled corticosteroid use, hypertension, sickle cell disease, and having no reliable contact information are not contraindications. If a patient has an intrauterine device (IUD) in place, it should be removed before taking medications. In these cases, ultrasound should be performed given the higher risk of ectopic pregnancy.[14]

If a patient is beyond the gestational limit for MAB, they should be offered or referred for procedural care.

Counseling and Informed Consent

All patients should undergo an informed consent process to confirm they understand the risks, benefits, and alternatives and are making a voluntary decision without coercion.

MAB is extremely safe. Risks include heavy bleeding, infection, continuing pregnancy, and the possible need for a follow-up procedure.

Patients should be counseled on how to take the pills and signs/symptoms necessitating return to care (**Table 4**) and who to contact after hours. If there is no 24-hour option for contact, patients should be given explicit instructions on when to seek emergency care.

Mifepristone can be taken in or out of the office. Patients should be advised that while some may experience nausea or spotting, most people continue their day as usual. After taking the misoprostol, patients will experience bleeding and cramping which will depend on the patient and their gestational age. Clinicians should advise patients to plan to have access to a bathroom and be home if possible. Work and school notes should be provided.

Ibuprofen should be prescribed for use 30 minutes before misoprostol and then every 6 to 8 hours as needed. Prescriptions for antiemetics and acetaminophen with an opioid may also be considered. While MAB is tolerated well by many, others will find it much more painful than a typical period.

All patients must sign the Mifepristone Patient Agreement which can be found on the Danco (earlyoptionpill.com) or Genbiopro (genbiopro.com) websites. They should also be provided with the Medication Guide that comes with the medication. Additional documentation or reporting may be required by your state or facility.

The mifepristone risk evaluation and mitigation strategy program outlines requirements for providers who wish to incorporate MAB in their practice.[30] The program requires providers to review the prescribing information for mifepristone and complete the Provider Agreement Form. Once certified, the provider may send mifepristone prescriptions to pharmacies that have completed the Pharmacy Agreement Form or stock mifepristone for in-clinic dispensing. These forms are available for both Danco and

Table 2
Evidence-based regimens for medication abortion

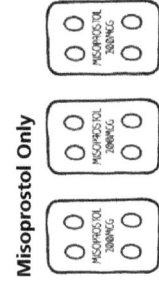

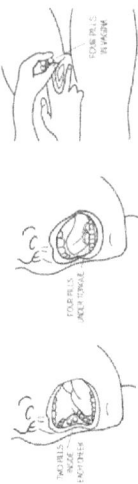

Regimen	Mifepristone + Misoprostol	Misoprostol Only
	MIFEPRISTONE 200MG + MISOPROSTOL 200MCG +/- MISOPROSTOL 200MCG	MISOPROSTOL 200MCG MISOPROSTOL 200MCG MISOPROSTOL 200MCG
Gestational age <64 d	24–48 h later, 800 mcg misoprostol via preferred route (vaginal*, buccal, sublingual)	800 mcg misoprostol 3 h later, 800 mcg misoprostol 3 h later, 800 mcg misoprostol Repeat until the pregnancy passes
	*if vaginal, can insert 0–72 h later	
Gestational age 64–70 d	Swallow 200 mg mifepristone	• 24–48 h later, 800 mcg misoprostol via preferred route (vaginal, buccal or sublingual)[25]	
Gestational age 71–77 d		• 4 h after first dose, take a second dose	
		• 24–48 h later, 800 mcg misoprostol via preferred route (buccal or sublingual)	
		• 4 h after first dose, take a second dose	

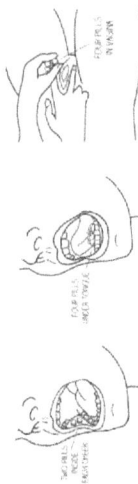

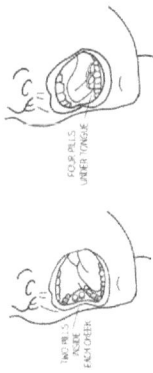

(continued on next page)

Table 2
(continued)

	Mifepristone + Misoprostol	Misoprostol Only
Regimen		
Analgesics & antiemetics	Take 30 min prior to starting misoprostol and throughout the process.	
Efficacy	94%–98%[14]	89%–99%, increased side effects[26,27]

Source Images adapted from Reproductive Health Access Project "How to Use Abortion Pills" Fact Sheet. https://www.reproductiveaccess.org/resource/mabfactsheet/. Accessed September 10, 2024.

Table 3
Medical contraindications to medication abortion

Medical Condition	Potential Concern	Comments
Long-term oral steroid use/chronic adrenal failure	Adrenal crisis[28]	Mifepristone can block cortisol receptors precipitating adrenal crisis. Can consider misoprostol-only regimens.
Inherited porphyria	Porphyria storm[29]	Mifepristone is a cytochrome P-350 inducer
Hemorrhagic disorder or blood thinner use (except Aspirin)	Hemorrhage[16]	Procedural abortion is generally preferred in this scenario
IUD in situ	Uterine damage/perforation, infection, retained products of conception[14]	If IUD can be removed, can proceed with medication abortion
Known ectopic pregnancy	Ongoing ectopic pregnancy[14]	Mifepristone and misoprostol are not effective for treatment of ectopic pregnancy.

Table 4	
Signs/symptoms that should prompt patients to return to care	
Bleeding	>2 maxi pads per h × 2 h ± symptomatic anemia
	No bleeding by 24 h after misoprostol
Pain	Severe one sided
	Not relieved by analgesics/heat
Vomiting	<30 min from taking pills (*consider redosing*)
	Not relieved by antiemetics
Fever	>24 h after last misoprostol dose
Persistent pregnancy symptoms	>1 wk from taking pills (*nausea first to go, breast sensitivity last*)

GenBioPro. Toolkits for integrating abortion into primary care practice are available through organizations such as the Reproductive Health Access Project (RHAP).[31]

Self-Managed Medication Abortion

Self-managed abortion, also known as self-sourced medication abortion, is becoming increasingly common given the current legal landscape.[32] Primary care clinicians should create a safe space for follow-up as needed. Many patients self-manage past 84 days gestation. While complications are rare, some patients may need in-person care. Many patients may not disclose they took pills. Management of early pregnancy loss and abortion are the same and should not matter clinically for management. If patients do disclose, clinicians are protected by HIPPAA (Health Insurance Portability and Accountability Act) and should not report patients to law enforcement.

Follow-Up

Clinicians should offer a plan to confirm the abortion is complete. Clinicians should ask patients if they took the medication as scheduled, if they bled and passed tissue and clots, if they think the abortion is complete, and if they are still having pregnancy symptoms.

Patients who experienced cramping, bleeding, and resolution of pregnancy symptoms can confirm completion with an at-home high-sensitivity urine pregnancy test at 4 to 6 weeks. Roughly 20% of patients will have a positive test at 4 weeks.[33] If a patient has a positive test but answers all following questions in a way to suggest their abortion is complete, they can repeat the test in 1 week.

Patients who have little or no bleeding, don't have symptoms of pregnancy, or prefer earlier confirmation may benefit from an ultrasound or beta hCG follow-up 1 to 2 weeks later. Those who desire lab follow-up must have a beta hCG drawn on or close to the day of they start the pills. Different criteria exist, but a drop of 80% at 2 weeks is commonly used to confirm completion. A heterogeneously thickened endometrial lining is a normal finding after an MAB and does not require treatment in the absence of symptoms. Caution should be taken when ordering official ultrasounds as "cannot rule out retained products of conception" is often noted in an abundance of caution.

Light bleeding can be expected for 4 to 8 weeks after an MAB and the next menstrual cycle may be heavier and mistimed.

If a patient is found to have a continuing pregnancy, they should be offered a procedural abortion. Some patients may prefer repeating the process with medications which is also a reasonable option.

Some patients may decide to forgo formal clinician-led follow-up which is appropriate given the safety of self-managed abortion.[34]

PROCEDURAL ABORTION

PAB, also commonly referred to as a uterine aspiration, can be completed in the first trimester with manual or electric suction. For this article, we will be discussing procedural abortion care for up to 12 weeks. PAB is commonly performed in outpatient settings and can be completed in primary care facilities with appropriate equipment and training. PAB can be provided by clinicians with appropriate training including physicians from various specialties and advanced practice clinicians.[35]

Counseling and Safety

As with MAB, informed consent should occur prior to the procedure. PAB complications are rare, with similar outcomes in office-based clinics compared to ambulatory surgical centers and hospital-based clinics. Rare serious risks including hemorrhage, infection, incomplete abortion/retained products of conception, perforation, and damage to surrounding organs, must be discussed with patients, but are more common with childbirth than with abortion. Mortality associated with childbirth is 14 times that of abortion.[36]

Medical history and vitals should be collected prior to PAB. As with MAB, clinicians must confirm that the patient is certain of their decision to end a pregnancy and is not being coerced.

Sedation/Pain Management

Many different elements including physical, emotional, and psychosocial contribute to pain perception during procedural abortion. Pain perception varies between individuals, and it is important to discuss comfort management options with patients before a procedure. Studies have shown disparities in pain management for people with substance use disorder as well as Black patients.[37,38] Clinicians must work to minimize their own biases to improve patient care, experience, and equity.

Nonpharmacologic pain management is closely linked with trauma-informed, person-centered care, starting with creating a comforting, nonjudgmental environment for patients. Often called "verbicaine," supportive verbal communication methods have been shown to improve comfort. Including relaxing imagery can also decrease pain and anxiety during gynecologic examinations and procedures.[39] Other helpful components include having a support person (per patient preference), playing music in the room, and use of heating pads during the procedure[40,41] It can be helpful to describe in general terms the steps of the procedure and what the clinician is doing rather than what a patient might feel.

Pharmacologic pain management during procedures includes the use of nonsteroidal anti-inflammatory drugs (NSAIDs), local anesthetic, and a variety of medications including anxiolytics, analgesics, or anesthesia. Premedication with NSAIDs should be offered to all patients who do not have a contraindication, as it is shown to decrease pain during the procedure.[42] Local anesthesia, often administered as a paracervical block (PCB), improves perceived pain scores during uterine aspiration.[43] Vaginal lidocaine gel can also be considered as an alternative to PCB in first-trimester uterine aspiration.[44]

Minimal or moderate sedation are also options in outpatient first trimester uterine aspiration. It is important to ensure appropriate monitoring parameters and staff are available for each sedation option.

Antibiotics

Prophylactic antibiotic use in procedural abortion has demonstrated decreased rates of postsuction infection.[45] Antibiotics (metronidazole, azithromycin, or doxycycline) should be given within 12 hours before the procedure.[46]

Equipment and Supplies

Procedural abortion is an in-office procedure, often done with no sedation or minimal to moderate sedation, that takes approximately 5 to 15 minutes. The procedure consists of a PCB (as mentioned earlier), cervical dilation with rigid cervical dilators, and suction aspiration with a manual vacuum aspirator or electric vacuum aspirator.

For review of procedural steps in detail refer to the TEACH workbook.[47]

MANAGEMENT OF COMMON PROCEDURAL ABORTION COMPLICATIONS

First-trimester PAB is very safe with a major complication rate of <1%. The most common complication is hemorrhage with a risk of significant bleeding of <5%.[48] Treatment of hemorrhage commonly includes verification of completion by ultrasound and/or examining products of conception for completeness, repeat aspiration to remove any retained products of conception or clot, and use of uterotonics such as misoprostol and methergine.

Postabortion endometritis occurs in fewer than 2% of patients. It should be suspected with postprocedure pelvic pain, fever, unusual bleeding, and/or foul-smelling vaginal discharge. Ultrasound should be done to evaluate for retained POC or clot which should be evacuated if present. Systemic antibiotics should be administered/prescribed, aligning with the Center for Disease Control's recommendation for pelvic inflammatory disease.[49]

Uterine perforation is a rare complication of first trimester PAB (0.3%).[49] Patients should be monitored postprocedurally for signs of hemodynamic instability or severe abdominal pain/peritoneal signs indicating internal bleeding. Patients with these signs/symptoms should be transferred to a setting where laparoscopy/laparotomy can be performed. There is no good-quality evidence on additional antibiotic prophylaxis in these cases.

Asherman's Syndrome, characterized by intrauterine adhesions and scarring, is exceedingly rare after PAB, especially when done with suction aspiration. It is more common after sharp curettage of uterus. Genetic and environmental factors play a role as well.[49]

Follow-Up

Routine follow-up after procedural abortion is not indicated. Patients should have access to follow-up if needed and need should be based on patient symptoms, preference, and concerns.

CONTRACEPTION AFTER ABORTION PROVISION

Offering contraception at the time of abortion is best practice to ensure access. However, many patients will not want to discuss contraception on the day of their abortion. The authors recommend asking permission to discuss contraception with patients.

For patients who elect MAB, the contraceptive implant can be administered on the day of mifepristone administration with negligible reduction in efficacy. Some studies have shown a slight reduction in MAB efficacy with medroxyprogesterone contraceptive injection on the same day as mifepristone.[50] However, given how effective MAB is, it is still reasonable to offer same day contraceptive injection to reduce barriers to care.

Combined hormonal contraceptive methods or progesterone-only pills can be started as soon as patients take misoprostol. Confirmation that the abortion is complete is required prior to IUD placement.

Patients who have procedures can receive the contraceptive injection on the same day or have IUDs or contraceptive implants placed immediately afterward. Other contraceptives can be started as soon as possible. No back up method is required if contraceptives are started within 5 - 7 days depending on the method.

DISCUSSION

Medication and procedural abortion are safe, effective, and within the scope of a primary care clinician. Major medical organizations such as The American Academy of Family Physicians and the American Medical Association support the provision of abortion services.[51,52]

Procedural abortion is an in-office procedure that builds the existing skill sets of many primary care clinicians, such as the placement of IUDs and endometrial biopsies.

Initiation and continuation of abortion in primary care require support and buy-in from leadership and the entire care team. Patients will interact with all staff and should feel respected and well-cared for throughout their visit. Clinicians should know their state-level restrictions and discuss them with their respective legal counsel. Even in states where abortion is illegal, patients need support pre or post abortion and there should be a plan in place to care for them.

CLINICS CARE POINTS

- Clinicians and patients can use shared decision-making to determine follow-up plans after medication abortion and procedural abortions generally do not require follow-up.
- For patients with pregnancy of unknown location, without signs or symptoms highly suspicious for ectopic pregnancy, abortion can be initiated while simultaneously determining the location of the pregnancy.
- Self-managed abortion and telehealth abortion are both safe and effective.
- Trauma-informed care should be practiced in all abortion and pregnancy-related care.
- A no-touch protocol has been shown to be safe for most patients, which allows for clinicians without access to ultrasound to provide medication and procedural abortion.
- Clinicians in all states should know how to triage concerns following an abortion, regardless of if they provide the service in their clinic currently.

DISCLOSURES

Dr M. Simmons receives honoraria from Organon for Nexplanon training. The findings and conclusions in this article are those of the authors and do not necessarily represent the views of Planned Parenthood Federation of America, Inc. All other authors report no disclosures.

REFERENCES

1. Jones R. An estimate of lifetime incidence of abortion in the United States using the 2021–2022 abortion patient survey. Contraception 2024;135:110445. Available at: https://www.contraceptionjournal.org/article/S0010-7824(24)00108-2/fulltext. Accessed August 29, 2024.
2. Korsmit K, Nguyen AT, Mandel MG, et al. Abortion surveillance — United States, 2021. MMWR Surveillance Summary Reports 2023;72:9.

3. Jones R, Philbin J, Kirstein M, et al. Long-term decline in US abortions reverses, showing rising need for abortion as supreme court is poised to overturn roe v. Wade, 2022, Guttmacher Institute, Washington (DC). Available at: https://www.guttmacher.org/article/2022/06/long-term-decline-us-abortions-reverses-showing-rising-need-abortion-supreme-court (Accessed 19 June 2024).

4. Yanow S. It is time to integrate abortion into primary care. Am J Publ Health 2013; 103(1):14–6.

5. Carvajal D, Cashman C, Lague I. "Primary care providers can help safeguard abortion." scientific American. Available at: https://www.scientificamerican.com/article/primary-care-providers-can-help-safeguard-abortion/. Accessed August 25, 2024.

6. Diamant J, Mohamed B, Leppert R. What the data says about abortion in the U.S. Pew Research Center; 2024. Available at: https://www.pewresearch.org/short-reads/2024/03/25/what-the-data-says-about-abortion-in-the-us/. Accessed June 19, 2024.

7. Sagar K, Rego E, Malhotra R, et al. Abortion providers in the United States: expanding beyond obstetrics and gynecology. AJOG Glob Rep 2023;3(2):100186.

8. "Reproductive Justice." sister song. Available at: https://www.sistersong.net/reproductive-justice. Accessed July 14, 2024.

9. Crear-Perry J, Correa-de-Araujo R, Lewis Johnson T, et al. Social and structural determinants of health inequities in maternal health. J Wom Health 2021;30(2): 230–5.

10. Vilda D, Wallace ME, Daniel C, et al. State abortion policies and maternal death in the United States, 2015–2018. Am J Publ Health 2021;111(9):1696–704.

11. Eliason EL. Adoption of medicaid expansion is associated with lower maternal mortality. Wom Health Issues 2020;30(3):147–52.

12. Upadhyay UD, Raymond EG, Koenig LR, et al. Outcomes and safety of history-based screening for medication abortion: a retrospective multicenter cohort study. JAMA Intern Med 2022;182(5):482–91. Available at: https://bit.ly/3a3d3yi.

13. Erlank CP, Lord J, Church K. Acceptability of No-test medical abortion provided via telemedicine during covid-19: analysis of patient-reported outcomes. BMJ Sex Reprod Health 2021;47(4):261–8.

14. Clinical policy guidelines for abortion care. National Abortion Federation 2024. Available at: https://prochoice.org/wp-content/uploads/2024-CPGs-FINAL-1.pdf. Accessed July 21, 2024.

15. Goldberg AB, Fulcher IR, Fortin J, et al. Mifepristone and misoprostol for undesired pregnancy of unknown location. Obstet Gynecol 2022;139(5):771–80.

16. Kerns JL, Brown K, Nippita S, et al. Society of family planning clinical recommendation: management of hemorrhage at the time of abortion. Contraception 2024; 129:110292.

17. Horvath S, Goyal V, Traxler S, et al. Society of family planning committee consensus on Rh testing in early pregnancy. Contraception 2022;114:1–5.

18. Karanth L, Jaafar SH, Kanagasabai S, et al. Anti-D administration after spontaneous miscarriage for preventing rhesus alloimmunisation. Cochrane Database Syst Rev 2013;3. https://doi.org/10.1002/14651858.CD009617.pub2.

19. Wiebe ER, Campbell M, Aiken AR, et al. Can we safely stop testing for Rh status and immunizing Rh-negative women having early abortions? A comparison of Rh alloimmunization in Canada and The Netherlands. Contraception 2019;X:1. https://doi.org/10.1016/j.conx.2018.100001.

20. Horvath S, Tsao P, Huang ZY, et al. The concentration of fetal red blood cells in first-trimester pregnant women undergoing uterine aspiration is below the calculated threshold for Rh sensitization. Contraception 2020;102(1):1–6.
21. "Medication abortion accounted for 63% of all US abortions in 2023—an increase from 53% in 2020" guttmacher institute. 2024. Available at: https://www.guttmacher.org/2024/03/medication-abortion-accounted-63-all-us-abortions-2023-increase-53-2020. Accessed July 14, 2024.
22. Kapp N, Eckersberger E, Lavelanet A, et al. Medication abortion in the late first trimester: a systematic review. Contraception 2019;99(2):77–86. Available at: https://bit.ly/2UMeu9e.
23. Creinin MD, Schreiber CA, Bednarek P, et al. Medical Abortion at the Same Time (MAST) Study Trial Group. Mifepristone and misoprostol administered simultaneously versus 24 hours apart for abortion: a randomized controlled trial. Obstet Gynecol 2007;109(4):885–94.
24. Crenin MD, Schreiber CA, Bednarek P, et al. Mifepristone and misoprostol administered simultaneously versus 24 hours apart for abortion: a randomized controlled trial. Obstet Gynecol 2007;109(4):885–94.
25. Hsia JK, Lohr PA, Taylor J, Creinin MD. Medical abortion with mifepristone and vaginal misoprostol between 64 and 70 days' gestation. Contraception 2019;100(3):178–81.
26. Raymond EG, Weaver MA, Shochet T. Effectiveness and safety of misoprostol-only for first-trimester medication abortion: an updated systematic review and meta-analysis. Contraception 2023;127:110132.
27. Moseson H, Jayaweera R, Egwuatu I, et al. Effectiveness of self-managed medication abortion with accompaniment support in Argentina and Nigeria (SAFE): a prospective, observational cohort study and non-inferiority analysis with historical controls. Lancet Global Health 2022;10(1):e105–13.
28. Molitch ME. Glucocorticoid receptor blockers. Pituitary 2022;25(5):733–6.
29. Cable EE, Pepe JA, Donohue SE, et al. Effects of mifepristone (RU-486) on heme metabolism and cytochromes P-450 in cultured chick embryo liver cells, possible implications for acute porphyria. Eur J Biochem 1994;225(2):651–7.
30. "Approved risk evaluation and mitigation strategies (REMS)" FDA. Available at: https://www.accessdata.fda.gov/scripts/cder/rems/index.cfm?event=RemsDetails.page&REMS=390. Accessed July 23, 2024.
31. "Abortion" reproductive health access Project. Available at: https://www.reproductiveaccess.org/abortion/. Accessed July 14, 2024.
32. Aiken ARA, Starling JE, Rebecca G. Factors associated with use of an online telemedicine service to access self-managed medical abortion in the US. JAMA Netw Open 2021;4:5.
33. Aiken ARA, Romanova EP, Morber JR, et al. Safety and effectiveness of self-managed medication abortion provided using online telemedicine in the United States: a population based study. Lancet Regional Health. Americas 2022;10:100200.
34. Raymond EG, Anger HA, Chong E, et al. False positive urine pregnancy test results after successful medication abortion. Contraception 2021;103(6):400–3.
35. Sagar K, Rego E, Malhotra R, et al. Abortion providers in the United States: expanding beyond obstetrics and gynecology. AJOG Glob Rep 2023;3(2):100186.
36. Raymond EG, Grimes DA. The comparative safety of legal induced abortion and childbirth in the United States. Obstet Gynecol 2012;119(2 Pt 1):215–9.
37. Sabin JA. How we fail Black patients in pain. AAMC Insights 2020. Available at: https://bit.ly/3tTlgeO. Accessed September 1, 2024.

38. Meghani SH, Byun E, Gallagher RM. Time to take stock: a meta-analysis and systematic review of analgesic treatment disparities for pain in the United States. Pain Med 2012;13(2):150–74.
39. Carwile JL, Feldman S, Johnson NR. Use of a simple visual distraction to reduce pain and anxiety in patients undergoing colposcopy. J Low Genit Tract Dis 2014; 18(4):317–21.
40. Altshuler AL, Ojanen-Goldsmith A, Blumenthal PD, et al. "Going through it together": being accompanied by loved ones during birth and abortion. Soc Sci Med 2021;284.
41. Wu J, Chaplin W, Amico J, et al. Music for surgical abortion care study: a randomized controlled pilot study. Contraception 2012;85(5):496–502.
42. Jackson E, et al. Clinical updates in reproductive health. Ipas; 2023. Available at: https://bit.ly/3KiUR0M. Accessed September 1, 2024.
43. Regina-Maria R, Edelman AB, Nichols MD, et al. Refining paracervical block techniques for pain control in first trimester surgical abortion: a randomized controlled noninferiority trial. Contraception 2016;94(5):461–6.
44. Liu SM, Shaw KA. Pain management in outpatient surgical abortion. Curr Opin Obstet Gynecol 2021;33(6):440–4.
45. Low N, Mueller M, Van Vliet HAAM, et al. Perioperative antibiotics to prevent infection after first-trimester abortion. Cochrane Database Syst Rev 2012; 2012(3). https://doi.org/10.1002/14651858.CD005217.pub2.
46. Achilles SL, Reeves MF, Society of Family Planning. Society of family planning "prevention of infection after induced abortion: release date october 2010: SFP guideline 20102". Contraception 2011;83(4):295–309.
47. Fleming M, Shih G, Goodman S, the TEACH Collaborative Working Group*. TEACH abortion training curriculum. 7th edition. San Francisco (CA): UCSF Bixby Center for Global Reproductive Health; 2022. Bixby Doc: 2020-001(07/22.
48. McLaren H, Hennessey C. First-trimester procedural abortion. Clin Obstet Gynecol 2023;66(4):676–84.
49. Dreisler Eva, Kjer J. Asherman's Syndrome: current perspectives on diagnosis and management. Int J Womens Health 2019;11:191–8.
50. Raymond EG, Weaver MA, Louie KS, et al. Effects of depot medroxyprogesterone acetate injection timing on medical abortion efficacy and repeat pregnancy: a Randomized controlled trial. Obstet Gynecol 2016;128(4):739–45.
51. "Reproductive and maternity health services. "AAFP. Available at: https://www.aafp.org/about/policies/all/reproductive-maternity-health-services.html. Accessed July 14, 2024.
52. "Advocacy in action: protecting reproductive health." American Medical Association. Available at: https://www.ama-assn.org/delivering-care/public-health/advocacy-action-protecting-reproductive-health. Accessed July 14, 2024.

Integrative Medicine in Women

Check for updates

Anne Kennard, DO[a],*, Erin Gillespie, MD[b],
Reagan McKendree, MD[c]

KEYWORDS

- Integrative medicine • Lifestyle medicine • Alternative and complementary medicine
- Nutrition • Endometriosis • Polycystic ovary syndrome

KEY POINTS

- Integrative therapies are evidence-based and offered alongside conventional medication and surgery for common gynecologic conditions.
- For dysmenorrhea, mild exercise, mind–body therapies, calcium, magnesium, and ginger are recommended.
- For polycystic ovary syndrome, nutrition, sleep, stress management, exercise, and supplements including myoinositol, vitamin D, n-acetyl-cysteine, and chromium help restore menses and improve metabolic profile.
- For premenstrual syndrome, vitex, magnesium, and calcium, along with mind–body movement, nutrition, and stress management are evidence-based modalities.
- Several evidence-based and emerging integrative therapies for endometriosis, such as nutrition, sleep, stress management, acupuncture, low-dose naltrexone, melatonin, curcumin, and vitamin D, can alleviate symptoms.

INTRODUCTION

Integrative medicine (IM) is a whole-person, healing-oriented approach to health care. It integrates complementary and alternative therapies with conventional Western medicine utilizing nutrition, exercise, mind–body therapies, spiritual healing, manual medicine, herbs, supplements, and other systems of medicine (traditional Chinese medicine and Ayurveda) with pharmacotherapy and surgery. Several common women's health conditions are amenable to an integrative approach, including

[a] Integrative and Lifestyle Medicine, Department of Obstetrics and Gynecology, Marian Regional Medical Center, Santa Maria, CA 93454, USA; [b] Integrative Medicine, Internal Medicine, Obesity Medicine, Leap Medical Writing and Editing LLC, Tijeras, NM 87059, USA; [c] Department of Family Medicine, Marian Regional Medical Center, 1400 E Church Street, Santa Maria, CA 93454, USA
* Corresponding author. Department of Obstetrics and Gynecology, Marian Regional Medical Center, 1400 E Church Street, Santa Maria, CA 93454.
E-mail address: anne.kennard@commonspirit.org

Prim Care Clin Office Pract 52 (2025) 291–306
https://doi.org/10.1016/j.pop.2025.01.003 **primarycare.theclinics.com**
0095-4543/25/© 2025 Elsevier Inc. All rights reserved, including those for text and data mining, AI training, and similar technologies.

Abbreviations	
CBT	cognitive behavioral therapy
CBT-I	cognitive behavioral therapy for insomnia
EPA	eicosapentanoic acid
IL	interleukin
IM	integrative medicine
LDN	low-dose naltrexone
MBSR	mindfulness-based stress reduction
NAC	N-acetyl cysteine
NSAIDs	nonsteroidal anti-inflammatories
PCOS	polycystic ovarian syndrome
PFPT	pelvic floor physical therapy
PMDD	premenstrual dysphoric disorder
PMS	premenstrual syndrome

dysmenorrhea, premenstrual syndrome (PMS), polycystic ovarian syndrome (PCOS), and endometriosis.

Dysmenorrhea: Integrative Approaches and Therapeutic Insights

Introduction

Dysmenorrhea occurs in 50% to 90% of women of reproductive age and is a significant cause of morbidity. The condition commonly presents with nausea, vomiting, headaches, muscle cramps, low back pain, fatigue, insomnia, and diarrhea.[1] Given the underlying mechanism of inflammation, dysmenorrhea is a prime target for integrative therapies such as nutrition, supplements, mind–body interventions, exercise, and acupuncture.

Nutrition

Patients with dysmenorrhea can benefit from nutritional interventions that address inflammatory mediators.[2] An anti-inflammatory or Mediterranean-style diet pattern rich in magnesium, calcium, and omega-3 fatty acids improves symptoms.[2] Omega-3 fatty acids obtained by supplementation or eating cold-water fish 2 to 3 times per week are effective at decreasing inflammation and pain, and supplementing with omega-3 fatty acids can reduce the amount of ibuprofen needed compared to placebo.[3] Sugars, fried foods, and other processed foods should be avoided as they increase inflammation and can worsen dysmenorrhea. Dietary changes must be implemented throughout the cycle rather than during menses to confer the most benefit.

Supplements

Supplementation with calcium, magnesium, and ginger addresses inflammation and the propagation of pain signals in the myometrium. Magnesium has been studied in several pain syndromes due to its antagonistic action at the N-methyl-D-aspartate receptor, with blockade of this receptor can prevent central sensitization and hypersensitivity.[4] Moreover, it is postulated that women with dysmenorrhea have lower levels of magnesium.[5] Magnesium is also helpful for treating bloating and menstrual migraine. Migraine prophylaxis is achieved with all forms of magnesium, with at 400 to 600 mg daily. It should be taken during the luteal phase, and further benefits may be noted with continuous use.[6] Magnesium is a simple and cost-effective supplement that improves pain scores and addresses the associated symptoms of dysmenorrhea.

Calcium reduces premenstrual pain by inhibiting uterine muscle contraction. Increases in dairy consumption are inversely associated with dysmenorrhea, illustrating the utility of nutritional interventions or supplementation. Effective doses range between 1000 and 1200 mg daily. Calcium should be taken continuously throughout the cycle.

Adding vitamin D to calcium supplementation further reduces symptoms of dysmenorrhea due to its inhibition of prostaglandin synthesis.[7] When calcium and magnesium are combined, a calcium-to-magnesium ratio 2:1 is preferred (1200 mg calcium to 600 mg magnesium).

Ginger, *Zingiber officinale*, is effective at treating dysmenorrhea due to its modulating effect on prostaglandin synthesis via arachidonic acid inhibition. Ginger's anti-inflammatory properties reduce pain and the need for medications.[8] At 1 to 2 g daily, ginger is more effective than placebo and equivalent to nonsteroidal anti-inflammatories (NSAIDs).[9] This herb is a helpful adjunct in the treatment of dysmenorrhea owing to its anti-inflammatory action and inhibition of multiple hormonal symptoms. **Table 1** lists the supplements for dysmenorrhea, adverse effects, and recommended dosages.

Mind–body
Mind–body interventions such as mindfulness, yoga, Tai Chi, Qigong, and breath regulation can alter dysmenorrhea's underlying mechanisms and associated inflammation.[11] These practices decrease perception of pain and help manage stress.[11]

Exercise
While yoga exerts positive effects via the mind–body connection, aerobic exercise helps patients manage pain and improves well-being through other mechanisms. Exercising at varying intensities at least 3 times weekly for 45 to 60 minutes decreased pain. Notably, moderate-intensity to high-intensity exercise modulates pain via anti-inflammatory cytokines and reduced the release of prostaglandins. Low-intensity exercise such as yoga or walking decreases the secretion of cortisol, a hormone that can increase the production of prostaglandins.[12] However, patients benefit from exercise regardless of the intensity or chosen activity.

Acupuncture
Acupuncture is known to improve dysmenorrhea. In 13 randomized controlled clinical trials, acupuncture and moxibustion relieved pain and had fewer adverse events than controls.[13] However, timing the treatments before menses resulted in more significant reductions in pain scores than at the onset of menses.[14] Given its efficacy and safety profile, acupuncture should be considered in for dysmenorrhea.

Table 1
Supplements for dysmenorrhea[10]

Supplement	Indications	Potential Adverse Effects	Recommended Dose
Calcium	Cramps	Caution in renal disease	1000–1200 mg per day
Magnesium	Cramps, bloating, migraine, and constipation	Diarrhea, nausea, hypotension, confusion, and caution in renal disease	400–600 mg per day
Ginger	Nausea and headaches	Diarrhea, reflux, stomach pain, and increased bleeding risk	1–2 g per day

Clinics care points

- A balanced diet rich in fruits, vegetables, whole grains, and fish, such as the anti-inflammatory or Mediterranean diet, can reduce symptoms.
- Omega-3 fatty acid supplementation or increased consumption of cold-water fish (2–3 times per week) offers anti-inflammatory benefits.
- Magnesium (400–600 mg daily) and calcium (1000–1200 mg daily) supplementation addresses deficiencies and alleviates pain, especially during the luteal phase. Consider adding vitamin D.
- Ginger (1–2 g per day) has anti-inflammatory properties and effectiveness comparable to NSAIDs.
- Mind–body interventions can help manage pain and reduce stress.
- Regular aerobic exercise (at least 3 times weekly for 45–60 minutes) reduces symptoms.
- Acupuncture before the onset of menses can result in significant pain relief.

Polycystic Ovarian Syndrome

Introduction

PCOS is a common disorder in women's health, affecting 6% to 10% of premenopausal women, with endocrinologic, metabolic, and reproductive implications.[13] The diagnosis is classically made if 2 of the 3 Rotterdam Criteria are met (oligo-ovulation or anovulation, hyperandrogenism, and ultrasound findings), but individual presentations can be heterogeneous,[14] with increasing recognition of other complications, including elevated cardiovascular disease risk, sleep apnea, infertility, and a high prevalence of mental or psychological health conditions. Addressing the driving factors of PCOS by reducing circulating insulin, improving insulin sensitization, balancing ovarian androgen production, and addressing stress and inflammation is key to improving patient outcomes, and the focus of integrative therapies.

Nutrition

A low-glycemic diet increases insulin sensitivity and improves metabolic parameters and reproductive health. The recommended dietary pattern is plant-forward, heavy in nonstarchy vegetables, low-glycemic fruits, and low in processed foods. It incorporates healthy fats or proteins to minimize blood sugar spikes and promote satiety. It also supports a healthy microbiome with adequate fiber (40 g/d) and prebiotics. Impaired glucose tolerance is common in PCOS, and continuous glucose monitors may play a future role in management by allowing patients to identify patterns in glucose swings and develop a sense of empowerment.[15]

Exercise and mind–body

Physical activity meeting the recommended guidelines of 150 to 200 minutes of moderate-intensity exercise per week can reduce markers of inflammation, promote weight maintenance, improve body composition and metabolic parameters, and regulate sleep, appetite, and mood.[16] Mind–body approaches address comorbid anxiety, depression, and stress and benefit mood, quality of life, and weight management. Studied modalities include cognitive behavioral therapy (CBT), mindfulness-based stress reduction (MBSR), yoga, and progressive muscle relaxation.[17,18]

Supplements

The literature supports the use of several supplements in PCOS. Chromium is a mineral that improves insulin sensitization and resistance in both PCOS and diabetes and is typically dosed at 200 μg daily.[19] Inositol at 3 to 4 g divided daily can improve

Table 2
Supplements for polycystic ovarian syndrome[19]

Supplement	Indications	Potential Adverse Effects	Recommended Doses
Vitamin D	PCOS, hyperlipidemia, and elevated testosterone	Nausea, vomiting, and constipation	3200–7000 IU daily
Inositol	PCOS	Nausea and diarrhea	3–4 g daily
NAC	PCOS and infertility	Nausea, vomiting, and diarrhea	1200–1800 mg daily, divided doses
Omega-3 fatty acids	PCOS and hyperlipidemia	Fish aftertaste, nausea, and diarrhea	2–3 g daily
Chromium	PCOS, obesity, elevated testosterone, and insulin resistance	Headaches, insomnia, mood changes, and caution in liver or kidney disease	200–400 µg daily

hyperandrogenism, insulin sensitization, fasting insulin, ovarian function, and spontaneous or augmented fertility outcomes.[20] Vitamin D deficiency is prevalent in patients with PCOS, especially those with comorbid obesity, and supplementation may improve metabolic disturbances and the success of ovulation induction.[21] N-acetyl cysteine (NAC) is an antioxidant used in multiple conditions to address oxidative stress, inflammation, and hepatic detoxification. In PCOS, it decreases the inflammatory burden, improves insulin sensitivity, and supports fertility by increasing ovulation, oocyte quality, and odds of successful live birth.[15,16,22] Doses studied for PCOS are typically around 600 mg 2 to 3 times daily. **Table 2** lists the supplements used for PCOS, adverse effects, and recommended dosages.

Acupuncture
The benefits of acupuncture in PCOS include improved ovulatory function and fertility, hormonal regulation with decreased hyperandrogenism and hypothalamus-pituitary-ovarian axis effects, healthy insulin and lipid metabolism, and improved stress and psychological comorbidities.[23,24]

Clinics care points

- A low glycemic-index diet rich in nonstarchy vegetables, low-glycemic fruits, healthy fats, and proteins can improve PCOS. Highlight the importance of fiber and prebiotics in supporting a healthy microbiome.

- Physical activity consistent with recommended guidelines (150–200 minutes of moderate-intensity weekly exercise) improves metabolic parameters and overall well-being.

- Refer for CBT or MBSR as needed.

- Inositol (3–4 g daily) can improve hyperandrogenism and insulin sensitivity.

- Vitamin D (3200–7000 IU daily) addresses deficiency and improves metabolic health.

- N-acetylcysteine (600–1800 mg daily, divided doses) has antioxidant properties and supports ovulation and fertility.

- Chromium (200–400 µg daily) enhances insulin sensitivity.

- Omega-3 fatty acids (2–3 g daily) have potential cardiovascular benefits.

Premenstrual Syndrome: Integrative Strategies for Management

Introduction

PMS consists of a constellation of symptoms that can vary in intensity and severity during the late luteal phase of the menstrual cycle. The syndrome affects up to 40% of menstruating women, and 90% of women experience premenstrual symptoms. Premenstrual dysphoric disorder (PMDD) involves symptoms that are greater in severity, and 8% of women are diagnosed with this condition. Addressing PMS not only improves well-being and quality of life but can also be life-saving because some women with PMS and PMDD are at a greater risk of suicide.[25] The etiology of PMS is unknown, and treatment of the disorder often involves hormonal manipulation or antidepressants.[26] Due to the significant burden and the complexity of symptoms affecting multiple organ systems, PMS is a prime target for integrative treatment strategies.

Nutrition

A Western dietary pattern is associated with a higher frequency of PMS symptoms, while a healthy and traditional plant-forward diet pattern has an inverse correlation with the syndrome. Intermittent fasting can decrease cortisol during the luteal phase and improve symptoms.[27] Sugars, simple fats, fried foods, coffee, and alcohol positively correlate with symptoms. Although women typically crave carbohydrates during the luteal phase due to the effect on serotonin levels, a diet rich in fruits, vegetables, and fiber can reduce PMS symptoms.[26] A whole-food, plant-forward dietary pattern addresses underlying inflammation and abnormal oxidative activity.[28] Nutritional considerations are essential for improving the symptoms of PMS as part of an integrative approach.

Supplements

Although several supplements are marketed for the treatment of PMS symptoms, few high-quality studies confirm their efficacy. Calcium has good-quality evidence for preventing the symptoms of PMS, such as bloating, anxiety, and cramping.[29] Calcium levels are lower in those with symptoms, and supplementation can decrease the syndrome's incidence. A suggested mechanism for the low calcium levels is related to estrogen's antagonistic effect on serum calcium levels and receptors. Fluctuating levels of estrogen can also affect the binding of serotonin at its receptor, resulting in mood symptoms typical of PMS.[30] A dose of 1200 mg daily from combined food and supplement sources appears most effective. Calcium citrate is best absorbed, compared with other forms.

Patients with PMS and PMDD often have lower serum magnesium levels. Magnesium supplementation can correct these deficiencies and has helped control symptoms of anxiety, irritability, bloating, mastalgia, and cramping at a dose of 300 to 600 mg per day; combining magnesium and vitamin B6 at 50 mg daily is more effective than magnesium alone.[31] However, studies on magnesium have been conflicting, so more robust evidence is needed.

Chaste tree berry, or *Vitex agnus-castus*, appears to be a safe and effective supplement for symptoms of PMS and PMDD.[32] This native Mediterranean plant has been used to treat several gynecologic disorders for centuries, including irregular menstruation and PMS. *V agnus-castus* operates as a dopamine agonist at the hypothalamic-pituitary axis. This results in more robust gonadotropin-releasing hormone signaling, increasing luteinizing hormone secretion and progesterone. Progesterone's effects may prolong the luteal phase in some patients, particularly those with an otherwise unexplained short luteal phase. Due to the dopamine agonist effects, it may interact with antipsychotics. It is particularly effective for mastalgia but can also improve irritability, anxiety, and bloating.[33] A typical dose is 500 mg of crude herb or 50 mg extract daily, and results are typically seen after 3 months of continuous use.[34]

Saint John's wort, *Hypericum perforatum*, is a supplement that has a similar mechanism of action to the selective serotonin reuptake inhibitor class of medications, and it alleviates the depressive symptoms of PMS and PMDD.[35] Similar to antidepressants, it is more effective if taken continuously.[2] The combination of *H perforatum* and *V agnus-castus* is more effective than placebo at treating the symptoms of PMS.[36] This supplement has several drug interactions and can cause photosensitivity.[37] **Table 3** lists the supplements used for PMS, adverse effects, and recommended dosages.

Mind–body

Patients with PMS may have alterations in the stress response and improved symptomology with mind–body interventions. Progressive muscle relaxation is a safe and effective technique that enhances quality of life.[39] Yoga, combining movement and breathing techniques, is also beneficial for managing symptoms.[40]

Exercise

Aerobic exercise may alleviate the behavioral and physical symptoms of PMS by regulating the stress response and the release of dopamine, estrogen, endorphins, and endogenous opiate peptides.[41] The frequency of exercise is more beneficial than the intensity, necessitating an enjoyable activity one can engage in regularly.[2] Regular exercise modulates neurotransmitters including serotonin, explaining the positive effects on mood and anxiety.[41] Exercise throughout the cycle is beneficial, but PMS benefits are noted when performed during the luteal phase.

Acupuncture

Acupuncture can be a safe and effective means of managing symptoms of PMS. Acupuncture treatments are superior to sham acupuncture or treatment with medication. The ideal timing of treatment during the menstrual cycle is unclear because

Table 3
Supplements for premenstrual syndrome[38]

Supplement	Indications	Possible Adverse Effects	Recommended Dosages
Calcium	Bloating, anxiety, and cramping	Caution in kidney disease	1200 mg daily
Magnesium	Anxiety, irritability, bloating, mastalgia, and cramping	Caution in kidney disease, low blood pressure, nausea, vomiting, and diarrhea	400–600 mg daily
Chasteberry (*V agnus-castus*)	Mastalgia, irritability, anxiety, and bloating	Fatigue, insomnia, and stomach pain	500 mg crude herb daily or 80 mg extract
Chamomile (*Matricaria chamomilla*)	PMS	Caution with severe ragweed allergy	100 mg 3 times daily
Saint John's wort (*H perforatum*)	Mood symptoms	Diarrhea, dizziness, insomnia, and restlessness	600–900 mg in 2–3 divided doses

treatments are equally effective at varying intervals during the cycle.[42] Acupuncture is thought to regulate the autonomic nervous system by promoting the release of neuropeptides and shifting the body toward a parasympathetic state. Additionally, treatment involving a particular point used in treating PMS, an acupuncture point (SP6), can alter sensory transduction pathways in the brain on functional MRI.[43] Acupuncture has minimal adverse effects, can alter the response to pain locally and centrally, can improve mood symptoms, and is a recommended tool for managing PMS.

Clinics care points

- A whole food, plant-forward diet should be recommended. Avoid sugars, simple fats, fried foods, excess caffeine, and alcohol.
- Calcium 1200 mg daily can alleviate bloating, anxiety, and cramping. Calcium citrate is the best-absorbed form.
- Magnesium 300 to 600 mg daily can alleviate anxiety, irritability, bloating, and cramping. Combine magnesium with vitamin B6 (50 mg daily) to enhance its effectiveness.
- Chasteberry (*V agnus-castus*) can relieve mastalgia, irritability, and bloating. Use 500 mg of the crude herb or 50 to 80 mg of extract daily. Caution in combination with antipsychotic medications.
- Saint John's wort (*H perforatum*) 600 to 900 mg daily can relieve mood symptoms in divided doses. Monitor for potential drug interactions and photosensitivity.
- Muscle relaxation techniques, yoga, and acupuncture can improve PMS symptoms and overall quality of life.

Endometriosis: An Integrative Approach to Pain Management

Introduction

Endometriosis affects more than 11% of women worldwide and is a chronic inflammatory condition that results from endometrial tissue growing outside of the uterus. Patients with endometriosis have decreased quality of life due to pain, infertility, menstrual dysfunction, and mood effects.[44] About 70% of patients suffer from unresolved pain and reduced quality of life despite conventional therapies, making an integrative approach vital to well-being.[45]

Understanding endometriosis and pain

The implants from endometriosis can cause several painful symptoms, including dysmenorrhea, dyspareunia, dyschezia, dysuria, and chronic pelvic pain. Retrograde menstruation of stem cells within the abdominal cavity and bone marrow-derived stem cells outside of the abdominal cavity are thought to initiate the development of these lesions, which bleed cyclically, causing endometriosis-associated pain.[46] Production of growth factors and cytokines such as interleukin (IL)-1, IL-2, IL-6, IL-8, IL-4, vascular endothelial growth factor, and tumor necrosis factor that create inflammation and angiogenesis. Due to the presence of immune cells and angiogenesis factors that enhance the invasion of endometriotic cells, endometriosis is increasingly thought of as an autoimmune-type disorder acted upon by the hormonal milieu of reproductive-age female individuals.[47]

The pathogenesis of neuropathic pain in endometriosis is both local due to hyperinnervation of the implants and central because of central sensitization. Patients have an increased concentration of nerve growth factor in the peritoneum, which can lead to neurogenic inflammation, neuroangiogenesis, and neuropathic pain.[48] It increases the pain modulation at the level of the spinal cord, leading to somatic hyperalgesia and referred pain.[49] The brain responds with altered neurotransmission, including glutamate upregulation, which leads to increased nociception. The increased levels of pain can lead to pelvic floor dysfunction, dyspareunia, complex chronic pain syndrome, bladder dysfunction, irritable bowel syndrome, and vulvodynia.[48] Increased connectivity between areas within the anterior insula and medial prefrontal cortex and elevated levels of glutamate contributed to anxiety, depression, and pain intensity.[50] Given the complexity of pain syndromes, particularly centralized pain, endometriosis presents an opportunity for comprehensive integrative care.

Diet and supplements

The integrative management of endometriosis should target the underlying mechanism of inflammation with diet and supplements. Women who consume proinflammatory diets are more likely to develop endometriosis, and women who eat red meat and processed meat have a higher rate of the disease. Alcohol, sugar, salt, saturated fat, and dairy should be avoided.[51] Omega-6 fatty acids derived from proinflammatory diets are more likely to induce pain. Foods rich in antioxidant vitamins such as D, E, and B-group and foods rich in calcium and omega-3 protect against developing endometriosis and associated pain.[52] A whole-food, plant-forward diet high in phytonutrients can help control symptoms and improve quality of life.

Omega-3 fatty acids, magnesium, and curcumin can decrease pain and improve the inflammation of endometriosis. Omega-3 fatty acids can be consumed in 2 to 3 servings of salmon or other high-quality cold-water fish per week or in supplement form with 2 g of docahexanoic acid (DHA)/eicosapentanoic acid (EPA) daily, with at least 1500 mg EPA form.[2] Supplementation with omega-3 fatty acids can decrease the medications needed to control pain, likely due to reducing inflammatory cytokines.[3] Magnesium is a more effective than a placebo for pain relief.[53] Curcumin, a supplement known for its potent anti-inflammatory properties, can help alleviate endometriosis symptoms. A supplement containing quercetin, curcumin, parthenium, nicotinamide, 5-methyltetrahydrofolate, and omega-3 decreased serum levels of prostaglandin E2 (PGE2) and cancer antigen 125 (CA-125) and reduced symptoms.[54]

An inverse correlation exists between serum vitamin D levels and the risk of endometriosis. Vitamin D has anti-inflammatory and immunomodulatory effects that may play a role in attenuating the dysregulation and inflammation of endometriosis.[55] Vitamin D is involved in cellular signaling pathways, gene expression, and cytokines common to endometriosis.[56] Maintaining adequate levels may reduce the risk and severity of endometriosis.

NAC has shown benefit in reducing pain, endometrioma size, and CA-125 levels in patients with endometriosis due to anti-inflammatory and antioxidant properties.[57] NAC may also be a suitable alternative for women trying to achieve pregnancy and is relatively well tolerated. This supplement has antiproliferative effects on cells, decreasing implant invasiveness, and is promising for treating ovarian endometriosis.[58]

Melatonin can improve pain scores in patients with endometriosis.[2] It has analgesic, antioxidant, and anti-inflammatory effects. At a dose of 10 mg, it can also increase brain-derived neurotrophic factor levels, decrease the need for analgesics, and improve sleep.[59] It can also regulate angiogenesis and immune response locally in the uterus, targeting endometriosis lesions. It may help suppress the growth of endometriotic lesions, relieve pelvic pain, and improve sleep quality.[60] **Table 4** lists the supplements used for endometriosis, adverse effects, and recommended dosages.

Mind–body

Mind–body medicine can often help those who have endometriosis to manage pain more effectively and modulate pain perception. Meditative techniques benefit mood

Table 4
Dietary supplements for treatment of endometriosis[61]

Supplement	Indications for Endometriosis	Potential Adverse Effects	Recommended Dose
Omega-3 fatty acids	Anti-inflammatory effects may help reduce pain and inflammation associated with endometriosis	Mild gastrointestinal discomfort	2–3 g daily, at least 1500 mg of which is EPA form
Magnesium	May help reduce pain and inflammation, potential to improve muscle relaxation	Diarrhea, nausea; caution in renal disease	300–800 mg daily, with most patients benefitting from 600 mg daily
Curcumin	Anti-inflammatory and antioxidant properties, may help reduce pain and inflammation	Gastrointestinal discomfort, potential interaction with anticoagulants	1 g daily
NAC	Antioxidant properties may help reduce oxidative stress and inflammation	Nausea and dyspepsia	1500 mg daily, taken in divided doses 3 times a day
Vitamin D	May help modulate immune response and reduce inflammation	Rare: hypercalcemia, kidney stones (in very high doses)	To serum level of at least 30–50 ng/mL; 50,000 IU weekly to repletion; then 2000 IU daily
Melatonin	Analgesic and anti-inflammatory effects, improves sleep	Vivid dreams, headaches, drowsiness, and dizziness	5–10 mg nightly, as tolerated

and anxiety disorders, which are more common in those with endometriosis.[62] Virtual MBSR programs improve emotional well-being and pain.[63] While an MBSR program requires significant time and effort, brief mindfulness-based intervention programs improve pain scores and mental well-being.[64] Other mind–body therapies, such as yoga, Qi Gong, Tai Chi, somatic bodywork, and emotional freedom technique tapping could be helpful.

Exercise

Exercise can offer several benefits for patients with endometriosis, such as improving pain, reducing inflammation, improving mental health, and increasing physical fitness.[65] International guidelines recommend that women exercise to improve their quality of life and encourage self-management of symptoms.[66] Regular physical activity can decrease systemic levels of inflammatory cytokines, reduce estrogen levels, and possibly reduce the prevalence of endometriosis.[67]

Pelvic floor physical therapy

Pelvic floor physical therapy (PFPT) helps manage the pain and discomfort of endometriosis. Pelvic floor muscle tension is more significant in women with endometriosis than in controls without the condition, creating spasms and dyspareunia.[68] The lesions and adhesions themselves can cause contractions of the muscles, which can be relieved by techniques used in PFPT. Interventions include releasing myofascial trigger points, kinesiotherapy to improve muscle function, electrotherapy modalities, pulsed high-intensity laser therapy, and relaxation techniques.[69] PFPT should be included in every management plan for patients with endometriosis because it can decrease the use of medications and the need for surgery.[70]

Integrative therapies

Low-dose naltrexone (LDN) is a mu-opioid receptor antagonist approved for opioid and alcohol dependence. Lower doses of naltrexone than are typically used for treating drug dependence can inhibit the proliferation of T and B cells and block toll-like receptor 4. This results in pain relief and dampens the inflammatory cascade.[71] The low dose stimulates endorphin release, which decreases pain scores. Adverse effects include sleep disturbances, daydreaming, nausea, mucosal dryness, and headache.[72] It may also act on activated microglial cells, making it one of the first glial cell modulators for chronic pain.[73] Most available studies use a 4.5 mg daily dose of LDN alongside norethindrone, which shows improvement over norethindrone alone.

Cannabinoids are effective for pain, mood, and gastrointestinal symptoms of endometriosis. Cannabinoids can also target serotonin receptors (5HT1A), exerting anxiolytic and antidepressant activities.[74] They exhibit antiangiogenic, immunomodulating, and antiproliferative effects specific to the underlying pathogenesis of endometriosis. Adverse effects include anxiety, nausea, dizziness, drowsiness/fatigue, cognitive effects, and dry mouth.[74] Oral use of high terpene, full-spectrum products with at least 50 mg cannabidiol would be beneficial, with no to low tetrahydrocannabinol (THC) use (0 or 0.5–1 mg), depending on state legality and individual patient factors.

Acupuncture

Acupuncture can be a safe and effective adjunct treatment of endometriosis. However, the reduction in dysmenorrhea can return to baseline with the cessation of treatment.[75] Evidence for benefit on overall pelvic pain, menstrual pain, and nonspecific pelvic pain has been shown, with minimal adverse effects. Given the low risk and possible benefit, acupuncture should be considered as part of a comprehensive pain management plan.[76]

Optimizing sleep for pain management

Patients with endometriosis have a high prevalence of insomnia due to pain, mood disorders, hormone fluctuations, and inflammation. Treating insomnia can alter the disease progression, decrease pain, and improve the quality of life of patients.[77] The American College of Physicians recommends cognitive behavioral therapy for insomnia (CBT-I) as the first step in treating chronic insomnia, with sleep hygiene habits. If necessary, medications should only be given briefly, usually a few weeks, and integrative therapies may help.[78]

Melatonin, which may be beneficial for endometriosis inflammation and pain due to its potent antioxidant effects, may also assist the patient with sleep. Magnesium, while mixed evidence, may also improve sleep alongside the available data for decreasing endometriosis pain.

CLINICS CARE POINTS

- Magnesium supplementation (300–600 mg daily) aids muscle relaxation and pain reduction.
- Curcumin (1 g daily) has anti-inflammatory effects in endometriosis.
- PFPT reduces muscle spasms and dyspareunia.
- Ensure adequate vitamin D levels (30–50 ng/mL). Consider supplementation with 50,000 IU weekly for repletion, followed by 2000 daily.
- Recommend NAC (1500 mg daily) for its antioxidant and anti-inflammatory properties.
- Use melatonin (5–10 mg nightly) for pain management, improved sleep, and its potential anti-inflammatory effects in endometriosis lesions.
- Consider LDN (4.5 mg daily) as an adjunct therapy to reduce pain.
- Explore cannabinoids to manage pain, anxiety, and gastrointestinal symptoms. Use full-spectrum products with high terpene content and low THC (0.5–1 mg).
- Manage sleep disturbances with CBT-I. Encourage sleep hygiene practices.

DISCLOSURE

None of the authors report any disclosures.

REFERENCES

1. McKenna KA, Fogleman CD. Dysmenorrhea. Am Fam Physician 2021;104(2): 164–70.
2. Romm AJ. Botanical medicine for women's health. Churchill Livingstone: Elsevier; 2018.
3. Rahbar N, Asgharzadeh N, Ghorbani R. Effect of omega-3 fatty acids on intensity of primary dysmenorrhea. Int J Gynaecol Obstet 2012;117(1):45–7.
4. Shin HJ, Na HS, Do SH. Magnesium and pain. Nutrients 2020;12(8):2184.
5. Parazzini F, Di Martino M, Pellegrino P. Magnesium in the gynecological practice: a literature review. Magnes Res 2017;30(1):1–7.
6. Low DT. An integrative approach to women's health. Integrative Medicine Education 2000;1–12.
7. Abdi F, Amjadi MA, Zaheri F, et al. Role of vitamin D and calcium in the relief of primary dysmenorrhea: a systematic review. Obstet Gynecol Sci 2021;64(1): 13–26.

8. Khayat S, Kheirkhah M, Behboodi Moghadam Z, et al. Effect of treatment with ginger on the severity of premenstrual syndrome symptoms. ISRN Obstet Gynecol 2014;2014:792708.

9. Chen CX, Barrett B, Kwekkeboom KL. Efficacy of oral ginger (zingiber officinale) for dysmenorrhea: a systematic review and meta-analysis. Evid-Based Complement Altern Med ECAM 2016;2016:6295737.

10. Pattanittum P, Kunyanone N, Brown J, et al. Dietary supplements for dysmenorrhoea. Cochrane Database Syst Rev 2016;2016(3):CD002124.

11. Kanchibhotla D, Subramanian S, Singh D. Management of dysmenorrhea through yoga: a narrative review. Front Pain Res 2023;4:1107669.

12. Armour M, Ee CC, Naidoo D, et al. Exercise for dysmenorrhoea. Cochrane Database Syst Rev 2019;2019(9):CD004142.

13. Williams T, Mortada R, Porter S. Diagnosis and treatment of polycystic ovary syndrome. Am Fam Physician 2016;94(2):106–13.

14. Rotterdam ESHRE/ASRM-Sponsored PCOS Consensus Workshop Group. Revised 2003 consensus on diagnostic criteria and long-term health risks related to polycystic ovary syndrome. Fertil Steril 2004;81(1):19–25.

15. Xenou M, Gourounti K. Dietary patterns and polycystic ovary syndrome: a systematic review. Mædica 2021;16(3):516–21.

16. Kite C, Lahart IM, Afzal I, et al. Exercise, or exercise and diet for the management of polycystic ovary syndrome: a systematic review and meta-analysis. Syst Rev 2019;8(1):51.

17. Abdollahi L, Mirghafourvand M, Babapour JK, et al. Effectiveness of cognitive-behavioral therapy (CBT) in improving the quality of life and psychological fatigue in women with polycystic ovarian syndrome: a randomized controlled clinical trial. J Psychosom Obstet Gynaecol 2019;40(4):283–93.

18. Stefanaki C, Bacopoulou F, Livadas S, et al. Impact of a mindfulness stress management program on stress, anxiety, depression and quality of life in women with polycystic ovary syndrome: a randomized controlled trial. Stress Amst Neth 2015;18(1):57–66.

19. Alesi S, Ee C, Moran LJ, et al. Nutritional supplements and complementary therapies in polycystic ovary syndrome. Adv Nutr 2021;13(4):1243–66.

20. Unfer V, Facchinetti F, Orrù B, et al. Myo-inositol effects in women with PCOS: a meta-analysis of randomized controlled trials. Endocr Connect 2017;6(8):647–58.

21. Rashidi B, Haghollahi F, Shariat M, et al. The effects of calcium-vitamin D and metformin on polycystic ovary syndrome: a pilot study. Taiwan J Obstet Gynecol 2009;48(2):142–7.

22. Kilic-Okman T, Kucuk M. N-acetyl-cysteine treatment for polycystic ovary syndrome. Int J Gynaecol Obstet 2004;85(3):296–7.

23. de Oliveira NM, Machado J, Lopes L, et al. A review on acupuncture efficiency in human polycystic ovary/ovarian syndrome. J Pharmacopuncture 2023;26(2):105–23.

24. Ye Y, Zhou CC, Hu HQ, et al. Underlying mechanisms of acupuncture therapy on polycystic ovary syndrome: evidences from animal and clinical studies. Front Endocrinol 2022;13:1035929.

25. Prasad D, Wollenhaupt-Aguiar B, Kidd KN, et al. Suicidal risk in women with premenstrual syndrome and premenstrual dysphoric disorder: a systematic review and meta-analysis. J Womens Health 2021;30(12):1693–707.

26. Siminiuc R, Țurcanu D. Impact of nutritional diet therapy on premenstrual syndrome. Front Nutr 2023;10:1079417.

27. Ohara K, Okita Y, Kouda K, et al. Cardiovascular response to short-term fasting in menstrual phases in young women: an observational study. BMC Wom Health 2015;15:67.
28. Modzelewski S, Oracz A, Żukow X, et al. Premenstrual syndrome: new insights into etiology and review of treatment methods. Front Psychiatry 2024;15:1363875.
29. Whelan AM, Jurgens TM, Naylor H. Herbs, vitamins and minerals in the treatment of premenstrual syndrome: a systematic review. Can J Clin Pharmacol 2009; 16(3):e407–29.
30. Beneficial role of calcium in premenstrual syndrome: a systematic review of current literature - PMC. Available at: https://www.ncbi.nlm.nih.gov/pmc/articles/PMC7716601/. Accessed July 7, 2024.
31. Fathizadeh N, Ebrahimi E, Valiani M, et al. Evaluating the effect of magnesium and magnesium plus vitamin B6 supplement on the severity of premenstrual syndrome. Iran J Nurs Midwifery Res 2010;15(Suppl1):401–5.
32. Cerqueira RO, Frey BN, Leclerc E, et al. Vitex agnus castus for premenstrual syndrome and premenstrual dysphoric disorder: a systematic review. Arch Womens Ment Health 2017;20(6):713–9.
33. Sureja VP, Kheni DB, Dubey VP, et al. Efficacy and tolerability evaluation of a nutraceutical composition containing Vitex agnus-castus extract (EVX40™), pyridoxine, and magnesium in premenstrual syndrome: a real-world, interventional, comparative study. Cureus 2023;15(8):e42832.
34. Verkaik S, Kamperman AM, van Westrhenen R, et al. The treatment of premenstrual syndrome with preparations of Vitex agnus castus: a systematic review and meta-analysis. Am J Obstet Gynecol 2017;217(2):150–66.
35. Canning S, Waterman M, Orsi N, et al. The efficacy of Hypericum perforatum (St John's wort) for the treatment of premenstrual syndrome: a randomized, double-blind, placebo-controlled trial. CNS Drugs 2010;24(3):207–25.
36. van Die MD, Bone KM, Burger HG, et al. Effects of a combination of Hypericum perforatum and Vitex agnus-castus on PMS-like symptoms in late-perimenopausal women: findings from a subpopulation analysis. J Altern Complement Med 2009;15(9):1045–8.
37. Kapusta M, Dusek J. [Therapeutic and toxicologic aspects of biological effects of Saint John's wort (Hypericum perforatum L.)]. Ceska Slov Farm Cas Ceske Farm Spolecnosti Slov Farm Spolecnosti 2003;52(1):20–8.
38. Sultana A, Heyat MBB, Rahman K, et al. A systematic review and meta-analysis of premenstrual syndrome with special emphasis on herbal medicine and nutritional supplements. Pharmaceuticals 2022;15(11):1371.
39. Abic A, Dag-Canatan S, Er-Korucu A, et al. The effects of yoga and progressive muscle relaxation exercises on premenstrual syndrome: a randomized controlled trial. Women Health 2024;64(3):261–73.
40. Pal A, Nath B, Paul S, et al. Evaluation of the effectiveness of yoga in management of premenstrual syndrome: a systematic review and meta-analysis. J Psychosom Obstet Gynaecol 2022;43(4):517–25.
41. Vaghela N, Mishra D, Sheth M, et al. To compare the effects of aerobic exercise and yoga on Premenstrual syndrome. J Educ Health Promot 2019;8:199.
42. Zhang J, Cao L, Wang Y, et al. Acupuncture for premenstrual syndrome at different intervention time: a systemic review and meta-analysis. Evid-Based Complement Altern Med ECAM 2019;2019:6246285.
43. Pang Y, Liu H, Duan G, et al. Altered brain regional homogeneity following electro-acupuncture stimulation at sanyinjiao (SP6) in women with premenstrual syndrome. Front Hum Neurosci 2018;12:104.

44. Ellis K, Munro D, Clarke J. Endometriosis is undervalued: a call to action. Front Glob Womens Health 2022;3:902371.

45. Agarwal SK, Foster WG, Groessl EJ. Rethinking endometriosis care: applying the chronic care model via a multidisciplinary program for the care of women with endometriosis. Int J Womens Health 2019;11:405–10.

46. Horne AW, Missmer SA. Pathophysiology, diagnosis, and management of endometriosis. BMJ 2022;379:e070750.

47. Abramiuk M, Grywalska E, Małkowska P, et al. The role of the immune system in the development of endometriosis. Cells 2022;11(13):2028.

48. Gruber TM, Mechsner S. Pathogenesis of endometriosis: the origin of pain and subfertility. Cells 2021;10(6):1381.

49. Bajaj P, Bajaj P, Madsen H, et al. Endometriosis is associated with central sensitization: a psychophysical controlled study. J Pain 2003;4(7):372–80.

50. As-Sanie S, Kim J, Schmidt-Wilcke T, et al. Functional connectivity is associated with altered brain chemistry in women with endometriosis-associated chronic pelvic pain. J Pain 2016;17(1):1–13.

51. Hudson T. Menstrual cramps (dysmenorrhea): an alternative approach. Townsend Lett Exam Altern Med 2006;279:130–5.

52. Habib N, Buzzaccarini G, Centini G, et al. Impact of lifestyle and diet on endometriosis: a fresh look to a busy corner. Przeglad Menopauzalny Menopause Rev 2022;21(2):124–32.

53. Proctor ML, Murphy PA. Herbal and dietary therapies for primary and secondary dysmenorrhoea. Cochrane Database Syst Rev 2001;3:CD002124.

54. Signorile PG, Viceconte R, Baldi A. Novel dietary supplement association reduces symptoms in endometriosis patients. J Cell Physiol 2018;233(8):5920–5.

55. Xie B, Liao M, Huang Y, et al. Association between vitamin D and endometriosis among American women: national health and nutrition examination survey. PLoS One 2024;19(1):e0296190.

56. Kahlon BK, Simon-Collins M, Nylander E, et al. A systematic review of vitamin D and endometriosis: role in pathophysiology, diagnosis, treatment, and prevention. FS Rev 2023;4(1):1–14.

57. Anastasi E, Scaramuzzino S, Viscardi MF, et al. Efficacy of N-acetylcysteine on endometriosis-related pain, size reduction of ovarian endometriomas, and fertility outcomes. Int J Environ Res Public Health 2023;20(6):4686.

58. Porpora MG, Brunelli R, Costa G, et al. A promise in the treatment of endometriosis: an observational cohort study on ovarian endometrioma reduction by N-acetylcysteine. Evid-Based Complement Altern Med 2013;2013:240702.

59. Schwertner A, Conceição Dos Santos CC, Costa GD, et al. Efficacy of melatonin in the treatment of endometriosis: a phase II, randomized, double-blind, placebo-controlled trial. Pain 2013;154(6):874–81.

60. Li Y, Hung SW, Zhang R, et al. Melatonin in endometriosis: mechanistic understanding and clinical insight. Nutrients 2022;14(19):4087.

61. Yalçin Bahat P, Ayhan I, Ureyen Ozdemir E, et al. Dietary supplements for treatment of endometriosis: a review. Acta Bio Medica Atenei Parm 2022;93(1):e2022159.

62. Arias AJ, Steinberg K, Banga A, et al. Systematic review of the efficacy of meditation techniques as treatments for medical illness. J Altern Complement Med N Y N 2006;12(8):817–32.

63. Miazga E, Starkman H, Schroeder N, et al. Virtual mindfulness-based therapy for the management of endometriosis chronic pelvic pain: a novel delivery platform

to increase access to care. J Obstet Gynaecol Can 2024;46(6). https://doi.org/10.1016/j.jogc.2024.102457.

64. de Franca Moreira M, Gamboa OL, Pinho Oliveira MA. A single-blind, randomized, pilot study of a brief mindfulness-based intervention for the endometriosis-related pain management. Eur J Pain Lond Engl 2022;26(5):1147–62.

65. Recommendations for research | Endometriosis: diagnosis and management | Guidance. NICE; 2017. Available at: https://www.nice.org.uk/guidance/ng73/chapter/Recommendations-for-research. Accessed July 2, 2024.

66. Tennfjord MK, Gabrielsen R, Tellum T. Effect of physical activity and exercise on endometriosis-associated symptoms: a systematic review. BMC Wom Health 2021;21(1):355.

67. Bonocher CM, Montenegro ML, Rosa E, et al. Endometriosis and physical exercises: a systematic review. Reprod Biol Endocrinol 2014;12(1):4.

68. dos Bispo APS, Ploger C, Loureiro AF, et al. Assessment of pelvic floor muscles in women with deep endometriosis. Arch Gynecol Obstet 2016;294(3):519–23.

69. Physiotherapy management in endometriosis - PMC. Available at: https://www.ncbi.nlm.nih.gov/pmc/articles/PMC9740037/. Accessed July 2, 2024.

70. Hunt J. Pelvic physical therapy for chronic pain and dysfunction following laparoscopic excision of endometriosis: case report. Internet J Allied Health Sci Pract 2019;17(3). https://doi.org/10.46743/1540-580X/2019.1684.

71. Patten DK, Schultz BG, Berlau DJ. The safety and efficacy of low-dose naltrexone in the management of chronic pain and inflammation in multiple sclerosis, fibromyalgia, Crohn's disease, and other chronic pain disorders. Pharmacotherapy 2018;38(3):382–9.

72. Maksym RB, Hoffmann-Młodzianowska M, Skibińska M, et al. Immunology and immunotherapy of endometriosis. J Clin Med 2021;10(24):5879.

73. Younger J, Parkitny L, McLain D. The use of low-dose naltrexone (LDN) as a novel anti-inflammatory treatment for chronic pain. Clin Rheumatol 2014;33(4):451–9.

74. Sinclair J, Abbott J, Proudfoot A, et al. The place of cannabinoids in the treatment of gynecological pain. Drugs 2023;83(17):1571–9.

75. Li PS, Peng XM, Niu XX, et al. Efficacy of acupuncture for endometriosis-associated pain: a multicenter randomized single-blind placebo-controlled trial. Fertil Steril 2023;119(5):815–23.

76. Giese N, Kwon KK, Armour M. Acupuncture for endometriosis: a systematic review and meta-analysis. Integr Med Res 2023;12(4):101003.

77. Ishikura IA, Hachul H, Pires GN, et al. The relationship between insomnia and endometriosis. J Clin Sleep Med JCSM 2020;16(8):1387–8.

78. Management of chronic insomnia disorder in adults: a clinical practice guideline from the American College of Physicians. Ann Intern Med 2016;165(2). https://doi.org/10.7326/P16-9016.

Infertility

Chelsea Faso, MD

KEYWORDS

- Infertility • Fertility • Pregnancy • Ovulation

KEY POINTS

- Primary care providers can offer initial infertility evaluation and medical treatments to their patients.
- Factors contributing to infertility include both female and male factors, with most factors possible to identify with an initial laboratory and imaging workup.
- Female infertility is most commonly caused by ovulatory dysfunction, but may also be caused by structural disease of pelvic organs.
- Medications such as letrozole can induce ovulation and increase fertility rates.
- Access to fertility care in primary and speciality care centers is limited by many barriers, and advocacy is needed to promote a person's ability to start a family.

DEFINITIONS

Infertility is clinically defined as the inability to achieve pregnancy within 12 months of trying to conceive for females under the age of 35, within 6 months if age 35 to 39, or sooner if age 40 and above.[1]

BURDEN OF DISEASE

Clinical infertility affects about 10% to 15% of heterosexual couples, and the CDC estimates about 11% of females and 9% of males of childbearing age struggle with infertility.[2–4] In the United States, approximately 12% of reproductive age females have received infertility services, and the use of assisted reproductive technology (ART), has increased approximately 25% in the last decade.[5,6]

BARRIERS TO CARE

Disparities exist in access to infertility care. Compared with White women in the United States, Black women experience higher rates of infertility, a longer time to evaluation, lower treatment utilization, and poorer treatment outcomes.[7,8] Sexual or gender minorities and unpartnered individuals may also need fertility assistance for family

Department of Family Medicine and Community Health, Mount Sinai Icahn School of Medicine, 690 Amsterdam Avenue, New York, NY 10025, USA
E-mail address: cfaso@institute.org

Prim Care Clin Office Pract 52 (2025) 307–316
https://doi.org/10.1016/j.pop.2025.01.004
0095-4543/25/© 2025 Elsevier Inc. All rights are reserved, including those for text and data mining, AI training, and similar technologies.
primarycare.theclinics.com

Abbreviations	
AMH	anti-Mullerian hormone
ART	assisted reproductive technology
CD	cycle day
FSH	follicle stimulating hormone
HSG	hysterosalpingogram
HyCoSy	hysterosalpingo-contrast sonography
IUI	intrauterine insemination
IVF	in vitro fertilization
LH	luteinizing hormone
MLP	mid-luteal progesterone
OPK	ovulation prediction kit
PCP	primary care physician
RJ	Reproductive Justice
TSH	thyroid stimulating hormone
TVUS	transvaginal ultrasound
WHO	World Health Organization

building but do not always meet definitions of clinical infertility to qualify them for infertility services.[9] Sexual and gender minorities, individuals who are not married, individuals with lower incomes, and individuals with disabilities face heightened barriers and discrimination in accessing infertility care.[9,10]

SisterSong defines Reproductive Justice (RJ) as "the human right to maintain personal bodily autonomy, have children, not have children, and parent the children we have in safe and sustainable communities."[11] In the United States, about 12 million people experience infertility, with only approximately 1500 fellowship trained reproductive endocrinologists available, although mostly concentrated in urban areas.[12] By expanding access to fertility care in the primary care setting, we support the full embodiment of RJ, by supporting those seeking to build families despite intersecting barriers to care.

Many primary care physicians (PCPs) currently provide a wide range of reproductive health care to patients who may not otherwise have access, including prenatal care, long acting reversible contraceptives, vasectomy procedures, and labor and delivery. Starting the conversation about fertility and first steps of diagnosis with a trusted PCP can increase access, equity, and alleviate barriers for our patients seeking to grow families.

Most insurances cover diagnostic workup of infertility, but because these services are not universally considered medically necessary, only 15 states require private insurers to cover some infertility treatment, with only one state requiring medicaid coverage for diagnostic workup and prescription drug coverage.[4,13] Experts in reproductive endocrinology (REI) and Obstetrics & Gynecology agree that in many cases, it is appropriate for PCPs to initiate the infertility evaluation. Lack of insurance coverage is still a barrier that prevents many PCPs from offering these services. In addition, lack of training in the diagnostic workup, medical treatment, and navigating insurance barriers also contributes to barriers in access to fertility care in the primary care setting.

ETIOLOGY

Causes of infertility include a broad range of factors including female factors (37%), male factors (8%), a combination of factors (35%), and unexplained factors (5%).[14,15] Common causes of female factor infertility are listed in **Table 1**.

Table 1
Causes of female factor infertility

Uterine factor (6%)	Endometrial polyps Leiomyomas (submucosal) Uterine synechiae Congenital uterine malformations
Tubal factor (14%)	Tubal obstruction or impaired tubal motility (secondary to sexually transmitted infections, pelvic inflammatory disease, abdominal or pelvic surgery, endometriosis)
Cervical factor (3%)	Stenosis Postsurgical scarring Decreased cervical mucus
Ovulatory dysfunction (21%)	WHO Class 1 (5%–10%)—hypogonadotropic hypogonadal anovulation (ie, excess/low body weight, decreased gonadotropin-releasing hormone [GnRH]) WHO Class 2 (70%–85%)—normogonadotropic normoestrogenic anovulation (ie, PCOS) WHO Class 3 (10%–30%)—hypergonadotropic hypoestrogenic anovulation (ie, primary gonadal failure)

Data from Refs.[15,26,27]

INFERTILITY WORKUP
Indications for Infertility Workup

Given 85% of infertility cases have an identifiable cause, workup should be offered once a patient meets clinical criteria for infertility.[16] Workup should begin[15–17]:

- After 12 months of trying to conceive if the female is younger than 35 years
- After 6 months of trying to conceive if the female is between age 35 and 40 years
- Immediately for females aged 40 and older
- Immediately for those in need of sperm donors (single people capable of pregnancy, same-sex couples)
- Immediately for those with risk factors for infertility (previous ovarian or tubal surgery, exposure to cytotoxic drugs such as chemotherapy, exposure to pelvic radiation, autoimmune disease, family history of early menopause or premature ovarian failure, endometriosis, testicular trauma, adult mumps, or evidence of sexual dysfunction)

For those who have not yet met the clinical definition of infertility, it is not recommended to initiate evaluation with laboratories or imaging. For females, evidence of functional ovulation is an excellent proxy for fertility. This is best demonstrated by regular monthly menstrual cycles with premenstrual symptoms such as chest tenderness, ovulatory pain, or bloating. General counseling on optimizing general health, preconception care, and counseling on timed intercourse should be offered.[16]

The workup for females is described later, but it is suggested to initiate workup for each couple trying to conceive simultaneously as about 35% of infertility cases are due to a combination of factors.[14]

Female Factor Infertility Workup

The general approach to clinical workup of female factor infertility involves evaluating 4 main physiologic and anatomic factors[16]:

- Ovulation

- Ovarian reserve
- Uterine anatomy
- Tubal patency

Elements of history gathering and physical examination are shown in **Table 2**.[16]

Laboratory infertility workup involves evaluation of ovulation and ovarian reserve as summarized in **Table 3**. A history of oligomenorrhea or amenorrhea is clinically sufficient to establish anovulation, and further testing of ovulatory status is not needed.[16] Ovulation can be confirmed by measuring serum mid-luteal progesterone (MLP). This test is best measured 1 week prior to menses, around cycle day (CD) 19 through CD 23. An MLP level above 3 to 5 ng/mL suggests the presence of ovulation. MLP levels above 10 to 12 ng/mL are usually needed to sustain pregnancy.[18] A urinary home ovulation prediction kit (OPK) is another tool to confirm ovulation by measuring the physiologic surge in luteinizing hormone (LH) that occurs about 2 days prior to ovulation.[19] If an MLP level or OPK does not suggest ovulation has occurred, laboratory workup for anovulation should follow, including a thyroid stimulating hormone (TSH), prolactin level, and workup for hyperandrogenism or polycystic ovarian syndrome (PCOS).[20]

Ovarian reserve can be assessed by measuring serum follicle stimulating hormone (FSH) and estradiol (E2) on CD 3 to 5 or a measurement of anti-Mullerian hormone (AMH) at any point in a cycle. Adequate reserve is evidenced by an FSH less than 10 mIU/L, E2 less than 80 pg/mL, or AMH greater than 1 but less than 3.5 ng/mL. Greater FSH values may suggest premature ovarian failure, and AMH levels above range may suggest PCOS.[21,22]

Imaging workup includes determination of ovarian reserve as noted above and serves to determine tubal patency and uterine anatomy (**Table 4**). Ovarian reserve may also be assessed on imaging, by measuring an antral follicle count on transvaginal transvaginal ultrasound (TVUS)/intracavitary ultrasound. This is a measurement of

---

Table 2
History and examination elements for female factor infertility workup

History	Elements of Examination
Medical history: sexually transmitted infections, pelvic inflammatory disease, abnormal pap smears and any follow-up treatment, hyper/hypothyroid symptoms, galactorrhea, hirsutism, chemo/radiation therapy, autoimmune disease, uterine fibroids, ovarian cysts, uterine polyps	*BMI Extremes*
	Hypogonadic hypogonadism: primary amenorrhea with incomplete secondary sexual characteristics
Surgical history: prior abdominal, uterine, or pelvic surgery	*Turner syndrome:* short body habitus, square chest, absent periods
Obstetric History	*Endocrinopathy:* thyroid examination, breast examination for galactorrhea
Menstrual history: menarche, cycle length, presence of molimina, dysmenorrhea, oligo/amenorrhea, menopausal symptoms	*Androgen excess:* hirsutism, acne, male pattern baldness, virilization
Sexual history: frequency of sperm introduction, dyspareunia	*Chronic pelvic inflammatory disease or endometriosis:* tenderness/masses in adnexae/posterior cul-de-sac, uterosacral ligaments, or rectovaginal septum
Family history: Fragile X, premature ovarian failure, infertility	*Mullerian anomaly:* vaginal/structural abnormality
Lifestyle: occupational/environmental exposures, exercise, stress, diet, smoking, alcohol	*Uterine anatomic anomaly:* uterine enlargement, irregularity, lack of mobility

Data from Refs.[2,3,16]

Table 3
Diagnostic laboratories for female factor infertility—assessment of ovulation and ovarian reserve

Laboratory	When to Check	Interpretation
TSH	Baseline[a]	
Prolactin	Baseline—CD2-4 (if regular cycles)	Inhibits release of GnRH from pituitary, prevents ovulation
FSH	Baseline—CD2-4 (if regular cycles)	Good ovarian reserve = FSH < 10 IU/L Increased level = reproductive aging
LH	Baseline—CD2-4 (if regular cycles)	
E2	Baseline—CD2-4 (if regular cycles)	Elevated E2 will suppress FSH, if >60–80 pg/mL, then FSH is unreliable per ACOG
AMH	Baseline/Any CD	Marker of ovarian reserve Low AMH (<1 ng/mL) = poor ovarian reserve <0.5 is premature ovarian failure or menopause Elevated is >3.5, consider PCOS
MLP	CD19–23	>3–5 ng/mL = ovulation present >12 level to sustain pregnancy

Abbreviations: ACOG, American College of Obstetricians and Gynecologists; AMH, anti-Mullerian hormone; CD, cycle day; E2, estradiol; FSH, follicle stimulating hormone; LH, luteinizing hormone; MLP, mid-luteal serum progesterone; TSH, thyroid stimulating hormone.
 [a] If amenorrhea/irregular menses, can check baseline laboratories at any point.
Data from Refs.[3,16,18,20–22]

the number of follicles that measure 2 to 10 mm in both ovaries and counts above 5 to 7 are suggestive of adequate reserve.[23]

Hysterosalpingogram (HSG, aka fluorosonogram) is a fluoroscopy contrast-enhanced X ray view of the uterus and fallopian tubes and is the standard of care for determining tubal patency and identifying occlusions or adhesions. This study has 65% sensitivity and 83% specificity to detect tubal patency. An HSG transmits fluoroscopic dye through a transcervical catheter that outlines the ovarian cavity and tubal patency as the dye passes through fallopian tubes and spills into the abdomen. It is most ideal to perform this study within 7 days of menses to avoid interrupting a desired pregnancy.[24]

Table 4
Diagnostic imaging for female factor infertility—assessment of uterine anatomy and tubal patency

Imaging	When to Check	Interpretation
Transvaginal Ultrasound (TVUS)	Baseline for antral follicle count, anatomy	Antral follicle count. Count all follicles b/t 2–10 mm in both ovaries <5–7 = low
Hysterosalpingogram/ Fluorosonogram (HSG)	CD7-10	Uterine anomalies Tubal patency
Saline Histogram (SHG), Hysterosalpingo-contrast sonography (HyCoSy)	CD7-10	Uterine anomalies Tubal patency

Data from Refs.[3,23–25]

Saline-infused sonohysterography or hysterosalpingo-contrast sonography is an ultrasound study that uses infusion of saline fluid and air bubbles via transcervical catheter to view anatomy of uterus and adnexa. This imaging modality is increasingly utilized, as it has high diagnostic accuracy for tubal occlusion (sensitivity 92% and specificity 95%), is thought to be better tolerated than HSG, and can be more useful than HSG to identify intrauterine structures such as uterine polyps. This study is also most ideal to perform within 7 days of menses.[25]

When available, follicle monitoring may be able to identify successful recruitment of a dominant follicle for ovulation. A TVUS can be used on CD 11 through 13 to identify any follicle >11 mm.[23] Coordinating this ultrasound at the ideal moment in a menstrual cycle may provide a significant barrier, and therefore, is not routinely recommended in ovulation induction protocols discussed later in this article.

Any detection of tubal obstruction or atypical uterine anatomy (septate uterus, uterine fibroids distorting uterine cavity) may warrant MRI for further evaluation, and referral to REI would be indicated, as in vitro fertilization (IVF) is generally the preferred pathway for infertility treatment when these factors are identified.[3]

MEDICAL MANAGEMENT OF FEMALE FACTOR INFERTILITY

Management of female factor infertility depends on the root cause, and most causes can be categorized into ovulatory dysfunction (21%), tubal damage (14%), uterine factors (6%), or cervical factors (3%).[26]

Treatment of ovulatory dysfunction can be offered in the primary care setting. The World Health Organization (WHO) classifies infertility due to ovulatory dysfunction into 4 types seen in **Table 1**.[27] Females who have a body mass index (BMI) outside of target range (20–25 kg/m^2) may benefit from weight loss or weight gain to restore ovulatory function. In those with PCOS and BMI above 29, a 5% to 10% body weight loss can restore ovulation in 55% to 100% of people within 6 months, and offers an inexpensive low-intervention method for restoration of ovulatory function.[28] It is important to note that trials of weight loss intervention for infertility have not shown improvements in live birth rates, and therefore, obesity should not be a criteria to deny access to fertility care or treatment, and readiness for weight loss interventions should be assessed using shared decision making, balancing evidence-based medical risks, and patient autonomy.[29]

Insulin sensitizing agents like metformin increase regular menstrual cyclicity and enhance spontaneous ovulation in PCOS, but do not increase live birth rates compared with ovulation induction.[30] Metformin is, therefore, not recommended as routine for ovulation induction except in females with glucose intolerance, as it could be used to facilitate weight loss and regular menstrual cycles.

Ovulation Induction

Clinicians may attempt to induce ovulation medically in anovulatory people (WHO Class 2) using letrozole or clomiphene citrate.[31,32] These agents can be used with timed intercourse or intrauterine insemination (IUI) to increase pregnancy rates. Medications that induce ovulation increase the risk of multiple pregnancy (up to 15%) and ovarian hyperstimulation syndrome (1%).[33,34] Patients using these agents should be counseled about these risks. Patients who do not achieve ovulation after 3 to 6 cycles should be referred to an infertility specialist for further treatment.

Letrozole has become the preferred method for ovulation induction in PCOS.[31] As an aromatase inhibitor, letrozole blocks estrogen biosynthesis, therefore, reducing negative estrogenic feedback at the pituitary, promoting FSH secretion, ovarian follicular development, and ovulation. Compared with ovulation induction with other agents (namely clomiphene), letrozole has a shorter half-life, therefore has less anti-estrogenic effect, and by allowing natural negative feedback mechanisms to kick in sooner, letrozole is more likely to promote mono-follicular ovulation (lower risk of multiple gestation), and has reduced anti-estrogen effects on endometrium (thinned lining) and cervical mucus (prevents development of mucus consistency optimal for sperm transport)—factors that aid in optimal pregnancy conditions. Letrozole demonstrates clinical superiority for ovulation induction compared with clomiphene. A randomized control trial comparing ovulation induction with letrozole versus clomiphene citrate in PCOS demonstrated that letrozole induction was superior in measured birth rates (27.5% vs 19.1%) and ovulation rates (27.5% vs 19.1%).[35,36]

Letrozole is given as a 2.5 mg daily dose for 5 days on CD 3 through CD 7 following spontaneous menstruation or progestin-induced bleed. If ovulation is achieved (as measured by MLP on CD 19–23), the 2.5 mg dose can be continued for the following cycles. If there is no evidence of ovulation, the dose may be increased to 5 mg daily for the next cycle. The maximum recommended dose is 7.5 mg, as higher doses are associated with thinning of endometrium, which may limit success of implantation. Once ovulation is achieved on an effective dose, the dose can be continued for 3 to 6 cycles. Encourage sperm introduction every other day starting 5 days after the last cycle dose of letrozole (CD 11). Patients can target CDs of highest fertility by using an OPK to detect urinary LH surge. The day of LH surge and the 2 days following are the days of highest fertility. Common side effects of letrozole include mild hot flashes and arthralgias. Typical cost for letrozole ranges from $10 to $18 per tablet.[37]

Further Management of Female Factor Infertility

IUI is a procedure used for the treatment of infertility caused by severe sexual dysfunction (ie, vaginismus), cervical factor infertility, and certain male infertility factors (ie, ejaculatory dysfunction). This procedure involves placing processed and concentrated motile sperm directly into the uterine cavity at time of spontaneous or triggered ovulation. IUI is sometimes used as an adjunctive procedure to ovulation induction to increase pregnancy rates, especially in unexplained infertility.[38] Treatment is generally limited for 3 cycles. In the United States, various types of health care professionals are permitted to perform and bill for IUI depending on state regulations, including physicians, certified nurse midwives, and nurse practitioners.

Cases of infertility due to tubal occlusion, uterine anomalies, endometriosis, and unidentified causes should be managed by OB/GYN and REI colleagues, usually with ART including IVF.

ROUTINE FERTILITY COUNSELING

For anyone attempting pregnancy or undergoing infertility workup and treatment, counseling about general fertility practices is recommended.[39] This includes teaching of timed sperm introduction/timed intercourse (every 1–2 days around expected time of ovulation), folic acid supplementation, prenatal vitamins, and avoidance of teratogenic agents. Although not supported by strong evidence, there are some recommendations for fertility counseling including: encourage healthy weight and consider target BMI (>19 and <30 kg/m^2), limiting caffeine intake (less than 3 cups/day), avoid smoking, alcohol, and recreational drugs, and checking if commercially available vaginal lubricants interfere with fertility as most lubricants are toxic to sperm. Counseling about ovulation tracking and fertility awareness is also recommended. Patients should be counseled on ovulation tracking using apps. OPKs can offer home point of care testing for tracking ovulation as described previously. Monitoring for cervical mucus changes can also identify highest fertility days, as high estrogen at midcycle produces clear, copious, elastic quality mucus optimal for sperm transport. Monitoring basal body temperature can detect when ovulation has already occurred and may not be useful at identifying when to introduce sperm.[39]

MOOD DISORDERS IN FERTILITY CARE

Patients undergoing infertility evaluation should also be screened and monitored for signs and symptoms of mood disorders, as females with fertility issues are twice as likely to have coexisting mood disorders compared with females without fertility issues, with the risk of fertility treatment increasing severity of anxiety and depression.[40,41]

FURTHER AREAS OF RESEARCH/ADVOCACY

Further research is needed to better understand the demand and accessibility for infertility services in cis-gendered and in gender minority populations. As the diagnosis of infertility has been recently recognized as an insurance billable medical diagnosis, more advocacy for expansive insurance coverage of fertility care diagnostic and treatment coverage is needed, as even fertility medication can still prove costly when used for multiple cycles. Grants may exist locally to support those with financial need for fertility care services, but these can vary by state and can have restrictions on who qualifies, highlighting equity concerns (excluding single persons for example).

SUMMARY

Diagnostic workup for infertility and medical management of ovulatory dysfunction can be accessible in the primary care setting. The ability to have and care for the family that you wish for is a fundamental tenet of RJ. PCPs have the opportunity to provide fertility workup, offer patient centered infertility care, and advocate for expanded access to fertility care for our communities.

CLINICS CARE POINTS

- Infertility workup should begin after 12 months of trying to conceive if the female partner younger than 35 years, after 6 months if age greater than 35, or immediately if age 40 or older or any risk factors for infertility.
- Infertility workup for females should begin by confirming ovulation with a serum progesterone level around day 21 of a menstrual cycle.
- Letrozole demonstrates superiority over clomiphene citrate to increase ovulation rates and live birth rates when used for infertility caused by PCOS.
- Metformin is not recommended as routine for infertility treatment except in females with glucose intolerance, as it could be used to facilitate weight loss and regular menstrual cycles.
- Workup for male partners should be initiated simultaneously, and should begin with a history and semen analysis.

DISCLOSURE

The author has nothing to disclose.

REFERENCES

1. Phillips K, Olanrewaju RA, Omole F. Infertility: evaluation and management. Am Fam Physician 2023;107(6):623–30.
2. Jose-Miller AB, Boyden JW, Frey KA. Infertility. Am Fam Physician 2007;75(6): 849–56.
3. Lindsay TJ, Vitrikas KR. Evaluation and treatment of infertility. Am Fam Physician 2015;91(5):308–14.
4. Weigel G, Ranji U, Long M, et al. Coverage and use of fertility services in the U.S. Kaiser Family Foundation: Women's Health Policy; 2020. Available at: https://www.kff.org/womens-health-policy/issue-brief/coverage-and-use-of-fertility-services-in-the-u-s/.
5. Jewett A., Mardovich S., Zhang Y., et al., 2020 Assisted Reproductive Technology Fertility Clinic and National Summary Report. Centers for Disease Control and Prevention. Available at: https://stacks.cdc.gov/view/cdc/148215.
6. National survey of family growth 2015-2019. Centers for Disease Control and Prevention; 2024.
7. Wiltshire A, McConnell R, Ghidei L. Addressing disparities in infertility care. Am Fam Physician 2023;107(6):573–4.
8. Craig LB, Peck JD, Janitz AE. The Prevalence of Infertility in American Indian/Alaska Natives and Other Racial/Ethnic groups: national survey of family growth. Peadiatr Perinat Epidemiol 2019;33(2):119–25.
9. Ethics Committee of the American Society for Reproductive Medicine. Access to fertility treatment irrespective of marital status, sexual orientation, or gender identity: an ethics committee opinion. Fertil Steril 2021;116(2):326–30.
10. ACOG committee opinion No. 749: marriage and family building equality for lesbian, gay, bisexual, transgender, queer, intersex, asexual, and gender nonconforming individuals. Obstet Gynecol 2018;132(2):e82–6.
11. SisterSong. Retrieved august 2024, from SisterSong: women of color reproductive Justice collective. 1997. Available at: https://www.sistersong.net/reproductive-justice/.
12. Adeleye AJ, Kawwass JF, Brauer A, et al. The mismatch in supply and demand: reproductive endocrinology and infertility workforce challenges and controversies. Fertil Steril 2023. S0015-0282(23):00045-00046.
13. New York State Department of Financial Services. IVF and fertility preservation law Q&A guidance. Available at: https://www.dfs.ny.gov/consumers/health_insurance/infertility_consumer_faq_052621 (Accessed 1 August 2024).
14. Recent advances in medically assisted conception. Report of a WHO Scientific Group. World Health Organ Tech Rep Ser 1992;820:1–111.
15. ACOG committee opinion no. 781: infertility workup for the women's health specialist. Obstet Gynecol 2019;133(6):e377–84.
16. Practice committee of the American Society for Reproductive Medicine, Practice Committee of the American Society for Reproductive Medicine. Fertility evaluation of infertile women: a committee opinion. Fertil Steril 2015;116(5):1255–65.
17. ACOG committee opinion no. 589: female age-related fertility decline. Obstet Gynecol 2014;101(3):633–4.
18. Wathen NC, Perry L, Lilford RJ, et al. Interpretation of single progesterone measurement in diagnosis of anovulation and defective luteal phase: observations on analysis of the normal range. Br Med J 1984;288(6410):7.
19. Hsiu-Wei S, Yi YC, Wei TY, et al. Detection of ovulation, a review of currently available methods. Bioen Transl Med 2017;2(3):238–46.

20. National Collaborating Centre for Women's and Children's Health. Fertility: assessment and treatment for people with fertility problems. London: National Institute for Health and Clinical Excellence (NICE); 2013. p. 1–63.
21. Practice Committee of the American Society for Reproductive Medicine. Testing and interpreting measures of ovarian reserve: a committee opinion. Fertil Steril 2015;103(3):e9.
22. ACOG committee opinion no. 618: ovarian reserve testing. Obstet Gynecol 2015; 125(1):268.
23. Ecochard R, Boehringer H, Rabilloud M, et al. Chronological aspects of ultrasonic, hormonal, and other indirect indices of ovulation. BJOG 2001;108(8):822–9.
24. Swart P, Mol BW, van der Veen F, et al. The accuracy of hysterosalpingography in the diagnosis of tubal pathology: a meta-analysis. Fertil Steril 1995;64(3):486.
25. Saunders RD, Shwayder JM, Nakajima ST. Current methods of tubal patency assessment. Fertil Steril 2011;95(7):2171.
26. Hull MG, Glazener CM, Kelly NJ, et al. Population study of causes, treatment, and outcome of infertility. Br Med J 1985;291(6510):1693.
27. Advances in methods of fertility regulation: report of a WHO scientific group. World Health Organization Tech Rep Ser 1973;527:1–42.
28. Crosignani PG, Colombo M, Vegetti W, et al. Overweight and obese anovulatory patients with polycystic ovaries: parallel improvements in anthropometric indices, ovarian physiology and fertility rate induced by diet. Hum Reprod 2003;18(9):1928.
29. Practice committee of the American Society for Reproductive Medicine, Practice Committee of the American Society for Reproductive Medicine. Obesity and reproduction: a committee opinion. Fertil Steril 2021;116(5):1266–85.
30. Thessaloniki ESHRE/ASRM-Sponsored PCOS Consensus Workshop Group. Consensus on infertility treatment related to polycystic ovary syndrome. Fertil Steril 2008;89(3):505.
31. ACOG committee Opinion No. 738 Summary: aromatase inhibitors in gynecologic practice. Obstet Gynecol 2018;131(6):1.
32. Gorlitsky GA, Kase NG, Speroff L. Ovulation and pregnancy rates with clomiphene citrate. Obstet Gynecol 1978;51(3):265.
33. Schenker JG, Weinstein D. Ovarian hyperstimulation syndrome: a current survey. Fertil Steril 1978;30(3):255.
34. Scialli AR. The reproductive toxicity of ovulation induction. Fertil Steril 1986; 45(3):315.
35. Legro RS, Brzyski RG, Diamond MP, et al. Letrozole versus clomiphene for infertility in the polycystic ovary syndrome. N Engl J Med 2014;371(2):119–29.
36. Franik S, Eltrop SM, Kremer JA, et al. Aromatase inhibitors (letrozole) for subfertile women with polycystic ovary syndrome. Cochrane Database Syst Rev 2018;5: CD010287.
37. Medi-Span price rx online pricing tool, Available at: https://www.wolterskluwer.com/en/solutions/medi-span/price-rx (Accessed 1 August, 2024).
38. Carson SA, Kallen AN. Diagnosis and management of infertility: a review. JAMA 2021;326(1):65–76.
39. Practice Committee of the American Society for Reproductive Medicine. Optimizing natural fertility: a committee opinion. Fertil Steril 2022;117(1):53–63.
40. Wdowiak A, Makara-Studzińska M, Raczkiewicz D, et al. Reproductive problems and intensity of anxiety and depression in women treated for infertility. Psychiatry Pol 2022;56(1):153–70.
41. Killen M. Addressing mood disorders in infertility care. Letter to the editor. Am Fam Physician 2024;109(4):296.

Cardiovascular Health in Women

Aury V. Garcia, MD[a,b,*], Yorgos Strangas, MD, MPH[a,c]

KEYWORDS

- Cardiovascular disease • Sex • Gender • Women

KEY POINTS

- Cardiovascular disease (CVD) is a leading cause of morbidity and mortality in women.
- Sex/gender disparities exist in the diagnosis, treatment, and long-term management of traditional CVD risk factors including hypertension, diabetes, obesity, dyslipidemia, tobacco use, and physical activity.
- Emerging literature shows unique CVD contributors across a woman's lifespan such as polycystic ovary syndrome, menopause, breast cancer, depression, hypertensive disorders of pregnancy, and gestational diabetes mellitus.

INTRODUCTION

In this article, we use the terms "women" and "men" to refer to female and male sex assigned at birth (**Table 1**). We use the term gender to refer to self-reported identity and acknowledge that gender is a complex concept not limited to the binary of men and women. The epidemiology and presentation of cardiovascular disease (CVD) in intersex and trans populations are beyond the scope of this article and deserve further in depth study.

The World Health Organization (WHO) defines CVD as a group of conditions affecting the heart and blood vessels.[1] These encompass coronary heart disease, cerebrovascular disease, peripheral arterial disease (PAD), rheumatic heart disease, congenital heart disease, deep venous thrombosis, and pulmonary embolism.[1] CVD has been the leading cause of death in the United States since 1921[2] with nearly 128 million Americans aged ≥20 currently living with some form of CVD or risk factor.[3] CVD prevalence in women is 44.8% when including coronary heart disease, heart

[a] Department of Internal Medicine, Center for Family and Community Medicine; [b] Columbia University Irving Medical Center/New York Presbyterian Hospital, 610 West 158th Street, New York, NY 10032, USA; [c] Columbia University Irving Medical Center/New York Presbyterian Hospital, 720 West 173rd Street Apartment 42, New York, NY 10032, USA
* Corresponding author. Department of Internal Medicine, Center for Family and Community Medicine, Columbia University Irving Medical Center/New York Presbyterian Hospital, 610 West 158th Street, New York, NY 10032.
E-mail address: avg2117@cumc.columbia.edu

Prim Care Clin Office Pract 52 (2025) 317–328
https://doi.org/10.1016/j.pop.2025.01.005
0095-4543/25/© 2025 Elsevier Inc. All rights are reserved, including those for text and data mining, AI training, and similar technologies.

Abbreviations	
AHA	American Heart Association
cHTN	chronic hypertension
CVD	cardiovascular disease
DM	diabetes mellitus
GDM	gestational diabetes mellitus
HTN	hypertension
LDL	low-density lipoprotein
PAD	peripheral arterial disease
PCOS	polycystic ovary syndrome
T2DM	type 2 diabetes mellitus
WHO	World Health Organization

failure, stroke, and hypertension.[3] Since 2010, there has been a nearly 20% increase in mortality attributable to atherosclerotic CVD in women suggesting significant opportunity for further exploration and intervention.[3] Disparities abound between sexes[4] in self-recognition of symptoms,[5] risk factor management,[6] referral for invasive and noninvasive testing,[7] and in-hospital mortality.[7,8] Emerging literature suggests that consideration of traditional and unique sex-based factors across a woman's lifespan may be key to screening, early intervention, and mitigation of downstream sequelae.[9]

Table 1
Relative risk for sex-specific risk factors for cardiovascular disease

Risk Factor	Relative Risk	Reference
Pregnancy-related complications		
History of preeclampsia without severe features	Relative risk (RR) of 2, $P < .05$	38,60,78
History of preeclampsia with severe features	RR of 5.36, $P < .001$	38,60,78
History of gestational diabetes	RR ranging from 1.23 (ischemic heart disease) to 3.16 (coronary artery bypass graft), $P < .05$	66,79
History of preterm delivery	Cardiovascular disease (CVD) (RR 1.43), $P < .05$ CVD death (RR 1.78), $P < .05$ Coronary heart disease (RR 1.49), $P < .05$ Cardiac death from coronary heart disease (RR 2.10), $P < .05$ Stroke (1.65), $P < .05$	68–71
Gynecologic risk factors		
Polycystic ovarian syndrome	RR 1.3, $P < .05$	38,39
Early menopause prior to age 45	RR 1.50 (1.28–1.76) for overall coronary heart disease (CHD), RR 1.11 (1.03–1.20) for fatal CHD, $P < .05$	46,47

The table demonstrates CVD relative risk for pregnancy-related and gynecologic risk factors.
95% confidence intervals used for all relative risks with $P <0.05$ with the exception of history of preeclampsia with severe features, $P < .001$.

CARDIOVASCULAR DISEASE PRESENTATION

Though women with acute coronary syndrome often report chest pain, they have lower odds of endorsing chest pain or diaphoresis when compared to their male counterparts.[10] Additionally, while both sexes may report atypical symptoms including shortness of breath, left arm and shoulder pain, and nausea and vomiting, women are more likely to present with these symptoms.[10] Prodromal symptoms in women are more likely to be attributed to anxiety or stress by both patients and health care providers.[11] From a pathophysiologic perspective, increased frequency of plaque erosion has been proposed as a mechanism for the higher proportion of unstable angina and non-ST-elevation myocardial infarctions in women.[12,13] Similar sex difference trends and disparities have been observed in women with cerebral vascular disease,[14] PAD,[15,16] and rheumatic heart disease.[17]

TRADITIONAL CARDIOVASCULAR RISK FACTORS
Hypertension

High blood pressure poses a significant risk for coronary heart disease, heart failure, and stroke in both men and women.[18] While a higher percentage of males have hypertension (HTN) up to age 64, for those ≥65 years of age, the percentage of females with HTN is higher.[19] Proposed mechanisms for this difference include hypertensive disorders in pregnancy, interactions between the renin-angiotensin-aldosterone axis and sex hormones, and socioeconomic disparities.[20] One study found that women were less likely to receive HTN medication despite having similar blood pressure values compared to their male counterparts.[21] A separate meta-analysis found that women were 15% less likely to be prescribed angiotensin-converting enzyme inhibitors and 30% more likely to receive diuretics.[22] Despite these differences and many published guidelines,[23] no major societies have recommended sex-specific thresholds for blood pressure control.

Diabetes Mellitus

Diabetes mellitus (DM) has been linked to coronary heart disease, heart failure, PAD, and stroke.[24] Overall, men have a higher prevalence of type 2 DM, but women have a higher prevalence of undiagnosed DM after age 60 and overall DM prevalence after age 70.[25] Men are diagnosed at a younger age and lower body mass index, whereas women have higher rates of excess weight and HTN at the time of diagnosis.[25] Women with DM have myocardial infarctions younger, lower rates of revascularization, higher risk of developing heart failure, and worse outcomes for PAD compared to their male counterparts.[26] Moreover, men have a greater net benefit with lifestyle modifications and pharmacotherapy compared to women.[25] Changes in insulin resistance, body fat distribution, sex hormones, pregnancy, and psychosocial factors have all been linked to disparities in diabetes prevalence, diagnosis, management, morbidity, and mortality in women.[25]

Obesity

The 2024 American Heart Association (AHA) reports increased prevalence for obesity in females from 33.4% in 1999 to 2000 to 41.9% in 2017 to 2018.[3] Obesity disproportionately contributes to coronary artery disease risk in women (64%) compared to men (46%).[27] Explanations for these differences include differing fat distribution, sex hormone changes, genetic susceptibility, and gut microbiome makeup.[28] Females are more likely to both be offered and to pursue lifestyle changes, be prescribed weight loss medications, and undergo bariatric surgery.[28] In contrast to other risk factors, it appears that management of obesity is lagging in men compared to women. However, it is important to note the disparate role that sociocultural norms play. For example, the perceived link between physical attractiveness and thinness in western societies and greater body dissatisfaction in women compared to men contributing to higher rates of depression and eating disorders in the former.[28]

Tobacco Use

Tobacco use is an independent risk factor for CVD and a major contributor to dyslipidemia, HTN, and DM.[3] Prevalence estimates show that among adults 18 years of age or older, 13.1% of males and 10.1% of females reported cigarette use every day or some days.[3] Additionally, 6.9% of females who gave birth in 2017 reported cigarette use during pregnancy, with greater prevalence in those aged 20 to 24.[29] In those who concurrently use oral contraceptives and tobacco products, there is a 10-fold increase in myocardial infarction risk and 3-fold increase in stroke risk.[29] When looking at CVD specifically, one meta-analysis found a 25% increase in risk of coronary artery disease in women compared to men.[30] Despite greater attempts to stop smoking, women experience disparate challenges with cessation.[31,32] The literature emphasizes the importance of addressing gendered experiences including trauma and violence, imbalances with caregiver roles, income disparities, and second-hand exposure to increase cessation success.[31,32]

Physical Activity

Physical inactivity is a major risk factor for CVD.[3] Overall, women are less likely to meet the aerobic physical activity (PA) guidelines ($\geq$150 min/wk of moderate PA, $\geq$75 min/wk of vigorous PA, or an equivalent combination) recommended by the AHA compared to their male counterparts.[3] Interestingly, one study found a greater all-cause mortality benefit in women compared to men with both aerobic exercise and strength training.[33] Moreover, women had a peak benefit in all-cause mortality at lower duration of moderate to vigorous exercise (140 min/wk in women compared to 300 min/wk in men) and higher duration of exercise before seeing plateau of these benefits (300 min/wk in women compared to 110 min/wk in men) compared to men.[33]

Dyslipidemia

Cholesterol has been classified as a causal risk factor for atherosclerosis and CVD.[3] While females compared to males are more likely to have a high protective high-density lipoprotein greater than 40, they are also more likely to have a total cholesterol greater than 200 and just as likely to have low-density lipoprotein (LDL) greater than 130, increasing CVD risk.[3] A myriad of mechanisms contribute to sex differences in dyslipidemia including sex hormone-driven lipoprotein metabolism, lipid profile type across the lifespan (ie, menstrual cycle, menopause, pregnancy, contraception use), and unique comorbidities like polycystic ovarian syndrome (PCOS).[34] Moreover, data show that women are less likely to have LDL assessed,[35] receive recommended lipid-lowering therapy,[36] and reach target LDL goals,[34] contributing to disparities in CVD prevention.

GENDER/SEX-SPECIFIC CARDIOVASCULAR DISEASE RISK FACTORS

The following section outlines unique gender/sex-specific risk factors.

Polycystic Ovarian Syndrome

PCOS is a sex-specific syndrome defined by the presence of 2 of 3 criteria, including anovulation and/or oligomenorrhea; excess androgen production; and characteristic imaging findings of many small ovarian cysts on pelvic ultrasound.[37] Women with PCOS have insulin resistance (50%–70%) and increased risk of metabolic syndrome.[38] One study found that women with PCOS have increased risk of HTN, DM, higher concentration of total cholesterol, and increased risk of nonfatal cerebrovascular disease compared to women without PCOS.[39] Though data regarding the relationship between PCOS and CVD remain controversial,[40] one meta-analysis found a small but statistically significant increase in risk of coronary heart disease, with a relative risk of 1.3 to develop CVD and 1.44 for coronary heart disease.[41]

MENOPAUSE

Women develop CVD several years later than men, often coinciding with the transition to menopause.[42] Symptoms of menopause including hot flashes, sleep difficulties, and depression have been associated with CVD and its risk factors.[43] One study found that women with higher total cholesterol and blood pressure were more likely to develop menopause earlier.[44] Additionally, a first cardiovascular event before age 35 was linked to a 2-fold increased risk of early menopause.[45] In numerous other studies, women who reached menopause at younger ages had increased risk of coronary heart disease[46] and heart failure.[47] Overall, the relationship between changes in sex hormone, body fat distribution, lipid profile, and menopause have been well documented and represent a critical stage for close monitoring and intervention.[43]

BREAST CANCER TREATMENT

The strongest risk factor for breast cancer is female gender with roughly 99% of cases occurring in women.[48] Existing literature supports a link between breast cancer and cardiovascular health.[49] CVD (namely heart failure and myocardial infarction) and CVD risk factors (ie, dyslipidemia, obesity, HTN) are increased in breast cancer survivors.[49] Breast cancer treatments including chemotherapeutic agents[50] and radiation therapy[51] have been associated with cardiotoxicity. This underscores the importance of monitoring patients with breast cancer for CVD risks and therapy-related cardiac effects.

DEPRESSION

According to the WHO, depression is 50% more common in women compared to men.[52] Women with depression have a 30% to 50% higher risk of CVD compared to men.[53] One study found that in women with CVD, depression is a predictor of death and all-cause mortality even after adjusting for demographic factors and CVD risk factors.[54] Moreover, women with depression are more likely to experience recurrent ischemia, cardiogenic shock, cardiac arrest, and in-hospital mortality.[55] Mechanistically speaking, persistent low-grade pro-inflammatory states influenced by variations in sex hormones across the lifespan contribute to both depression and CVD in women.[56]

PREGNANCY-RELATED RISK FACTORS

Multiple studies have found correlations between common complications of pregnancy and both cardiovascular risk and future all-cause mortality.[57] Hypertensive disorders of pregnancy, gestational diabetes, and preterm birth have also been associated with increased all-cause mortality decades later, with CVD being the predominant cause of death.[57] In shorter time frames, complications of pregnancy are repeatedly associated with higher risk scores on established cardiovascular risk calculators, implying greater CVD risk later in life.[58,59] Despite these findings, many women with complications of pregnancy are unaware of their risk. One study found that up to 96% of women were unaware of the relationship between preeclampsia and CVD.[60]

HYPERTENSIVE DISORDERS IN PREGNANCY: CHRONIC HYPERTENSION, GESTATIONAL HYPERTENSION, AND PRE-ECLAMPSIA

Hypertensive disorders of pregnancy include a continuum of syndromes ranging from chronic hypertension (cHTN) (blood pressure >140/90 mm Hg prior to 20 weeks gestation) to gestational hypertension (new-onset blood pressure >140/90 mm Hg after 20 weeks gestation), pre-eclampsia (new onset blood pressure >140/90 mm Hg after 20 weeks gestation with proteinuria and/or signs of end-organ damage), and cHTN with superimposed PEC (preeclampsia).[61] According to the Centers for Disease Control and Prevention (CDC), between 2017 and 2019 prevalence of hypertensive disorders in pregnancy increased from 13.3% to 15.9% with the highest prevalence among women aged 35 to 44 (18%) and 44 to 55 (31%) and those who identified as Black (20.9%).[62] Hypertensive disorders of pregnancy both predispose individuals to other CVD risk factors and act as independent CVD risk factors themselves.[38] Literature shows an increased risk of future maternal myocardial infarction, heart failure, cHTN, and stroke with history of hypertensive disorders of pregnancy.[63] One study of 4273 women found that hypertensive disorders of pregnancy conferred an almost 2-fold risk of progressing to an elevated risk for CVD, based on Framingham 30 criteria, 2 to 7 years after delivery.[57] Early identification of women at risk for CVD based on reproductive history of hypertensive disorders of pregnancy may help reduce associated morbidity and mortality.[61]

Gestational Diabetes Mellitus

Gestational diabetes mellitus (GDM) is most commonly diagnosed based on 2 or more abnormal values on a 3-hour oral glucose tolerance test, often following an abnormal 1 hour screening test between 24 and 28 weeks of gestation.[64] Women with GDM have an increased risk of developing hypertensive disorders of pregnancy and type 2 diabetes mellitus (T2DM) later in life, both CVD risk factors.[64] One study with 90,000 women found a 43% increased risk of CVD (myocardial infarction or stroke) in women with a history of GDM with a median follow-up of nearly 26 years.[65] In addition to increasing the risk of T2DM, GDM has been associated with early atherosclerosis and endothelial dysfunction further contributing to downstream CVD risk.[66] In conjunction with managing GDM, providers should prioritize postpartum counseling to mitigate the CVD risk that persists for decades after this diagnosis.

Preterm Delivery

Preterm deliveries (<37 weeks gestational age) affect 11% of pregnancies worldwide.[67] One systematic review and meta-analysis of 338,000 women with preterm deliveries found an increased relative risk (RR) of future maternal CVD (RR 1.43), CVD death (RR 1.78), coronary heart disease (RR 1.49), coronary heart disease death (RR 2.10), and stroke (RR 1.65).[68] Women with a history of preterm birth have been noted to have higher atherogenic lipids and carotid arterial wall thickening predisposing them to future CVD compared to women with term births.[69] Moreover, studies show an inverse relationship between weeks of pregnancy prior to delivery and insulin resistance[70] and blood pressure values.[71] Overall, health care providers should consider detailed history of prior deliveries to identify and offer interventions for CVD at risk patients.

PREVENTION AND SURVEILLANCE

Current guidelines recommend screening for 10-year atherosclerotic CVD risk in patients 40 to 75 years of age using the joint American College of Cardiology/AHA guidelines.[72,73] Adults are encouraged to prioritize a healthy diet (minimal trans fats, processed foods, refined carbohydrates, and sweetened beverages) and engage in 150 minutes per week of moderate-intensity or 75 minutes per week of vigorous-intensity exercise to reduce CVD risk.[73] Strong evidence supports the discussion of tobacco cessation at every health care visit.[73] Based on clinician evaluation of CVD risk, consideration is made for pharmacotherapy including antihypertensives, metformin, statins, and/or aspirin in addition to lifestyle modifications.[73]

Women routinely undergo screening mammography,[74] which may provide insight into cardiovascular health and an opportunity for risk stratification. Recent evidence has found the presence of breast arterial calcification, an incidental finding, to confer a 2.06 relative risk of cardiac death, with similarly elevated risk ratios for ischemic stroke, PAD, and heart failure.[75] The updated 2011 AHA risk stratification guidelines take into account nontraditional risk factors such as autoimmune diseases and pregnancy-related complications.[76] Moreover, the fourth trimester or postpartum period has been identified as a key stage to screen for and address CVD risks.[77] The AHA has recently published extensive recommendations including an early postpartum visit to counsel on hypertensive disorders of pregnancy, GDM, contraception, and lactation followed by a 6-week visit for screening of other essential health parameters conferring CVD risk.[77] From a pharmacotherapy standpoint, the AHA found "not useful/effective and maybe harmful" evidence for use of hormone replacement therapy, selective estrogen receptor modulators, antioxidant supplements, folic acid, and aspirin in women less than 65 years of age for primary CVD prevention.[76]

DISCUSSION

Further investigation is needed in identifying causal factors, treatments, and prevention strategies for gynecologic disease and complications of pregnancy. The identification and quantification of cardiovascular risk conferred by gynecologic syndromes or pregnancy complications have been studied in the context of existing risk assessment tools. Identifying sex-specific risks thus allows for early identification of patients who are likely to be high enough risk to merit pharmacologic intervention, perhaps years before traditional risk calculators such as the atherosclerotic cardiovascular disease (ASCVD) risk calculator.

Early capture of risk represents an opportunity for the health care system and individual patients to intervene and forestall future CVD. Moreover, the ability to enact meaningful lifestyle changes is largely determined outside of the health care system. For example, access to healthy diet and exercise is often driven largely by external circumstances such as what food sources are available, what employment opportunities exist, and the availability, affordability, and safety of facilities for physical exercise and exposure to chronic stressors. The addition of pregnancy-related risk factors further complicates the social determinants, with childcare support systems now also affecting maternal stress and ability to enact recommended behavioral changes.

Incorporating sex-based risk factors may also allow providers to have more nuanced discussions with patients around a shared decision regarding interventions, acting as a tiebreaker in cases where there is ambiguity regarding the patient's degree of cardiovascular risk or around the risk/benefit of pharmacologic intervention.

CLINICS CARE POINTS

- Health care providers should take into consideration both traditional and unique sex-based factors when screening women for cardiovascular disease.

- Though there is a paucity of sex-specific guidelines, all women aged 40 to 75 should be screened for 10-year atherosclerotic CVD risk, counseled on the specifics of a healthy diet, exercise frequency, and tobacco cessation per the AHA guidelines, and offered evidence-based pharmacotherapy when indicated.

- Further research is needed to better quantify the CVD risk conferred by disorders of pregnancy and gynecologic syndromes in addition to the role of sex-specific structural determinants of health to better enact change and decrease existing disparities.

DISCLOSURES

The authors of this publication have no disclosures.

REFERENCES

1. Cardiovascular diseases (CVDs). World Health Organization. 2021. Available at: https://www.who.int/news-room/fact-sheets/detail/cardiovascular-diseases-(cvds. Accessed July 10, 2024.
2. Centers for Disease Control and Prevention. Achievements in public health, 1900-1999: decline in deaths from heart disease and stroke–United States, 1900-1999. MMWR (Morb Mortal Wkly Rep) 1999;48:649–56.
3. Martin SS, Aday AW, Almarzooq ZI, et al. 2024 Heart disease and stroke statistics: a report of US and global data from the American Heart Association. Circulation 2024;149(8):e347–913.
4. Rodriguez F, Foody JM, Wang Y, et al. Young Hispanic women experience high in-hospital mortality following an acute myocardial infarction. J Am Heart Assoc 2015;4(9).
5. Cushman M, Shay CM, Howard VJ, et al. Ten year differences in women's awareness related to coronary heart disease: results of the 2019 American Heart Association national survey: a special report from the American Heart Association. Circulation 2021;143(7):e239–48.
6. Mosca L, Kinfante AH, Benjamin EJ, et al. National study of physician awareness and adherence to cardiovascular disease prevention guidelines. Circulation 2005;111(4):499–510.
7. Roger VL, Farkouh ME, Weston SA, et al. Sex differences in evaluation and outcome of unstable angina. JAMA 2000;283(5):646–52.
8. Gupta A, Wang Y, Spertus JA. Trends in acute myocardial infarction in young patients and differences by sex and race 2001 to 2010. J Am Coll Cardiol 2014;64(4):337–45.
9. Westfall E, Viere AB, Genewick JE. Preventing CVD in women: common questions and answers. Am Fam Physician 2023;108(6):595–604.
10. van Oosterhout REM, de Boer AR, Maas AHEM, et al. Peters SAE. Sex differences in symptom presentation in acute coronary syndromes: a systematic review and meta-analysis. J Am Heart Assoc 2020;9(9):e014733.

11. Lichtman JH, Leifheit EC, Safdar B, et al. Sex differences in the presentation and Perception of symptoms among young patients with myocardial infarction: evidence from the VIRGO study (variation in Recovery: role of gender on outcomes of young AMI patients). Circulation 2018;137(8):781–90.

12. Yahagi K, Davis HR, Arbustini E, et al. Sex differences in coronary artery disease: pathological observations. Atherosclerosis 2015;239(1):260–7.

13. Akhter N, Milford-Beland S, Roe MT, et al. Gender differences among patients with acute coronary syndromes undergoing percutaneous coronary intervention in the American College of Cardiology-National Cardiovascular Data Registry (ACC-NCDR). Am Heart J 2009;157(1):141–8.

14. Shajahan S, Sun L, Harris K, et al. Sex differences in the symptom presentation of stroke: a systematic review and meta-analysis. Int J Stroke 2023;18(2):144–53.

15. Cartland SP, Stanley CP, Bursill C, et al. Sex, endothelial cell functions, and peripheral artery disease. Int J Mol Sci 2023;24(24):17439.

16. Pabon M, Cheng S, Altin SE, et al. Sex differences in peripheral artery disease. Circ Res 2022;130(4):496–511.

17. DesJardin JT, Chikwe J, Hahn RT, et al. Sex differences and similarities in valvular heart disease. Circ Res 2022;130(4):455–73.

18. Clark D, Colantonio LD, Min YI, et al. Population-attributable risk for cardiovascular disease associated with hypertension in Black adults. JAMA Cardiol 2019;4: 1194–202.

19. Centers for Disease Control and Prevention and National Center for Health Statistics. National health and nutrition examination survey (NHANES) public use data files. Available at: https://cdc.gov/nchs/nhanes/. Accessed August 7, 2023.

20. Connelly PJ, Currie G, Delles C. Sex differences in the prevalence, outcomes and management of hypertension. Curr Hypertens Rep 2022;24(6):185–92.

21. Pana TA, Luben RN, Mamas MA, et al. Long term prognostic impact of sex-specific longitudinal changes in blood pressure. The EPIC-Norfolk Prospective Population Cohort Study. Eur J Prev Cardiol 2021;44. https://doi.org/10.1093/eurjpc/zwab104.

22. Zhao M, Woodward M, Vaartjes I, et al. Sex differences in cardiovascular medication prescription in primary care: a systematic review and meta-analysis. J Am Heart Assoc 2020;9. https://doi.org/10.1161/JAHA.119.014742.

23. Reboussin DM, Allen NB, Griswold ME, et al. Systematic review for the 2017 ACC/AHA/AAPA/ABC/ACPM/AGS/APhA/ASH/ASPC/NMA/PCNA guideline for the prevention, detection, evaluation, and management of high blood pressure in adults. Hypertension 2023;71(6):e116–35.

24. Sarwar N, Gao P, Seshasai SR, et al, Emerging Risk Factors Collaboration. Diabetes mellitus, fasting blood glucose concentration, and risk of vascular disease: a collaborative meta-analysis of 102 prospective studies. Lancet 2010;375: 2215–22.

25. Kautzky-Willer A, Leutner M, Harreiter J. Sex differences in type 2 diabetes. Diabetologia 2023;66(6):986–1002 [published correction appears in Diabetologia 2023;66(6):1165. doi:10.1007/s00125-023-05913-8].

26. Garcia M, Mulvagh SL, Merz CN, et al. Cardiovascular disease in women: clinical perspectives. Circ Res 2016;118(8):1273–93.

27. Wilson PW, D'Agostino RB, Sullivan L, et al. Overweight and obesity as determinants of cardiovascular risk: the Framingham experience. Arch Intern Med 2002; 162(16):1867–72.

28. Koceva A, Herman R, Janez A, et al. Sex- and gender-related differences in obesity: from pathophysiological mechanisms to clinical implications. Int J Mol Sci 2024;25(13):7342.

29. Kaminski P, Szpotanska-Sikorska M, Wielgos M. Cardiovascular risk and the use of oral contraceptives. Neuroendocrinol Lett 2013;34(7):587–9.

30. Huxley RR, Woodward M. Cigarette smoking as a risk factor for coronary heart disease in women compared with men: a systematic review and meta-analysis of prospective cohort studies. Lancet 2011;378(9799):1297–305.

31. Greaves L. The meanings of smoking to women and their implications for cessation. Int J Environ Res Publ Health 2015;12(2):1449–65.

32. Smith PH, Bessette AJ, Weinberger AH, et al. Sex/gender differences in smoking cessation: a review. Prev Med 2016;92:135–40.

33. Ji H, Gulati M, Huang T, et al. Sex differences in association of physical activity with all-cause and cardiovascular Mortality. JACC (J Am Coll Cardiol) 2024; 83(8):783–93.

34. Zimodro JM, Mucha M, Berthold HK, et al. Lipoprotein metabolism, dyslipidemia, and lipid-lowering therapy in women: a comprehensive review. Pharmaceuticals 2024;17(7):913.

35. Rachamin Y, Grischott T, Rosemann T, et al. Inferior control of low-density lipoprotein cholesterol in women is the primary sex difference in modifiable cardiovascular risk: a large-scale, cross-sectional study in primary care. Atherosclerosis 2021;324:141–7.

36. Peters S, Colantonio L, Zhao H, et al. Sex differences in high-intensity statin use following myocardial infarction in the United States. JACC (J Am Coll Cardiol) 2018;71(16):1729–37.

37. Stener-Victorin E, Teede H, Norman RJ, et al. Polycystic ovary syndrome. Nat Rev Dis Primers 2024;10(1):27.

38. Young L, Cho L. Unique cardiovascular risk factors in women. Heart 2019; 105(21):1656–60.

39. Wekker V, van Dammen L, Koning A, et al. Long-term cardiometabolic disease risk in women with PCOS: a systematic review and meta-analysis. Hum Reprod Update 2020;26(6):942–60.

40. Profili NI, Castelli R, Gidaro A, et al. Possible effect of polycystic ovary syndrome (PCOS) on cardiovascular disease (CVD): an update. J Clin Med 2024;13(3):698.

41. Zhao L, Zhu Z, Lou H, et al. Polycystic ovary syndrome (PCOS) and the risk of coronary heart disease (CHD): a meta-analysis. Oncotarget 2016;7(23): 33715–21.

42. Maas AH, Appelman YE. Gender differences in coronary heart disease. Neth Heart J 2010;18(12):598–602.

43. El Khoudary SR, Aggarwal B, Beckie TM, et al. Menopause transition and cardiovascular disease risk: implications for timing and early prevention: a scientific statement from the American Heart Association. Circulation 2020;142(25): e506–32.

44. Kok HS, van Asselt KM, van der Schouw YT, et al. Heart disease risk determines menopausal age rather than the reverse. J Am Coll Cardiol 2006;47(10):1976–83.

45. Zhu D, Chung HF, Pandeya N, et al. Premenopausal cardiovascular disease and age at natural menopause: a pooled analysis of over 170,000 women. Eur J Epidemiol 2019;34(3):235–46.

46. Muka T, Oliver-Williams C, Kunutsor S, et al. Association of age at onset of menopause and time since onset of menopause with cardiovascular outcomes,

Intermediate vascular traits, and all-cause mortality: a systematic review and meta-analysis. JAMA Cardiol 2016;1(7):767–76.

47. Appiah D, Schreiner PJ, Demerath EW, et al. Association of age at menopause with incident heart failure: a prospective cohort study and meta-analysis. J Am Heart Assoc 2016;5(8):e003769.

48. Breast cancer. World Health Organization. 2024. Available at: https://www.who.int/news-room/fact-sheets/detail/breast-cancer#:~:text=Femalegenderisthestrongest,breastcancersoccurinmen. Accessed August 11, 2024.

49. Mehta LS, Watson KE, Barac A, et al. Cardiovascular disease and breast cancer: where these entities intersect: a scientific statement from the american heart association. Circulation 2018;137(8):e30–66.

50. McGowan JV, Chung R, Maulik A, et al. Anthracycline chemotherapy and cardiotoxicity. Cardiovasc Drugs Ther 2017;31(1):63–75.

51. Darby SC, Ewertz M, McGale P, et al. Risk of ischemic heart disease in women after radiotherapy for breast cancer. N Engl J Med 2013;368(11):987–98.

52. Depressive disorder (depression). World Health Organization. 2023. Available at: https://www.who.int/news-room/fact-sheets/detail/depression. Accessed August 12, 2024.

53. Vaccarino V, Badimon L, Bremner JD, et al. Depression and coronary heart disease: 2018 position paper of the ESC working group on coronary pathophysiology and microcirculation. Eur Heart J 2020;41(17):1687–96 [published correction appears in Eur Heart J 2020;41(17):1696. doi:10.1093/eurheartj/ehz811].

54. Wassertheil-Smoller S, Shumaker S, Ockene J, et al. Depression and cardiovascular sequelae in postmenopausal women. The Women's Health Initiative (WHI). Arch Intern Med 2004;164(3):289–98.

55. AbuRuz ME, Al-Dweik G. Depressive symptoms and complications early after acute myocardial infarction: gender differences. Open Nurs J 2018;12:205–14.

56. Rivera MAM, Rivera IR, Avila W, et al. Depression and cardiovascular disease in women. Int J Cardiovasc Sci 2022;35(4):537–45.

57. Hinkle SN, Schisterman EF, Liu D, et al. Pregnancy complications and long-term mortality in a diverse cohort. Circulation 2023;147(13):1014–25.

58. Venkatesh KK, Khan SS, Yee LM, et al. Adverse pregnancy outcomes and predicted 30-year risk of maternal cardiovascular disease 2-7 Years after delivery. Obstet Gynecol 2024;143(6):775–84.

59. Andersgaard AB, Acharya G, Mathiesen EB, et al. Recurrence and long-term maternal health risks of hypertensive disorders of pregnancy: a population-based study. Am J Obstet Gynecol 2012 Feb;206(2):143.e1–8.

60. Hussien NA, Shuaib N, Baraia ZA, et al. Perceived cardiovascular disease risk following preeclampsia: a cross-sectional study. Healthcare (Basel) 2023;11(16):2356.

61. Gestational hypertension and preeclampsia: ACOG practice bulletin, Number 222. Obstet Gynecol 2020;135(6):e237–60.

62. Ford ND, Cox S, Ko JY, et al. Hypertensive disorders in pregnancy and mortality at delivery Hospitalization - United States, 2017-2019. MMWR Morb Mortal Wkly Rep 2022;71(17):585–91.

63. Vahedi FA, Gholizadeh L, Heydari M. Hypertensive disorders of pregnancy and risk of future cardiovascular disease in women. Nurs Womens Health 2020;24(2):91–100.

64. ACOG practice bulletin No. 190: gestational diabetes mellitus. Obstet Gynecol 2018;131(2):e49–64.

65. Tobias DK, Stuart JJ, Li S, et al. Association of history of gestational diabetes with long-term cardiovascular disease risk in a large prospective cohort of US women. JAMA Intern Med 2017;177(12):1735–42.

66. Caliskan M, Turan Y, Caliskan Z, et al. Previous gestational diabetes history is associated with impaired coronary flow reserve. Ann Med 2015;47(7):615–23.

67. Blencowe H, Cousens S, Chou D, et al. Born too soon: the global epidemiology of 15 million preterm births. Reprod Health 2013;10(Suppl 1):S2.

68. Wu P, Gulati M, Kwok CS, et al. Preterm delivery and future risk of maternal cardiovascular disease: a systematic review and meta-analysis. J Am Heart Assoc 2018;7(2):e007809.

69. Catov JM, Dodge R, Barinas-Mitchell E, et al. Prior preterm birth and maternal subclinical cardiovascular disease 4 to 12 years after pregnancy. J Womens Health (Larchmt) 2013;22(10):835–43.

70. Perng W, Stuart J, Rifas-Shiman SL, et al. Preterm birth and long-term maternal cardiovascular health. Ann Epidemiol 2015;25(1):40–5.

71. Catov JM, Lewis CE, Lee M, et al. Preterm birth and future maternal blood pressure, inflammation, and intimal-medial thickness: the CARDIA study. Hypertension 2013;61(3):641–6.

72. US Preventive Services Task Force, Curry SJ, Krist AH, Owens DK, et al. Risk assessment for cardiovascular disease with nontraditional risk factors: US preventive Services Task Force recommendation statement. JAMA 2018;320(3): 272–80. PMID: 29998297.

73. Arnett DK, Blumenthal RS, Albert MA, et al. 2019 ACC/AHA guideline on the primary prevention of cardiovascular disease: a report of the American College of Cardiology/American heart association Task Force on clinical practice guidelines. J Am Coll Cardiol 2019;74(10):e177–232 [published correction appears in J Am Coll Cardiol 2019;74(10):1429–30. doi:10.1016/j.jacc.2019.07.011] [published correction appears in J Am Coll Cardiol 2020;75(7):840. doi:10.1016/j.jacc.2019.12.016].

74. US Preventive Services Task Force. Screening for breast cancer: US preventive services task force recommendation statement. JAMA 2024;331(22):1918–30.

75. Koh TJW, Tan HJH, Ravi PRJ, et al. Association between breast arterial calcifications and cardiovascular disease: a systematic review and meta-analysis. Can J Cardiol 2023 Dec;39(12):1941–50. Epub 2023 Jul 26. PMID: 37506765.

76. Mosca L, Benjamin EJ, Berra K, et al. Effectiveness-based guidelines for the prevention of cardiovascular disease in women–2011 update: a guideline from the american heart association. Circulation 2011;123(11):1243–62 [published correction appears in Circulation 2011;123(22):e624] [published correction appears in Circulation 2011;124(16):e427].

77. Lewey J, Beckie TM, Brown HL, et al. Opportunities in the postpartum period to reduce cardiovascular disease risk after adverse pregnancy outcomes: a scientific statement from the American heart association. Circulation 2024;149(7): e330–46.

78. McDonald SD, Malinowski A, Zhou Q, et al. Cardiovascular sequelae of preeclampsia/eclampsia: a systematic review and meta-analyses. Am Heart J 2008;156(5):918–30.

79. McKenzie-Sampson S, Paradis G, Healy-Profitós J, et al. Gestational diabetes and risk of cardiovascular disease up to 25 years after pregnancy: a retrospective cohort study. Acta Diabetol 2018;55(4):315–22.

Chronic Pain Syndromes in Women

Karen Muchowski, MD

KEYWORDS

- Women and chronic pain • Fibromyalgia • Interstitial cystitis/bladder pain syndrome
- Chronic migraines • Chronic pelvic pain

KEY POINTS

- Chronic pain and chronic pain syndromes are more common in women.
- Comorbid anxiety and depression frequently occur in chronic pain syndromes.
- Multidisciplinary care can decrease pain and improve quality of life for all the chronic pain syndromes.

Chronic noncancer pain is common in adults across the world and women have higher rates of chronic pain than men.[1,2] Data from the 2021 National Health Interview survey showed that 22% of women and 19.7% of men in the United States have chronic pain.[3] More importantly, 7.6% of women have high impact pain (pain that disrupts daily functioning). Higher rates of pain and painful conditions continue as women age.[4] Compared to patients with other chronic diseases, patients with chronic pain conditions have higher levels of psychological distress, lower health related quality of life scores and incur health care costs 3 times higher than matched controls.[5]

Chronic pain conditions (fibromyalgia, irritable bowel syndrome, and migraine) are more common in women. Many theories exist on why women have more pain than men, but no clear etiology has been found. Studies on gender differences in pain are often preclinical, contradictory or inconclusive without enough convincing evidence to change clinical practice.[6] Gender differences in pain are likely from a complex interaction of genetic, physiologic, psychological, and social factors.[7]

Gender bias in health care and research may also play a role in how studies are reported and how patients are treated. Few studies compare pain in men to women, but women are often compared to men (andronormativity).[8] Some studies also demonstrate hegemonic masculinity in which masculine attributes are idealized as the norm against which both men and women are judged.[7] Women are more often described as being hysterical, emotional, or complainers. Women with chronic pain are more often

Graybill Medical Group, 31795 Rancho California Road, Suite 102, Temecula, CA 92591, USA
E-mail address: Muchowski3684@msn.com

Prim Care Clin Office Pract 52 (2025) 329–340
https://doi.org/10.1016/j.pop.2025.01.006
0095-4543/25/© 2025 Elsevier Inc. All rights are reserved, including those for text and data mining, AI training, and similar technologies.
primarycare.theclinics.com

Abbreviations	
CGRP	calcitonin gene-related peptide
COC	combined oral contraceptives
CPP	chronic pelvic pain
IC/BPS	interstitial cystitis/bladder pain syndrome
SNRIs	selective norepinephrine reuptake inhibitors
TCA	tricyclic antidepressants

assigned psychological rather than somatic causes for their pain and their narratives often focus on having to prove they are in pain to health care providers.[5]

In most pain syndromes, no clear etiology exists so treatment cannot be standardized. Because women often have multiple coexisting pain syndromes, it can take longer to elicit a patient's full history and do a physical. Multidisciplinary treatment has consistently been shown to decrease pain scores and improve quality of life. Education about chronic pain is beneficial and often gives a patient reassurance that something horrible (ie, cancer, multiple sclerosis) is not present. Nonpharmaceutical treatments (exercise, dietary changes, mindfulness-based therapies, and physical therapy) are helpful in most chronic pain disorders and can provide substantial relief in some patients. Pharmaceutical medications are available but often do not provide complete pain relief, so setting patient expectations is important. Opioids are not recommended for most pain disorders because they are not helpful and have a poor benefit to risk ratio.[9] Comorbid anxiety and depression are common and when present, worsen pain's impact on daily life. Although specialty care may be required, primary care physicians are well trained to primarily manage most pain syndromes and comorbid disorders.

FIBROMYALGIA

Fibromyalgia is a common chronic pain syndrome with a prevalence of 2% to 5% in women in the United States.[10] The incidence of fibromyalgia increases with age, with the highest rates of incidence in patients more than 45 years of age.[11] Current data points to abnormal central pain processing as the etiology of the syndrome. Evidence supports an imbalance in inhibitory neurotransmitters (serotonin, norepinephrine) and excitatory neurotransmitters (Substance P, glutamate).[12] Because of abnormal pain processing, hyperalgesia (increased sensitivity to painful stimuli) as well as allodynia (sensitivity to normally nonpainful stimuli) are common in fibromyalgia.

Patients with fibromyalgia have widespread pain. Other common symptoms include fatigue (up to 90%), sleep disturbance (up to 75%), headaches, morning stiffness, and cognitive issues. Comorbidities are common, with higher rates of depression, anxiety, headache syndromes, and irritable bowel syndrome than seen in the general population.[13] Patients with fibromyalgia will have a normal physical examination without evidence of synovitis or inflammatory disease.

Either the 2016 American College of Rheumatology[14] (https://www.fpmx.com.au/resources/office/New_Clinical_Fibromyalgia_Diagnostic_Criteria.pdf) or the Analgesic, Anesthetic, and Addiction Clinical Trial Translations Innovations Opportunities and Networks-American Pain Society Taxonomy[15] criteria can be used to make the diagnosis of fibromyalgia. These are 80% sensitive and 74% sensitive respectively for diagnosing fibromyalgia.[16] Laboratory testing is not required for the diagnosis of fibromyalgia but is useful in excluding other disorders.

Nonpharmacologic treatments should be the focus of therapy because they are more effective than pharmacologic treatments.[17] Simply establishing the diagnosis of fibromyalgia can improve satisfaction with health and decrease health care utilization.[18,19] The National Fibromyalgia Foundation has helpful resources if patients desire web-based education (https://www.fmaware.org/).

Cognitive behavioral therapy is an effective treatment of fibromyalgia.[20,21] It reduces pain, disability, and fatigue and improves health related quality of life. Exercise should be recommended for all patients with fibromyalgia. Aerobic and resistance exercise decreases depression and pain and improves quality of life, fatigue and sleep.[22,23] Studies involving lower intensity exercise or having a goal of 50% maximum heart rate had lower attrition rates and better symptom improvement.[24,25] Meditative movement therapies (Tai Chi, yoga) improve overall function, sleep, depression, and fatigue[26–28] Studies support the benefits of mindfulness-based interventions, hypnosis, electromyographic (EMG) biofeedback, and hydrotherapy.[29] Although many patients use cannabis products for treatment of their fibromyalgia[30] more research needs to be done to see if these products are clinically effective.[31]

Pharmacologic therapy is available for patients who do not have desired improvement with nonpharmacologic interventions. However, the effect sizes of many medications are modest, with a small number of patients achieving a 30% reduction in pain. Cyclobenzaprine is a muscle relaxer, but the chemical structure is similar to tricyclic antidepressants (TCAs). It produces a modest improvement in global functioning.[32] TCAs offer effective treatment of fibromyalgia, with amitriptyline being the most studied. Three meta-analyses have found a moderate to large effect on pain reduction.[24,33,34] The selective norepinephrine reuptake inhibitors (SNRIs) duloxetine and milnacipran have a small to moderate effect on pain reduction.[24,35] A systematic review of 5 studies found that pregabalin reduces pain versus placebo. Opioids and nonsteroidal anti-inflammatory medications are not recommended because of side effect profile and ineffectiveness.[9]

CHRONIC PELVIC PAIN

Chronic pelvic pain (CPP) has a world-wide prevalence of up to 26%[36] In the United States, it accounts for 40% of laparoscopies and 12% of hysterectomies.[37] The American College of Obstetrics and Gynecology describes CPP as pain symptoms perceived to originate from the pelvic organs/structures typically lasting more than 6 months. It is often associated with negative cognitive, behavioral, sexual, and emotional consequences as well as with symptoms suggestive of lower urinary tract, sexual, bowel, pelvic floor, myofascial or gynecologic dysfunction.[38] Women with CPP have higher rates of sleep disorders, prior physical and/or sexual abuse and in a specialty CPP clinic, one-third screened positive for post-traumatic stress disorder (PTSD).[39] Comorbid anxiety and depression is also common.[37] Imaging studies show increased activation in pain centers and decreased gray matter volume, which is seen in other chronic pain conditions.[40,41]

The most common causes of CPP include musculoskeletal pelvic floor pain, irritable bowel syndrome, interstitial cystitis, chronic uterine pain (leiomyoma, endometriosis, adenomyosis) and peripheral neuropathy (nerve entrapment syndromes). Musculoskeletal disorders are often underdiagnosed and were found in 50% to 90% of patients at CPP centers.[37] In women who have no identifiable cause, their pain can be part of other pain syndromes like fibromyalgia.

Because of the broad differential, a standardized history and examination form can be helpful. https://osher.ucsf.edu/sites/osher.ucsf.edu/files/inline-files/Chronic_Pelvic_Pain.pdf. A psychosocial assessment using standardized questionnaires like the patient health questionnaire (PHQ) and general anxiety disorder (GAD) 7 can identify comorbid depression and anxiety.

Physical examinations can be painful and emotionally difficult for patients with CPP. The examination should be chaperoned and fully explained to the patient before beginning. The musculoskeletal examination should include a full examination of the spine, sacroiliac joints, and hips. The abdominal examination can evaluate tenderness and abdominal wall trigger points. The genitourinary examination begins with an external examination. A moistened cotton swab can be used to identify painful areas on the thighs or external genitalia. A single digit internal examination can evaluate tenderness of the pelvic floor muscles, urethra, and bladder. A bimanual examination should be done to evaluated uterine and adnexal abnormalities and finally a speculum examination can visualize the vagina and cervix.

Treatment of CPP should be multidisciplinary. Cognitive behavioral therapy is helpful for other pain syndromes but has not specifically been studied in CPP. Pelvic floor physical therapy can reduce pain.[42] Although TCAs, SNRIs, and SSRIs are beneficial in other pain syndromes, they have not been studied in women with CPP. A recent randomized controlled trial (RCT) with gabapentin did not reduce pain in women with CPP. Opioids remain controversial, with some experts recommending weaning all women off of opioids for management of CPP[38] and some recommending considering after multiple other treatment modalities have been tried.[43] Small studies of abdominal wall and pelvic floor trigger point injection or peripheral nerve blocks have limited effectiveness.[37,38] Laparoscopic lysis of adhesions for management of CPP alone is not effective,[44] and there is limited evidence for support of laparoscopic uterosacral nerve ablation and presacral neurectomy.[38]

INTERSTITIAL CYSTITIS/BLADDER PAIN SYNDROME

Interstitial cystitis/bladder pain syndrome (IC/BPS) is a chronic pain syndrome involving the urinary system. Although the term interstitial cystitis was previously used, there is no inflammation in most patients who have this disorder, therefore the new name IC/BPS is currently recommended. The American Urology Association defines IC/BPS as an unpleasant sensation (pain, pressure, and discomfort) perceived to be related to the urinary bladder, associated with lower urinary tract symptoms of more than 6 weeks duration, in the absence of infection or other identifiable cause.[45] Studies show a prevalence of 0.1% to 2.3% with a 5-fold women predominance.[46] Symptoms can be daily, affected by social stress, diet, intercourse and prolonged sitting. Women often describe suprapubic, urethral, lower back or abdominal pain with bladder filling which is relieved with bladder emptying. Patients often have multiple low-volume voids per day to avoid bladder pain (whereas women with overactive bladder void multiple times a day to avoid incontinence).

The etiology is unknown and only 5% to 10% of women have visual and/or histologic changes on cystoscopy (Hunner lesions). Women with IC/BPS have higher rates of fibromyalgia, CPP, IBS, and migraines; therefore the cause of this syndrome is likely an interplay of immunologic and neurologic abnormalities affected by patient's environment and genetics. As with other chronic pain syndromes, women should be evaluated and treated for anxiety and depression.

Using the genitourinary pain index (https://elevation-physio.com/files/pdf/OCM-Female-GUPI.pdf) and a voiding diary (file:///C:/Users/Owner/Downloads/diary_508.pdf) can be helpful to evaluate the extent of symptoms and to follow intervention efficacy. In a large survey, 96% of women with IC/BPS felt that foods could worsen their symptoms (citrus fruits, tomatoes, coffee, tea, carbonated beverages, artificial sweeteners, and spicy foods).[47]

Examination should include the abdominal wall, hips, pelvic floor, bladder base and urethra as well as uterus and adnexal structures. Urinalysis and urine cultures are normal in IC/BPS, and abnormal results should result in further workup and/or consideration of a different etiology. Urologic guidelines recommend evaluation for incomplete bladder emptying in all patients.[46] Cystoscopy is not required to make the diagnosis but should be considered if there are abnormal findings on examinations or urine evaluation or if patients do not respond to initial interventions. Urodynamics are not required for evaluation and can be painful for patients.

As with other chronic pain syndromes, there is not 1 treatment that will benefit all patients and patients often respond to multimodal care. In a large study of women, 45% had improvement with behavioral modifications (understanding bladder function, urge suppression techniques, management of fluid intake, avoiding dietary triggers).[48] Another study showed that education on dietary triggers was helpful in reducing symptoms.[49] Both the International Cystitis Association (https://www.ichelp.org/understanding-ic/diet/the-ic-plate/) and the Interstitial Cystitis Network (https://www.ic-network.com/) have dietary information on their websites. In women who have pelvic floor tenderness, pelvic floor physical therapy is recommended.[45] Mindfulness based stress reduction improved pain self-efficacy and symptoms in women with IC/BPS.[50]

Oral analgesics (phenazopyridine, acetaminophen, and non-steroidal anti-inflammatory drugs [NSAIDs]) can be prescribed. Although amitriptyline is recommended in guidelines[45,46] the studies show minimal improvement in symptoms.[48,51] Amitriptyline may be helpful in women who have other disorders that could benefit from a TCA. Although supported only by single small studies of low-quality evidence, some guidelines recommend gabapentin, montelukast, sildenafil, or hydroxyzine.[45,46]

Pentosan polysulfate is the only Food and Drug Administration (FDA) approved medication for IC/BPS. It takes 3 to 6 months before a benefit is seen and is associated with a rare retinal pigmentary maculopathy. Therefore, patients will need retinal examinations before and periodically during treatment. Intravesicular installations (dimethyl sulfoxide [DMSO], lidocaine, and heparin), hydrodistension under anesthesia during cystoscopy, and treatment of Hunner lesions can improve pain in some patients.[45] If other treatments are not helpful, intradetrussor injections of onobotulinum toxin A may help some.[45] Major surgeries are rarely recommended and only for women who have not responded to all other therapies.

CHRONIC MIGRAINE

World-wide, migraine headaches are the #2 cause of years lived with disability for women and the #1 cause for women aged 15 to 49.[52] 17% of women will have a migraine each year and the cumulative lifetime incidence is 43% (vs 6% and 18% in men).[53,54] Migraines often start at menarche and can increase in the mid-30s, and in perimenopause. Migraines often worsen with menstruation but can improve in pregnancy, breastfeeding women, and menopause. Women have longer migraines, higher rates of recurrence, more symptoms (nausea, vomiting, photophobia, and phonophobia) and more migraine with aura than men.[55,56]

Migraines are classified into migraine without aura, migraine with aura, chronic migraine (headaches for >15 days a month) and migraine-overuse headache (headaches for >15 days a month in patients who take medications for headaches 10–15 days a month). For full details on the International classification of headache disorders criteria, see https://ihs-headache.org/en/resources/guidelines/. This review will focus on chronic migraines. As with other chronic pain syndromes, higher rates of anxiety, depression, and sleep disorders are present, and these associations are more pronounced in women with chronic migraine versus episodic migraine.[57] Women with migraines also have higher rates of cardiovascular disease and cardiovascular mortality.[58]

The pathophysiology of migraine is unknown. Estrogen is a central neural stimulator. Migraines may occur with sudden decreases or fluctuating levels of estrogen as seen before menses or in perimenopause. Lower estrogen levels may make blood vessels more permeable to pain producing prostaglandins. In addition, estrogen increases serotonergic tone, and serotonin is an important pain modulator (decreases pain).[56,59] Other neuropeptides are likely involved, with calcitonin gene-related peptide (CGRP) levels increasing during migraines and returning to normal once migraines resolve.[60]

A thorough history is often all that is needed to diagnose a migraine. Many migraines have triggers (stress, hormone levels, not eating, weather, and sleep disturbance).[61] It is important to consider medication overuse headache in women with frequent headaches. This is often underdiagnosed and most often occurs with the following medicines (in order of frequency): opioids, butalbital containing analgesics, aspirin-acetaminophen-caffeine combinations, and triptans.[62] Although it can be seen with NSAIDs, this group of medications is the least likely to cause medication overuse headaches. Taking the above medications for less than 10 days a month (or 15 days a month for acetaminophen, aspirin, or NSAIDs) effectively prevents overuse headaches. The treatment is to stop the inciting medication.

Although women with migraines have higher rates of strokes (11/100,000), taking combined oral contraceptives (COC) does not increase this risk unless women have migraine with aura. Taking COC increases risk of stroke 6-fold and is therefore contraindicated in women with migraine with aura.[63] Women taking hormone replacement (either estrogen or estrogen and progesterone) have higher rates of migraine.[59] However, women with migraines have higher rates of menopausal symptoms. Small studies evaluated the route and dosing of postmenopausal estrogen but have variable results. Variations in progesterone do not seem to influence migraines.

A neurologic examination should be normal. Neuroimaging modalities should only be ordered if a secondary cause of headache (tumor, infection) is considered. MRI is recommended over CT because of higher resolution and avoidance of ionizing radiation.[57]

Table 1
Behavioral interventions for treatment of chronic migraine

Intervention	Strength of Evidence	Source
Biofeedback	Moderate	Nestoriuc et al,[65] 2008
Lifestyle education	Low	Holroyd et al,[66] 2010; Bond et al,[67] 2018
Weight loss (behavioral or surgical)	Moderate	Di Vincenzo et al,[68] 2020
Exercise	Moderate	Varangot-Reille et al,[69] 2022
Craniosacral Therapy	Moderate	Haleer et al,[70] 2020
External trigeminal nerve stimulation	Moderate	Tao et al,[71] 2018
Acupuncture	Moderate	Linde et al,[72] 2016; Xu et al,[73] 2018

Table 2
Medications for treatment of chronic migraine

Medication	Strength of Evidence	Source
Coenzyme Q	Low	Sândor et al,[74] 2005
Riboflavin	Low	Schoenen et al,[75] 1998
Feverfew	Insufficient	Wider et al,[76] 2015
Magnesium	Insufficient	Teign et al,[77] 2015
NSAIDs (naproxen has the strongest data)	High	Gray et al,[78] 2010
Candesartan	High	Messina et al,[79] 2020; Tronvik et al,[80] 2003; Stovner et al,[81] 2014
Metoprolol	High	Pringsheim et al,[82] 2010; Shamliyan et al,[83] 2013
Propranolol	High	Shamliyan et al,[83] 2013; Reuter et al,[84] 2018
Amitriptyline	High	Shamliyan et al,[83] 2013; Reuter et al,[84] 2018
Topiramate	High	Reuter et al,[84] 2018
Valproate	High	Shamliyan et al,[83] 2013; Reuter et al,[84] 2018
CGRP antagonists (erenumab, fremanezumab, galcanezumab, eptinezumab, rimegepant, atogepant)	High	Nestoriuc et al,[65] 2008

Effective treatments are available for chronic migraine. This is most likely to occur with multimodal care (behavioral treatments, nonpharmaceutical interventions, and pharmaceutical medications).[64] Please see **Table 1** for behavioral interventions and **Table 2** for a list of medications effective for chronic migraine. Although there are many medications that can decrease migraine frequency, only the CGRP targeting therapies are specifically made for the treatment of migraine. Multiple studies have shown that this class of medication is safe, is at least as effective as other preventative therapies and has less side effects. The American Headache Society recently recommended that this class be first-line for the treatment of chronic migraines.[60]

STRENGTH OF EVIDENCE SCALE
High

High confidence that the evidence reflects the true effect. Further research is very unlikely to change the confidence in the estimate of effect.

Moderate

Moderate confidence that the evidence reflects the true effect. Further research may change the confidence in the estimate of effect and may change the estimate.

Low

Low confidence that the evidence reflects the true effect. Further research is likely to change the confidence in the estimate of effect and is likely to change the estimate.

Insufficient

Evidence either is unavailable or does not permit a conclusion.

CLINICS CARE POINTS

- Behavioral and nonpharmacological interventions decrease pain and improve function and should be offered to all patients with chronic pain.
- Evidence-based pharmacologic medications improve functioning in patients with fibromyalgia, chronic pelvic pain, interstitial cystitis/bladder pain syndrome, and chronic migraine.
- Opioids are not recommended for most chronic pain syndromes.

DISCLOSURE

Dr K. Muchowski is on the medical advisory board and an investor in Defined Research, a company evaluating CBD products for the treatment of insomnia.

REFERENCES

1. Andrews P, Steultjens M, Riskowski J. Chronic widespread pain prevalence in the general population: a systematic review. Eur J Pain 2018;22(1):5–18.
2. Lamerato LE, Dryer RD, Wolff GG, et al. Prevalence of chronic pain in a large integrated healthcare delivery system in the USA. Pain Pract 2016;16(7):890–8.
3. https://www.cdc.gov/mmwr/volumes/72/wr/mm7215a1.htm.
4. Larsson C, Hansson EE, Sundquist K, et al. Chronic pain in older adults: prevalence, incidence, and risk factors. Scand J Rheumatol 2017;46(4):317–25.
5. Dukes E, Martin S, Edelsberg J, et al. Characteristics and healthcare costs of patients with fibromyalgia syndrome. Int J Clin Pract 2007;61(9):149801508.
6. Casale R, Atzeni F, Bazzichi L, et al. Pain in women: a perspective review on a relevant clinical issue that deserves prioritization. Pain and Ther 2021;10: 287–314.
7. Pieretti S, Di Giannuario A, Di Giovannandrea R, et al. Gender differences in pain and its relief. Ann Ist Super Sanita 2016;52(2):184–9.
8. Samulowitz A, Gremyr I, Eriksson E, et al. "Brave men" and "emotional women": a theory-guided literature review on gender bias in health care and gendered norms towards patients with chronic pain. Pain Res Manag 2018;2018.
9. Winslow BT, Vandal C, Dang L. Fibromyalgia: diagnosis and management. Am Fam Physician 2023;107(2):137–44.
10. Arnold LM, Clauw DJ, Dunegan LJ, et al. A framework for fibromyalgia management for primary care providers. Mayo Clin Proc 2012;87(5):488–96.
11. Weir P, Harlan G, Nkoy F, et al. The incidence of fibromyalgia and its associated comorbidities: a population-based retrospective cohort study based on international classification of diseases, 9th revision codes. J Clin Rheumatol 2006; 12(3):124–8.
12. Rahman A, Underwood M, Carnes D. Fibromyalgia, clinical review. BMJ 2014; 348:g1224.
13. Elvin A, Siosteen A, Nilsson A, et al. Decreased muscle blood flow in fibromyalgia patients during standardized muscle exercise: a contrasat media enhanced colour Doppler study. Eur J Pain 2006;10(2):137–44.

14. Wolfe F, Clauw DJ, Fitzcharles MA, et al. 2016 revisions to the 2010/2011 fibromyalgia diagnostic criteria. Semin Arthritis Rheum 2016;46(3). WB Saunders.
15. Arnold LM, Bennett RM, Crofford LJ, et al. AAPT diagnostic criteria for fibromyalgia. J Pain 2019;20(6):611–28.
16. Salaffi F, Di Carlo M, Farah S, et al. Diagnosis of fibromyalgia: comparison of the 2011/2016 ACR and AAPT criteria and validation of the modified Fibromyalgia Assessment Status. Rheumatology 2020;59(10):3042–9.
17. Nuesch E, Hauser W, Bernardy K, et al. Comparative efficacy of pharmacological and non-pharmacological interventions in fibromyalgia syndrome: network meta-analysis. Ann Rheum Dis 2013;72:955–62.
18. White KP, Nielson WR, Harth M, et al. Does the label "fibromyalgia" alter health status, function and health service utilization? A prospective, within-group comparison in a community cohort of adults with chronic widespread pain. Arthritis Rheum 2002;47(3):260–5.
19. Annemans L, Wessely S, Spaepen E, et al. Health economic consequences related to the diagnosis of fibromyalgia syndrome. Arthritis Rheum 2008;58(3):895–902.
20. Mascarenhas RO, Souza MB, Oliveira MX, et al. Association of therapies with reduced pain and improved quality of life in patients with fibromyalgia: a systematic review and meta-analysis. JAMA Intern Med 2021;181(1):104–12.
21. Bernardy K, Klose P, Welsch P, et al. Efficacy, acceptability and safety of cognitive behavioural therapies in fibromyalgia syndrome–A systematic review and meta-analysis of randomized controlled trials. Eur J Pain 2018;22(2):242–60.
22. Couto N, Monteiro D, Cid L, et al. Effect of different types of exercise in adult subjects with fibromyalgia: a systematic review and meta-analysis of randomised clinical trials. Sci Rep 2022;12(1):10391.
23. Estévez-López F, Maestre-Cascales C, Russell D, et al. Effectiveness of exercise on fatigue and sleep quality in fibromyalgia: a systematic review and meta-analysis of randomized trials. Arch Phys Med Rehabil 2021;102(4):752–61.
24. Dupree-Jones K, Adams D, Winters-Stone K, et al. A comprehensive review of 46 exercise treatment studies in fibromyalgia (1988-2005). Health Qual Life Outcome 2006;4(67).
25. 2012 Canadian guidelines for the diagnosis and management of fibromyalgia syndrome. Available at: www.canadianpainsociety.ca/pdf/Fibromyalgia_Guidelines_2012.pdf.
26. Mist S, Firestone K, Dupree Jones K. Complementary and alternative exercise for fibromyalgia: a meta-analysis. J Pain Res 2013;6:247–60.
27. Langhorst J, Klose P, Dobos G, et al. Efficacy and safety of meditative movement therapies in fibromyalgia syndrome: a systematic review and meta-analysis of randomized controlled trials. Rheumatol Int 2013;33:193–207.
28. Bravo C, Skjaerven LH, Guitard Sein-Echaluce L, et al. Effectiveness of movement and body awareness therapies in patients with fibromyalgia: a systematic review and meta-analysis. Eur J Phys Rehabil Med 2019;55(5):646–57.
29. Lauche R, Cramer H, Häuser W, et al. A systematic overview of reviews for complementary and alternative therapies in the treatment of the fibromyalgia syndrome. Evid base Compl Alternative Med 2015;1(2015):610615.
30. Singla A, Anstine CV, Huang L, et al. A cross-sectional survey study of cannabis use for fibromyalgia symptom management. Mayo Clin Proc 2024;99(4). Elsevier.
31. Bourke SL, Schlag AK, O'Sullivan SE, et al. Cannabinoids and the endocannabinoid system in fibromyalgia: a review of preclinical and clinical research. Pharmacol Ther 2022;240:108216.

32. Tofferi JK, Jackson JL, O'Malley PG. Treatment of fibromyalgia with cyclobenzaprine: a meta-analysis. Arthritis Rheum 2004;51(1):9–13.
33. Hauser W, Bernardy K, Uceyler N, et al. Treatment of fibromyalgia syndrome with antidepressants, a meta-analysis. JAMA 2009;301(2):198–209.
34. Hauser W, Wolfe F, Tolle T, et al. The role of antidepressants in the management of fibromyalgia syndrome: a systematic review and meta-analysis. CNS Drugs 2012; 26(4):297–307.
35. Hauser W, Urrutia G, Tort S, et al. Serotonin and norepinephrine reuptake inhibitors (SNRIs) for fibromyalgia syndrome. Cochrane Database Syst Rev 2013;4. Available at: http://www.thecochranelibrary.com.
36. Ahangari A. Prevalence of chronic pelvic pain among women: an updated review. Pain Physician 2014;17(2):E141–7.
37. Zaks N, Batuure A, Lin E, et al. Association between mental health and reproductive system disorders in women: a systematic review and meta-analysis. JAMA Netw Open 2023;6(4):e238685.
38. Pain, Chronic Pelvic. "ACOG practice bulletin" number 218. Obstet Gynecol 2020;3:e98–109.
39. Meltzer-Brody S, Leserman J, Zolnoun D, et al. Trauma and posttraumatic stress disorder in women with chronic pelvic pain. Obstet Gynecol 2007;109(4):902–8.
40. Hampson JP, Reed BD, Clauw DJ, et al. Augmented central pain processing in vulvodynia. J Pain 2013;14(6):579–89.
41. As-Sanie S, Harris RE, Napadow V, et al. Changes in regional gray matter volume in women with chronic pelvic pain: a voxel-based morphometry study. PAIN® 2012;153(5):1006–14.
42. FitzGerald MP, Anderson RU, Potts J, et al. Randomized multicenter feasibility trial of myofascial physical therapy for the treatment of urological chronic pelvic pain syndromes. J Urol 2009;182(2):570–80.
43. Jarrell JF, Vilos GA, Allaire C, et al. No. 164-consensus guidelines for the management of chronic pelvic pain. J Obstet Gynaecol Can 2018;40(11):e747–87.
44. van den Beukel BA, de Ree R, van Leuven S, et al. Surgical treatment of adhesion-related chronic abdominal and pelvic pain after gynaecological and general surgery: a systematic review and meta-analysis. Hum Reprod Update 2017;23(3):276–88.
45. Clemens JQ, Erickson DR, Varela NP, et al. Diagnosis and treatment of interstitial cystitis/bladder pain syndrome. J Urol 2022;208(1):34–42.
46. Homma Y, Akiyama Y, Tomoe H, et al. Clinical guidelines for interstitial cystitis/ bladder pain syndrome. Int J Urol 2020;27(7):578–89.
47. Bassaly R, Downes K, Hart S. Dietary consumption triggers in interstitial cystitis/ bladder pain syndrome patients. Urogynecology 2011;17(1):36–9.
48. Foster HE, Hanno PM, Nickel JC, et al. Effect of amitriptyline on symptoms in treatment naïve patients with interstitial cystitis/painful bladder syndrome. J Urol 2010;183(5):1853–8.
49. Oh-Oka H. Clinical efficacy of 1-year intensive systematic dietary manipulation as complementary and alternative medicine therapies on female patients with interstitial cystitis/bladder pain syndrome. Urology 2017;106:50–4.
50. Kanter G, Komesu YM, Qaedan F, et al. Mindfulness-based stress reduction as a novel treatment for interstitial cystitis/bladder pain syndrome: a randomized controlled trial. Int Urogynecol J 2016;27:1705–11.
51. van Ophoven ARNDT, Pokupic S, Heinecke A, et al. A prospective, randomized, placebo controlled, double-blind study of amitriptyline for the treatment of interstitial cystitis. J Urol 2004;172(2):533–6.

52. Steiner TJ, Stovner LJ, Jensen R, et al. Migraine remains second among the world's causes of disability, and first among young women: findings from GBD2019. J Headache Pain 2020;21:1–4.
53. Lipton RB, Bigal ME, Diamond M, et al. Migraine prevalence, disease burden, and the need for preventive therapy. Neurology 2007;68(5):343–9.
54. Stewart WF, Wood C, Reed ML, et al. Cumulative lifetime migraine incidence in women and men. Cephalalgia 2008;28(11):1170–8.
55. Allais G, Chiarle G, Sinigaglia S, et al. Gender-related differences in migraine. Neurol Sci 2020;41:429–36.
56. Todd C, Lagman-Bartolome AM, Lay C. Women and migraine: the role of hormones. Curr Neurol Neurosci Rep 2018;18:1–6.
57. Eigenbrodt AK, Ashina H, Khan S, et al. Diagnosis and management of migraine in ten steps. Nat Rev Neurol 2021;17(8):501–14.
58. Kurth T, Winter AC, Eliassen AH, et al. Migraine and risk of cardiovascular disease in women: prospective cohort study. BMJ 2016;353:i2610.
59. Ripa P, Ornello R, Degan D, et al. Migraine in menopausal women: a systematic review. Int J Wom Health 2015;7:773–82.
60. Charles AC, Digre KB, Goadsby PJ, et al. Calcitonin gene-related peptide-targeting therapies are a first-line option for the prevention of migraine: an American Headache Society position statement update. Headache J Head Face Pain 2024;64(4):333–41.
61. Kelman L. The triggers or precipitants of the acute migraine attack. Cephalalgia 2007;27(5):394–402.
62. Ljubisavljevic S, Ljubisavljevic M, Damjanovic R, et al. A descriptive review of medication-overuse headache: from pathophysiology to the comorbidities. Brain Sci 2023;13(10):1408.
63. Champaloux SW, Tepper NK, Monsour M, et al. Use of combined hormonal contraceptives among women with migraines and risk of ischemic stroke. Am J Obstet Gynecol 2017;216(5):489.e1–7.
64. Seok JI, Cho HI, Chung CS. From transformed migraine to episodic migraine: reversion factors. Headache J Head Face Pain 2006;46(7):1186–90.
65. Nestoriuc Y, Martin A, Rief W, et al. Biofeedback treatment for headache disorders: a comprehensive efficacy review. Appl Psychophysiol Biofeedback 2008;33:125–40.
66. Holroyd KA, Cottrell CK, O'Donnell FJ, et al. Effect of preventive (β blocker) treatment, behavioural migraine management, or their combination on outcomes of optimised acute treatment in frequent migraine: randomised controlled trial. BMJ 2010;341.
67. Bond DS, Thomas JG, Lipton RB, et al. Behavioral weight loss intervention for migraine: a randomized controlled trial. Obesity 2018;26(1):81–7.
68. Di Vincenzo A, Beghetto M, Vettor R, et al. Effects of surgical and non-surgical weight loss on migraine headache: a systematic review and meta-analysis. Obes Surg 2020;30:2173–85.
69. Varangot-Reille C, Suso-Martí L, Romero-Palau M, et al. Effects of different therapeutic exercise modalities on migraine or tension-type headache: a systematic review and meta-analysis with a replicability analysis. J Pain 2022;23(7):1099–122.
70. Haller H, Lauche R, Sundberg T, et al. Craniosacral therapy for chronic pain: a systematic review and meta-analysis of randomized controlled trials. BMC Muscoskel Disord 2020;21:1–14.

71. Tao H, Wang T, Dong X, et al. Effectiveness of transcutaneous electrical nerve stimulation for the treatment of migraine: a meta-analysis of randomized controlled trials. J Headache Pain 2018;19:1–10.
72. Linde K, Allais G, Brinkhaus B, et al. Acupuncture for the prevention of episodic migraine. Cochrane Database Syst Rev 2016;6.
73. Xu J, Zhang FQ, Pei J, et al. Acupuncture for migraine without aura: a systematic review and meta-analysis. J Integr Med 2018;16(5):312–21.
74. Sândor PS, Di Clemente L, Coppola G, et al. Efficacy of coenzyme Q10 in migraine prophylaxis: a randomized controlled trial. Neurology 2005;64(4):713–5.
75. Schoenen J, Jean J, Lenaerts M. Effectiveness of high-dose riboflavin in migraine prophylaxis A randomized controlled trial. Neurology 1998;50(2):466–70.
76. Wider B, Pittler MH, Ernst E. Feverfew for preventing migraine. Cochrane Database Syst Rev 2015;4.
77. Teigen L, Boes CJ. An evidence-based review of oral magnesium supplementation in the preventive treatment of migraine. Cephalalgia 2015;35(10):912–22.
78. Gray RN, Goslin RE, McCrory DC, et al. Drug treatments for the prevention of migraine headache. Rockville (MD): Agency for Health Care Policy and Research (US); 1999.
79. Messina R, Lastarria Perez CP, Filippi M, et al. Candesartan in migraine prevention: results from a retrospective real-world study. J Neurol 2020;267:3243–7.
80. Tronvik E, Stovner LJ, Helde G, et al. Prophylactic treatment of migraine with an angiotensin II Receptor Blocker: a randomized controlled trial. JAMA 2003; 289(1):65–9.
81. Stovner LJ, Linde M, Gravdahl GB, et al. A comparative study of candesartan versus propranolol for migraine prophylaxis: a randomised, triple-blind, placebo-controlled, double cross-over study. Cephalalgia 2014;34(7):523–32.
82. Pringsheim T, Davenport WJ, Becker WJ. Prophylaxis of migraine headache. CMAJ (Can Med Assoc J) 2010;182(7):E269–76.
83. Shamliyan TA, Choi JY, Ramakrishnan R, et al. Preventive pharmacologic treatments for episodic migraine in adults. J Gen Intern Med 2013;28:1225–37.
84. Reuter U, Goadsby PJ, Lanteri-Minet M, et al. Efficacy and tolerability of erenumab in patients with episodic migraine in whom two-to-four previous preventive treatments were unsuccessful: a randomised, double-blind, placebo-controlled, phase 3b study. Lancet 2018;392(10161):2280–7.

Mental Health Disorders in Women

William E. Michael, MD[1], Karina Atwell, MD, MPH[2],
Jennifer Svarverud, DO*

KEYWORDS

- Mental health • Women • Depression • Anxiety

KEY POINTS

- Depression and anxiety are more common in women. Women tend to respond better to SSRI/SNRI treatment than men.
- Women should be screened throughout pregnancy and following delivery for perinatal and postpartum mood disorders.
- It's estimated that women experience PTSD at two to three times the rate that men do.
- Somatic symptom disorders often coexist with anxiety and depression and have a 10:1 female predominance.
- Cognitive Behavioral Therapy for Insomnia (CBT-I) is considered first-line treatment for insomnia before considering sleep medications.

INTRODUCTION

Mental health conditions are more prevalent among women, with 27.2% of females experiencing any mental illness (AMI) compared to 18.1% of males, and a similar pattern observed with serious mental illness.[1] Additionally, women with AMI were more likely to receive mental health services (51.7%) than men (40.0%).[1] 40% of office visits for mental health concerns occur in primary care settings, with primary care physicians responsible for 47% of prescriptions for mental illness.[2] Over 36% of active psychiatrists are over age 65 and only 12.3% are under 40. As such, the reliance on primary care physicians to deliver mental health care is going to increase.[3] This chapter explores common mental health diagnoses and treatment in women.

ANXIETY DISORDERS

The lifetime prevalence for anxiety disorders is 30.5% for women and 19.2% for men.[4] Women with anxiety are more likely to engage the medical system than men through

Department of Family Medicine and Community Health, Family Medicine Residency Program, School of Medicine and Public Health, University of Wisconsin, Madison, WI, USA
[1] Present address: 1121 Bellwest Boulevard, Belleville, WI 53508.
[2] Present address: 100 North Nine Mound Road, Verona, WI 53593.
* Corresponding author. 100 North Nine Mound Road, Verona, WI 53593.
E-mail address: jennifer.svarverud@fammed.wisc.edu

Prim Care Clin Office Pract 52 (2025) 341–351
https://doi.org/10.1016/j.pop.2025.01.007
0095-4543/25/© 2025 Elsevier Inc. All rights are reserved, including those for text and data mining, AI training, and similar technologies.

Abbreviations	
AMI	any mental illness
BD	bipolar disorder
CBT	cognitive behavioral therapy
CBT-I	cognitive behavioral therapy for insomnia
EPDS	Edinburgh postpartum depression scale
MBSR	mindfulness-based stress reduction
PMDD	premenstrual dysphoric disorder
PMS	premenstrual syndrome
PPD	postpartum depression
PTSD	posttraumatic stress disorder
SNRIs	serotonin and norepinephrine reuptake inhibitors
SSRIs	selective serotonin reuptake inhibitors

emergency room (ER), urgent care, and doctor office visits (1.04 visits/month vs 0.71 visits/month) and more than half of the medical costs for individuals with anxiety are related to nonpsychiatric expenditures.[4] Women with anxiety are more likely to experience fatigue, lassitude, autonomic disturbances, sleep reduction and pain than men.[5]

Nonpharmaceutical approaches are as effective as monotherapy or as augmentation to pharmacologic treatments. Cognitive Behavioral Therapy (CBT) is particularly beneficial for treating anxiety, surpassing other forms of psychotherapy.[6] For women who want to minimize pharmacologic exposure during pregnancy or while trying to conceive, CBT is especially advantageous.[7] Regular exercise, stress management techniques (eg, yoga, mindfulness meditation, tai chi),[8] and certain diets like the Mediterranean diet have also demonstrated benefits in reducing anxiety and improving mood disorders.[9]

First-line pharmaceutical treatments for anxiety disorders include Selective Serotonin Reuptake Inhibitors (SSRIs) and Serotonin and Norepinephrine Reuptake Inhibitors (SNRIs).[10] Females respond better to serotonergic antidepressant medications than men, but this increase in effect wanes in postmenopausal women.[11] Benzodiazepines may be used short-term but have dose-dependent side effects and addiction risks; intermediate-acting (eg, chlordiazepoxide) or long-acting (eg, clonazepam) benzodiazepines carry a lower dependency risk.[12]

Sertraline, Fluoxetine, Escitalopram, and Citalopram are specifically recommended as first-line medications in pregnancy by ACOG, though previously effective anxiety medications should also be considered.[7] Benzodiazepines should be avoided or used sparingly during pregnancy due to their side effect profile, dependency risk, and potential for neonatal withdrawal.[7]

Managing anxiety in pregnant and postpartum patients is crucial, underscored by the United States Preventitive Services Task Force (USPSTF) and American College of Obstetricians and Gynecologists (ACOG) recommending anxiety screening during pregnancy and postpartum. Severe anxiety during pregnancy is an independent risk factor for mood and behavioral issues in offspring and is associated with pre-term delivery and low birth weight.[13,14] During perimenopause and menopause, anxiety symptoms are linked to vasomotor symptoms, though the effectiveness of hormone replacement therapy (HRT) in treating anxiety in these patients shows mixed results and is not recommended to solely treat anxiety symptoms.[15]

SLEEP DISORDERS

The percentage of adults taking sleep medications increases with age, and women are more likely to be prescribed medications than men (10.2% vs 6.6%).[16] The American

Academy of Sleep Medicine recommends CBT-I before prescribing sleep medications, and Brief Behavioral Therapy for Insomnia can be used in the primary care setting while awaiting CBT-I.[17] CBT-I combines traditional CBT methods with stimulus control and sleep restriction therapy.[10] While non-pharmacologic management is preferred for women, especially when pregnant or breastfeeding, medication use may be acceptable in certain cases (**Table 1**). During pregnancy, sleep disturbances are common with 80% of women reporting sleep concerns at some point.[18] A Danish study of over 1,300 pregnant women taking benzodiazepine receptor agonists, such as zolpidem, did not find an increased risk of teratogenicity.[19] However, transplacental transfer occurs, and neonatal withdrawal symptoms have been documented.[18] Benzodiazepines and benzodiazepine receptor agonists may be associated with increased risks of preterm labor, cesarean section, and low birth weight.[20] In breastfeeding women, discussing sleep medication use can be supported by internet-based resources, such as InfantRisk and LactMed. Poor sleep quality and sleep disorders are highly prevalent during menopause, independent of vasomotor symptoms.[21] As with other life stages, CBT-I should be the first-line intervention for menopausal patients.[22] For menopausal patients with or without vasomotor symptoms, hormone therapy has shown a small benefit on perceived sleep quality[23] and can be considered in select women.

SOMATIC SYMPTOM DISORDERS

Somatic symptom disorders are characterized by significant preoccupation with physical symptoms, leading to functional impairment.[24] Somatic symptom disorder is prevalent in 5% to 7% of the general population, with a notable female-to-male ratio of 10:1.[25] Unlike previous editions, the Diagnostic and Statistical Manual of Mental Disorders, 5th Edition (DSM-5) does not require these symptoms to be "unexplained", and may have chronic medical conditions with an abnormal, heightened response to the physical symptoms, potentially warranting an additional diagnosis of somatic symptom disorder.[10] Effective treatment combines psychotherapy, particularly cognitive-behavioral therapy (CBT) and mindfulness, with medication. Avoiding over-testing and maintaining frequent, short-interval follow-ups have been shown to be beneficial.[10] Cognitive-behavioral therapy is highly effective in addressing maladaptive thoughts and behaviors related to physical symptoms.[26] Mindfulness-

Table 1
Somatic symptom scale – 8 (SSS-8)

During the *past 7 d*, How Much Have You Been Bothered by Any of the following Problems?					
	Not at All	A Little Bit	Somewhat	Quite a Bit	Very Much
Stomach or bowel problems	0	1	2	3	4
Back pain	0	1	2	3	4
Pain in your arms, legs, or joints	0	1	2	3	4
Headaches	0	1	2	3	4
Chest pain or shortness of breath	0	1	2	3	4
Dizziness	0	1	2	3	4
Feeling tired or having low energy	0	1	2	3	4
Trouble sleeping	0	1	2	3	4

Based Stress Reduction (MBSR) techniques can help manage stress and reduce symptom severity.[27] SSRIs and SNRIs can be effective, especially when treating co-morbid anxiety and depression, with a number needed to treat (NNT) of 3.[10] Tricyclic antidepressants (TCAs), like amitriptyline, can also be used at lower doses but must be prescribed cautiously due to anticholinergic side effects and potential teratogenic risks in patients who are pregnant or planning pregnancy.[28] Treatment effectiveness can be monitored using the Somatic Symptom Scale-8 (SSS-8), a validated retrospective patient questionnaire (see **Table 1**).[29]

EATING DISORDERS

Between 2.6% and 8.4% of females experience an eating disorder during their life, including subthreshold or atypical eating disorders.[30] Anorexia nervosa and bulimia nervosa are estimated to be three times more likely in women than men.[31,32] Lesbian and bisexual women are more likely to engage in binge-eating behaviors than any other gender and sexuality. This population also reports a higher prevalence of purging and laxative use than heterosexual groups.[33,34]

Girls are at the greatest risk of developing eating disorders between late childhood into late adolescence.[35] Women's reproductive events, especially pregnancy and menopause, reflect a complex blend of biopsychosocial phenomena leaving women psychologically vulnerable.[36] Comparable levels of dieting and disordered eating are now found across young and elderly women.[37] In middle-aged women, aged 40 to 60, 4.6% met the full criteria for a clinical eating disorder, while another 4.8% met the subthreshold standards.[38] In US women over age 50, 79% report that weight/shape affects their self-image; 41% weigh themselves daily; 36% spent at least half of the last 5 years dieting; 13.3% report eating disorder symptoms; and 8% report purging.[39]

Eating disorders affect every system in the body, including electrolyte imbalances, endocrine dysfunction, increased risk for osteopenia and osteoporosis, and a compromised immune system. In adult women, eating disorders can deplete fat stores exacerbates the decline in estrogen level, accelerate natural neuromuscular decline, and raise mortality risk associated with low weight.[40]

Multiple validated screening tools exist for use in primary care settings to help identify possible disordered eating and indications for additional evaluation and treatment.[41,42]

TRAUMA RELATED DISORDERS

About half of all women in the U.S. will be exposed to at least one traumatic event in their lifetime.[43] While women are somewhat less likely to experience traumatic events overall, they are more vulnerable to high impact traumas, like sexual assault and childhood sexual abuse, than men.[44–47] It's estimated that women experience PTSD at two to three times the rate that men do.[48] U.S. prevalence estimates of lifetime PTSD from the National Comorbidity Survey Replication are 9.7% for women and 3.6% for men.[43]

Women may be more susceptible to mental health consequences of trauma because they are more like to experience trauma within established relationships, or their traumatic exposures are more chronic than those experienced by men (eg, ongoing interpersonal violence).[48] Women are more likely to report co-occurring internalizing disorders like anxiety and depression versus externalizing disorders like substance abuse.[44,47] They seek more social support after trauma, the lack of it being the most consistent predictor of negative outcome of trauma, and a more powerful resilience factor for women compared to men.[49]

Several psychosocial factors have been identified that increase the risk for PTSD following trauma exposure,[50,51] including:

- Pre-existing mental health problems
- Family history of mental health problems
- Experiencing additional life stressors
- Availability of post-trauma social support

The treatments of choice for PTSD are psychological interventions, such as trauma-focused cognitive behavioral therapy and eye movement desensitization and reprocessing (EMDR).[52,53] Several pharmacological approaches (fluoxetine, paroxetine, sertraline, and venlafaxine) reduce PTSD symptoms, but with a lower effect size than psychological treatments.[54] Evidence suggests women have greater reduction in clinician and patient-rated PTSD symptoms with trauma-focused psychological interventions.[55]

DEPRESSION

Depression is up to two times more common in women as compared to men in both the United States and elsewhere in the world.[56] Research shows that women have bimodal peaks of incidence across their lifetime, one at the beginning of adolescence and then again in the late 40s to early 50s. One theory correlates to sex hormone changes, as these ages are associated with onset of menarche and menopause respectively.[57] Potential mechanisms include the effect of estrogen on the hypothalamic-pituitary axis, specifically in regulation of neurotransmitters including serotonin, gaba-aminobutyric acid (GBA) and cortisol.[58] Other psychosocial risk factors include abuse and increased risk of development of depression after a serious life event.[59] Family history of depression significantly increases risk.[60] Notably, women present more with physical symptoms including appetite changes, sleep issues, sexual disturbance and loss of interest and pleasure and are less likely to report substance use/abuse as compared to men.[61] Rates of depression among women of different ethnic groups does vary; however, a study of women of differing ethnic backgrounds with intimate partner violence, supports that decreased education and lower income are associated with increased risk of depression, contributing to the health disparities seen in individuals with lower socioeconomic status.[62] Similar to anxiety, women have better response to serotonergic antidepressants (SSRI/SNRI) than men, and post-menopausal women tend to have decreased response to antidepressants as compared to younger women.[11] In post-menopausal women specifically, SSRIs and SNRIs remain first line therapy for treatment of depression, but hormone replacement therapy has been shown to improve mood and can be considered as an adjunct treatment option.[63] Exercise and behavioral therapy are supported as first line treatments along with medications; however, no difference has been seen in response to these interventions in women compared to men.[64]

Perinatal depression and postpartum depression (PPD) confer increased risk for both infant and maternal health. One study showed rates of minor depression in the perinatal period increased to 17% as compared to 11% in non-pregnant women; however, there was no difference in major depression between the two groups.[6] All pregnant women should be screened for depression at initial prenatal visit, later in pregnancy and during post-partum visits.[65] Although no specific guidelines exist regarding which screening tool should be utilized, the Edinburgh post-partum depression scale (EPDS) is commonly utilized.[65,66] Specifically in the post-partum period, rates of depression peak at two and 6 months.[67] The American Academy of Pediatrics recommends screening post-partum mothers at one, two and 4 months postpartum.[68] Multiple studies have shown an association with increased behavioral issues, poorer language and IQ development, and increased rates of gastrointestinal and lower respiratory tract infections in children of mothers with PPD.[69] Growing literature suggests that the EPDS may under diagnose post-partum depression in African American women who have higher rates of discrimination stress, systemic and structural racism stress and abuse by their partner, and that women with these exposures are at two-fold higher odds of developing depression during pregnancy.[70,71] One study of 261 African American women showed that an initial obstetric visit EPDS score $\geq$ 10 was associated with increased risk for preeclampsia, preterm birth and low birth weight.[72] ACOG guidelines recommend psychotherapy as first line treatment for mild to moderate perinatal depression.[7] Initial pharmacologic treatment for both perinatal and PPD is SSRIs; however, SNRIs are considered reasonable second line.[7]

PREMENSTRUAL SYNDROME/PREMENSTRUAL DYSPHORIC DISORDER

Premenstrual disorders encompasses both premenstrual syndrome (PMS) as well as the more severe form of premenstrual dysphoric disorder (PMDD), diagnostic criteria. The integrative medicine chapter reviews many of the nonpharmaceutical and diet approaches to treatment of premenstrual disorders and this section will focus on pharmaceutical treatment consideration. First line pharmacologic treatment includes SSRIs and can be dosed either continuously or intermittently (at onset of symptoms through menses) with similar efficacy.[73,74] Combined oral contraceptives have been shown to have moderate decrease in overall symptoms compared to placebo; however, evidence is low to moderate and has not shown improvement in mood specific symptoms.[73] For severe cases that fail these treatments, Gonadotropin-Releasing Hormone Agonists can be used to induce anovulation, and failing this surgical management with oophorectomy may be considered.[73] Other treatments recommended by ACOG with low quality evidence include acupuncture and nonsteroidal anti-inflammatory drugs during the luteal phase.[73]

BIPOLAR DISORDER

Bipolar disorder (BD) affects 0.5% to 1.0% of the world's population and is characterized by alterations in mood, levels of energy, and functioning.[10] Sex may affect epidemiology and clinical features at presentation (**Table 2**). For instance, hormonal oscillations related to the menstrual and reproductive cycle may influence clinical course and treatment and symptoms may worsen when gonadal hormone levels are low.[75] A recent meta-analysis found an overall postpartum relapse risk of 35%.[76] Discontinuation of psychopharmaceutical interventions during pregnancy may trigger a mood recurrence leading to disruption of daily functioning and ability to parent.[77] Clinicians must balance the risk-benefit analysis of pharmacotherapy for BD during pregnancy for each patient, considering illness severity, past pregnancy treatment outcomes, psychosocial supports, and key windows during fetal development.

Agents approved for the treatment of BD, mania, or both include lithium, the anticonvulsants carbamazepine, lamotrigine and valproate, and the second-generation antipsychotics aripiprazole, olanzapine, quetiapine, risperidone, and ziprasidone. Gender-specific considerations should be taken, such as teratogenicity (lithium and valproic acid), breastfeeding risks (lithium), interactions between mood stabilizers and oral contraceptives and HRT, and the risk of hyperprolactinemia with typical and atypical antipsychotics.[10]

Table 2
Gender differences in bipolar disorder

	Females	Males
Epidemiology	• Higher frequency of BD type 2 diagnosis	• Equal frequency of BD types 1 and 2 diagnosis
Features of clinical Presentation	• Depressive onset and recurrences • Hypomania • Mixed episodes • Rapid cycling • Suicide attempts • Longer time to first recurrence	• Manic onset • Childhood onset of mania • More deaths by suicide
Common comorbidities	• Personality disorders • Eating disorders • PTSD • Panic disorder • Organic disorders (eg, hypothyroidism) • Alcohol abuse (BD 2)	• Alcohol and other substance-related disorders • Pathologic gambling • Obsessive compulsive disorder (OCD)

Adapted from Ref.[78]

CLINICS CARE POINTS

- Depression and anxiety are up to two times more common in women compared to men.
- First line treatments for anxiety and depression in women include SSRI and SNRI medications, along with non-pharmaceutical treatments including Cognitive Behavioral Therapy (CBT), exercise, stress management and dietary modifications.
- Women respond better to serotonergic antidepressant medications than men, but this increase in effect wanes in post-menopausal women.
- For post-menopausal women, SSRI/SNRIs remain first line treatment for depression, however hormone replacement therapy can be considered if no improvement in symptoms with these medications.
- Treatment for somatic symptom disorders involves a combination of psychotherapy (particularly CBT and Mindfulness-Based Stress Reduction) and medication.
- Women are more likely than men to experience high-impact traumas, such as sexual assault and childhood sexual abuse, leading to higher rates of PTSD compared to men.
- First line treatment for PMDD includes SSRIs, dosed either continuously or intermittently.

DISCLOSURE

None.

REFERENCES

1. Mental illness, Available at: https://www.nimh.nih.gov/health/statistics/mental-illness (Accessed 6 August 2024).
2. Mental health services, Available at: https://www.aafp.org/about/policies/all/mental-health-services.html (Accessed 6 August 2024).
3. US physican workforce data, Available at: https://www.aamc.org/data-reports/report/us-physician-workforce-data-dashboard (Accessed 6 August 2024).

4. McLean CP, Asnaani A, Litz BT, et al. Gender differences in anxiety disorders: prevalence, course of illness, comorbidity and burden of illness. J Psychiatr Res 2011;45(8):1027–35.

5. Pesce L, van Veen T, Carlier I, et al. Gender differences in outpatients with anxiety disorders: the leiden routine outcome monitoring study. Epidemiol Psychiatr Sci 2016;25(3):278–87.

6. Papola D, Miguel C, Mazzaglia M, et al. Psychotherapies for generalized anxiety disorder in adults: a systematic review and network meta-analysis of randomized clinical trials. JAMA Psychiatr 2024;81(3):250–9.

7. Treatment and management of mental health conditions during pregnancy and postpartum: ACOG clinical practice guideline No. 5. Obstet Gynecol 2023; 141(6):1262–88.

8. Saeed SA, Cunningham K, Bloch RM. Depression and anxiety disorders: benefits of exercise, yoga, and meditation. Am Fam Physician 2019;99(10):620–7.

9. Firth J, Gangwisch JE, Borisini A, et al. Food and mood: how do diet and nutrition affect mental wellbeing? BMJ 2020;369:m2382.

10. McCarron RM. Association of medicine and psychiatry primary care psychiatry. 2nd edition. Philadelphia (PA): Lippincott Williams and Wilkins; 2019. p. 394, xvii.

11. Sramek JJ, Murphy MF, Cutler NR. Sex differences in the psychopharmacological treatment of depression. Dialogues Clin Neurosci 2016;18(4):447–57.

12. Locke AB, Kirst N, Shultz CG. Diagnosis and management of generalized anxiety disorder and panic disorder in adults. Am Fam Physician 2015;91(9):617–24.

13. O'Donnell KJ, Glover V, Barker ED, et al. The persisting effect of maternal mood in pregnancy on childhood psychopathology. Dev Psychopathol 2014;26(2): 393–403.

14. Ding XX, Wu YL, Xu SJ, et al. Maternal anxiety during pregnancy and adverse birth outcomes: a systematic review and meta-analysis of prospective cohort studies. J Affect Disord 2014;159:103–10.

15. Stute P, Lozza-Fiacco S. Strategies to cope with stress and anxiety during the menopausal transition. Maturitas 2022;166:1–13.

16. Reuben C, Elgaddal N, Black LI. Sleep medication use in adults aged 18 and over: United States, 2020. NCHS Data Brief 2023;462:1–8.

17. Edinger JD, Arnedt JT, Bertisch SM, et al. Behavioral and psychological treatments for chronic insomnia disorder in adults: an American Academy of Sleep Medicine clinical practice guideline. J Clin Sleep Med 2021;17(2):255–62.

18. Miller MA, Mehta N, Clark-Bilodeau C, et al. Sleep pharmacotherapy for common sleep disorders in pregnancy and lactation. Chest 2020;157(1):184–97.

19. Wikner BN, Källén B. Are hypnotic benzodiazepine receptor agonists teratogenic in humans? J Clin Psychopharmacol 2011;31(3):356–9.

20. Reichner CA. Insomnia and sleep deficiency in pregnancy. Obstet Med 2015; 8(4):168–71.

21. Baker FC, Lampio L, Saaresranta T, et al. Sleep and sleep disorders in the menopausal transition. Sleep Med Clin 2018;13(3):443–56.

22. McCurry SM, Guthrie KA, Morin CM, et al. Telephone-based cognitive behavioral therapy for insomnia in perimenopausal and postmenopausal women with vasomotor symptoms: a MsFLASH randomized clinical trial. JAMA Intern Med 2016; 176(7):913–20.

23. Cintron D, Lipford M, Larrea-Mantilla L, et al. Efficacy of menopausal hormone therapy on sleep quality: systematic review and meta-analysis. Endocrine 2017;55(3):702–11.

24. Löwe B, Levenson J, Depping M, et al. Somatic symptom disorder: a scoping review on the empirical evidence of a new diagnosis. Psychol Med 2022;52(4): 632–48.

25. Kurlansik SL, Maffei MS. Somatic symptom disorder. Am Fam Physician 2016; 93(1):49–54.

26. Kroenke K. Efficacy of treatment for somatoform disorders: a review of randomized controlled trials. Psychosom Med 2007;69(9):881–8.

27. Lakhan SE, Schofield KL. Mindfulness-based therapies in the treatment of somatization disorders: a systematic review and meta-analysis. PLoS One 2013;8(8): e71834.

28. O'Malley PG, Jackson JL, Santoro J, et al. Antidepressant therapy for unexplained symptoms and symptom syndromes. J Fam Pract 1999;48(12):980–90.

29. Gierk B, Kohlmann S, Kroenke K, et al. The somatic symptom scale-8 (SSS-8): a brief measure of somatic symptom burden. JAMA Intern Med 2014;174(3): 399–407.

30. Halbeisen G, Braks K, Huber TJ, et al. Gender differences in treatment outcomes for eating disorders: a case-matched, retrospective pre-post comparison. Nutrients 2022;14(11). https://doi.org/10.3390/nu14112240.

31. Statistics and Research on Eating Disorders. National eating disorders association, Available at: https://www.nationaleatingdisorders.org/statistics-research-eating-disorders (Accessed 26 June 2024).

32. Striegel-Moore RH, Rosselli F, Perrin N, et al. Gender difference in the prevalence of eating disorder symptoms. Int J Eat Disord 2009;42(5):471–4.

33. Nagata JM, Ganson KT, Austin SB. Emerging trends in eating disorders among sexual and gender minorities. Curr Opin Psychiatry 2020;33(6):562–7.

34. Parker LL, Harriger JA. Eating disorders and disordered eating behaviors in the LGBT population: a review of the literature. J Eat Disord 2020;8:51.

35. Smolak L, Levine MP, Striegel-Moore R. The developmental psychopathology of eating disorders : implications for research, prevention, and treatment. England, UK: Routledge; 1996. p. 438, xxiii.

36. Mangweth-Matzek B, Hoek HW, Rupp CI, et al. The menopausal transition–a possible window of vulnerability for eating pathology. Int J Eat Disord 2013; 46(6):609–16.

37. Lewis DM, Cachelin FM. Body image, body dissatisfaction, and eating attitudes in midlife and elderly women. Eat Disord 2001;9(1):29–39.

38. Mangweth-Matzek B, Hoek HW, Rupp CI, et al. Prevalence of eating disorders in middle-aged women. Int J Eat Disord 2014;47(3):320–4.

39. Gagne DA, Von Holle A, Brownley KA, et al. Eating disorder symptoms and weight and shape concerns in a large web-based convenience sample of women ages 50 and above: results of the Gender and Body Image (GABI) study. Int J Eat Disord 2012;45(7):832–44.

40. Maine MD, Samuels KL, Tantillo M. Eating disorders in adult women: biopsychosocial, developmental, and clinical considerations. Adv Eat Disord 2015;3(2):133–43.

41. Feltner C, Peat C, Reddy S, et al. Screening for eating disorders in adolescents and adults: evidence report and systematic review for the US preventive services task force. JAMA 2022;327(11):1068–82.

42. Cotton MA, Ball C, Robinson P. Four simple questions can help screen for eating disorders. J Gen Intern Med 2003;18(1):53–6.

43. Mitchell KS, Mazzeo SE, Schlesinger MR, et al. Comorbidity of partial and subthreshold ptsd among men and women with eating disorders in the national comorbidity survey-replication study. Int J Eat Disord 2012;45(3):307–15.

44. Kessler RC, Sonnega A, Bromet E, et al. Posttraumatic stress disorder in the national comorbidity survey. Arch Gen Psychiatry 1995;52(12):1048–60.

45. Breslau N, Davis GC, Andreski P, et al. Traumatic events and posttraumatic stress disorder in an urban population of young adults. Arch Gen Psychiatry 1991;48(3):216–22.

46. Norris FH, Foster JD, Weisshaar DL. The epidemiology of gender differences in PTSD across developmental, societal, and research contexts. Gender and PTSD. New York City (NY): The Guilford Press; 2002. p. 3–42.

47. Tolin DF, Foa EB. Sex differences in trauma and posttraumatic stress disorder: a quantitative review of 25 years of research. Psychol Bull 2006;132(6):959–92.

48. Kimerling R, Weitlauf JC, Iverson KM, et al. Gender issues in PTSD. Handbook of PTSD: science and practice. 2nd edition. New York City (NY): The Guilford Press; 2014. p. 313–30.

49. Olff M. Sex and gender differences in post-traumatic stress disorder: an update. Eur J Psychotraumatol 2017;8(sup4):1351204.

50. Brewin CR, Andrews B, Valentine JD. Meta-analysis of risk factors for posttraumatic stress disorder in trauma-exposed adults. J Consult Clin Psychol 2000;68(5):748–66.

51. Ozer EJ, Best SR, Lipsey TL, et al. Predictors of posttraumatic stress disorder and symptoms in adults: a meta-analysis. Psychological Trauma: Theory, Research, Practice, and Policy 2008;S(1):3–36.

52. Bisson JI, Olff M. Prevention and treatment of PTSD: the current evidence base. Eur J Psychotraumatol 2021;12(1):1824381.

53. Lewis C, Roberts NP, Andrew M, et al. Psychological therapies for post-traumatic stress disorder in adults: systematic review and meta-analysis. Eur J Psychotraumatol 2020;11(1). https://doi.org/10.1080/20008198.2020.1729633.

54. Hoskins MD, Bridges J, Sinnerton R, et al. Pharmacological therapy for post-traumatic stress disorder: a systematic review and meta-analysis of monotherapy, augmentation and head-to-head approaches. Eur J Psychotraumatol 2021;12(1). https://doi.org/10.1080/20008198.2020.1802920.

55. Wade D, Varker T, Kartal D, et al. Gender difference in outcomes following trauma-focused interventions for posttraumatic stress disorder: systematic review and meta-analysis. Psychol Trauma 2016;8(3):356–64.

56. Burt VK, Stein K. Epidemiology of depression throughout the female life cycle. J Clin Psychiatry 2002;63(Suppl 7):9–15.

57. Parker G, Brotchie H. Gender differences in depression. Int Rev Psychiatry 2010;22(5):429–36.

58. Labaka A, Goñi-Balentziaga O, Lebeña A, et al. Biological sex differences in depression: a systematic review. Biol Res Nurs 2018;20(4):383–92.

59. Keita GP. Psychosocial and cultural contributions to depression in women: considerations for women midlife and beyond. J Manag Care Pharm 2007;13(9 Suppl A):S12–5.

60. Colvin A, Richardson GA, Cyranowski JM, et al. Does family history of depression predict major depression in midlife women? Study of Women's Health Across the Nation Mental Health Study (SWAN MHS). Arch Womens Ment Health 2014;17(4):269–78.

61. Cavanagh A, Wilson CJ, Kavanagh DJ, et al. Differences in the expression of symptoms in men versus women with depression: a systematic review and meta-analysis. Harv Rev Psychiatry 2017;25(1):29–38.

62. Montalvo-Liendo N, Grogan-Kaylor A, Graham-Bermann S. Ethnoracial variation in depression symptoms. Hisp Health Care Int 2016;14(2):81–8.

63. Lumsden MA, Davies M, Sarri G, Guideline Development Group for Menopause: Diagnosis and Management (NICE Clinical Guideline No. 23). Diagnosis and management of menopause: the national institute of health and care excellence (NICE) guideline. JAMA Intern Med 2016;176(8):1205–6.

64. Farr SL, Dietz PM, Williams JR, et al. Depression screening and treatment among nonpregnant women of reproductive age in the United States, 1990-2010. Prev Chronic Dis 2011;8(6):A122.

65. Screening and diagnosis of mental health conditions during pregnancy and post-partum: ACOG clinical practice guideline No. 4. Obstet Gynecol 2023;141(6): 1232–61.

66. Lancaster CA, Gold KJ, Flynn HA, et al. Risk factors for depressive symptoms during pregnancy: a systematic review. Am J Obstet Gynecol 2010;202(1):5–14.

67. Pearlstein T, Howard M, Salisbury A, et al. Postpartum depression. Am J Obstet Gynecol 2009;200(4):357–64.

68. Earls MF, Committee on Psychosocial Aspects of Child and Family Health American Academy of Pediatrics. Incorporating recognition and management of perinatal and postpartum depression into pediatric practice. Pediatrics 2010;126(5): 1032–9.

69. O'Hara MW, McCabe JE. Postpartum depression: current status and future directions. Annu Rev Clin Psychol 2013;9:379–407.

70. Sroka AW, Mbayiwa K, Ilyumzhinova R, et al. Depression screening may not capture significant sources of prenatal stress for Black women. Arch Womens Ment Health 2023;26(2):211–7.

71. Bower KM, Geller RJ, Jeffers N, et al. Experiences of racism and perinatal depression: findings from the pregnancy risk assessment monitoring system, 2018. J Adv Nurs 2023;79(5):1982–93.

72. Kim DR, Sockol LE, Sammel MD, et al. Elevated risk of adverse obstetric outcomes in pregnant women with depression. Arch Womens Ment Health 2013; 16(6):475–82.

73. Management of Premenstrual Disorders: ACOG clinical practice guideline No. 7. Obstet Gynecol 2023;142(6):1516–33.

74. Marjoribanks J, Brown J, O'Brien PM, et al. Selective serotonin reuptake inhibitors for premenstrual syndrome. Cochrane Database Syst Rev 2013;2013(6): CD001396.

75. Gogos A, Ney LJ, Seymour N, et al. Sex differences in schizophrenia, bipolar disorder, and post-traumatic stress disorder: are gonadal hormones the link? Br J Pharmacol 2019;176(21):4119–35.

76. Vega P, Barbeito S, Ruiz de Azúa S, et al. Bipolar disorder differences between genders: special considerations for women. Womens Health (Lond) 2011;7(6): 663–74 [quiz: 675–4].

77. Wesseloo R, Kamperman AM, Munk-Olsen T, et al. Risk of postpartum relapse in bipolar disorder and postpartum psychosis: a systematic review and meta-analysis. Am J Psychiatry 2016;173(2):117–27.

78. Dell'Osso B, Cremaschi L, Macellaro M, Cafaro R, Gender and sex issues in bipolar disorder, Available at: https://www.psychiatrictimes.com/view/gender-and-sex-issues-in-bipolar-disorder (Accessed 22 June 2024).

Bone Health in Women

Brenna Gibbons, MD[1], Julia Lubsen, MD[1],
Andrea Ildiko Martonffy, MD*

KEYWORDS

• Osteoporosis • Fragility fracture • Bone density

KEY POINTS

• Clinicians should focus on bone health across the lifespan as almost 50% of women in the United States will sustain an osteoporotic fracture.
• To support bone health, recommend adequate calcium, vitamin D, and physical activity and avoidance of tobacco and alcohol use.
• Bone density testing should begin at age 65 for most women, and earlier for those at higher risk for osteoporosis.
• Once identified by bone density testing or history of fragility fracture, osteoporosis evaluation should include a laboratory evaluation to look for causes of secondary osteoporosis.
• Oral bisphosphonates are the first-line treatment for osteoporosis.

ARTICLE

Definition

Osteoporosis is a condition of decreased bone mass and altered bone architecture that results in weakened bones. This weakening increases risk for fracture with resultant morbidity and mortality.[1,2]

Pathophysiology

Osteoporosis is characterized by loss of bone mass through architectural deterioration on a microscopic level, which can be measured by a dual-energy x-ray absorptiometry (DEXA) scan to measure bone density at the femoral neck, lumbar spine, and sometimes the distal radius. Bone strength is affected by the bone turnover rate—the rate at which old bone is resorbed and new bone is created. These factors that determine bone quality mean that older women are particularly vulnerable to osteoporosis since menopause-related decreases in estrogen levels increase bone resorption and decrease new bone formation.

Department of Family Medicine and Community Health, University of Wisconsin, Madison, WI, USA
[1] Present address: 1121 Bellwest Boulevard, Belleville, WI 53508.
* Corresponding author. 610 N. Whitney Way, Suite 200, Madison, WI 53705.
E-mail address: ildi.martonffy@fammed.wisc.edu

Prim Care Clin Office Pract 52 (2025) 353–370
https://doi.org/10.1016/j.pop.2025.01.008
0095-4543/25/© 2025 Elsevier Inc. All rights are reserved, including those for text and data mining, AI training, and similar technologies.

Abbreviations	
ACP	American College of Physicians
AFF	atypical femoral fracture
DEXA	dual-energy x-ray absorptiometry
IV	intravenous
ONJ	osteonecrosis of the jaw
PTH	parathyroid hormone
VTE	venous thromboembolic disease

Osteoporosis is diagnosed when bone density is 2.5 or more standard deviations below that of a young adult (T score). Less severe bone loss, or osteopenia, is defined as bone density ranging between 1 and 2.5 standard deviations below that of a young adult. In both cases, fracture risk increases as bone loses density and strength.[3]

Epidemiology

Worldwide, osteoporosis is thought to affect over 200 million women with osteoporotic fractures causing significant pain, morbidity, and mortality.[4] One-year mortality post hip fracture is estimated to be as high as 14% to 58%, with significant burden to finances and independence even to those who thrive clinically.[5] Of the 10 million people in the United States who have osteoporosis, approximately 80% are women, and approximately half of American women older than age 50 will break a bone due to osteoporosis.[3] In the United States, the cost of osteoporosis-related fracture treatment and resultant care needs is estimated at $17.9 billion annually.[6]

Presentation

Hip fractures, vertebral fractures, and distal forearm fractures are the most common types of osteoporotic fractures, often occurring after simple mechanical falls. Screening is particularly important because many women do not become aware that they have osteoporosis until they experience a fracture.

Osteoporosis Screening

Newly updated US Preventive Services Task Force guidelines recommend screening for osteoporosis using bone density testing in all women age 65 and over as well as postmenopausal women under age 65 who are at increased risk for an osteoporotic fracture (grade B recommendations).[7] The level of risk for women under age 65 should be determined using a formal clinical risk assessment tool such as the fracture risk assessment tool (FRAX) fracture risk assessment tool.[8,9] There are no consistent guidelines for screening transgender patients.[10]

Good quality evidence to inform screening and follow-up intervals for bone density testing is lacking. For patients on osteoporosis treatment, expert recommendations suggest repeating DEXA after 1 year of initiating medication therapy and after 1 year of changing medication therapy.[11] In those not qualifying for treatment, the American College of Preventive Medicine and the American Academy of Family Physicians (AAFP) Choosing Wisely Campaign recommend bone density screening no more frequently than every 2 years while the National Osteoporosis Foundation and the Bone Health and Osteoporosis Foundation recommend screening every 2 years[12]

Data from a single cohort study of 4,957 women age 67 and older indicate that consideration should be given to adjusting screening intervals based on a woman's bone density on initial screening. This study found that in women with normal bone density or mild osteopenia on initial testing, osteoporosis would develop in just 10%

of postmenopausal women over 15 years. For women with moderate osteopenia and advanced osteopenia, this 10% threshold was reached at 5 years and 1 year, respectively.[13]

Indications for early screening for osteoporosis are outlined in **Box 1**.

For postmenopausal women, lower T scores correlate with higher fracture risk. For premenopausal women, a Z score is reported which is a measure of the difference between the patient's bone density and an average bone density of healthy age, sex, and ethnicity matched peers.[14]

The American Association of Clinical Endocrinologists/American College of Endocrinology Clinical Practice (AACE/ACE) recommends pharmacologic treatment for people who are in 1 of 3 categories: those with osteopenia and history of a fragility fracture of the hip or spine; those with T score −2.5 even in absence of fracture history; and those with T score −1.0 to −2.5 with 10-year FRAX probability of major osteoporotic fracture greater than 20% or hip fracture greater than 3% with other groups setting forth similar recommendations.[15] Tools for shared decision-making can be used to facilitate an informed discussion about risks and benefits of treatment with patients using graphical models that represent the impact of treatment decisions based on the patients' own fracture risk data.[16,17] Clinicians should be aware that the FRAX tool has received some criticism for underestimating fracture risk in minoritized people and thus creating risk for undertreatment of osteoporosis in these patients.[18]

OSTEOPOROSIS EVALUATION

Patients who have osteoporosis should have a comprehensive evaluation looking for modifiable risk factors and medical conditions that affect bone health.[15]

History and Physical

The clinician should ask about prior fractures and how they were sustained. Low-impact (fragility) fractures are fractures that occur due to a fall from standing height or less, or a similar force, excluding fractures of the face, skull, fingers, and toes. Low-impact injuries generally would not be expected to cause a fracture in normal bone. A history of height loss, kyphosis, or spinal tenderness on examination suggests the possibility of vertebral fractures that may not have previously come to clinical attention. The history should identify risk factors for low bone density including smoking, excessive alcohol intake (3 or more drinks per day), early menopause, and a family history of osteoporosis. It is also important to assess fall risk using validated tools such as those described in the Centers for Disease Control and Prevention Stopping Elderly

---

Box 1
Indications for early screening for osteoporosis[15]

All postmenopausal women:
  With a history of fracture(s) without major trauma
  With osteopenia identified radiographically
  Starting or taking long-term systemic glucocorticoid therapy ($\geq$3 months)

Other perimenopausal or postmenopausal women with risk factors for osteoporosis if willing to consider pharmacologic interventions:
  BMI <20 kg/m^2
  Family history of osteoporotic fracture
  Premature menopause
  Current smoking status
  Alcohol use >2 drinks/day

Accidents, Deaths & Injuries (CDC STEADI) algorithm, and to assess gait, lower extremity strength, and balance as contributors to fall risk and therefore fracture risk.[19] The history and physical examination should look for medical conditions and medications that can cause osteoporosis, and comorbidities that could affect osteoporosis treatment decisions (see **Box 1**), including a history of chronic kidney disease, dental disease, gastroesophageal reflux disease, and esophageal disease.

Medications and medical conditions that contribute to osteoporosis are listed in **Table 1**.

Table 1
Medications and medical conditions that contribute to osteoporosis

Medications
  Antiepileptic drugs (phenobarbital,
    phenytoin, primidone, valproate,
    carbamazepine)
  Aromatase inhibitors
  Androgen deprivation therapy
  Chemotherapy
  Depot medroxyprogesterone acetate
    (Depo-Provera)
  Glucocorticoids
  Gonadotropin-releasing
    hormone agonists and antagonists
  Heparin
  Immunosuppressants
    (cyclosporin A, tacrolimus)
  Lithium
  Methotrexate
  Proton pump inhibitors
  Selective serotonin
    reuptake inhibitors
  Sodium-Glucose Cotransporter-2 (SGLT2)-
    inhibitors
  Tamoxifen
  Thiazolidinediones
  Thyroid hormone (excess dosing)
Lifestyle Factors
  Alcohol use
  Immobilization
  Physical inactivity
  Smoking
Gastrointestinal/Nutrition
  Anorexia nervosa
  Calcium deficiency
  Celiac disease
  Chronic liver disease
  Gastrointestinal surgery
    including bariatric surgery
  High salt intake
  Inflammatory bowel disease
  Low calcium intake
  Malabsorption syndromes
  Pancreatic disease
  Total parenteral nutrition
  Vitamin A excess
  Vitamin D deficiency

Endocrine
  Acromegaly
  Cushing's syndrome
  Diabetes mellitus (type 1 and 2)
  Female athlete triad
  Growth hormone deficiency
  Hyperparathyroidism
  Hyperprolactinemia
  Hyperthyroidism
  Hypogonadism
  Premature menopause
Genetic disorders
  Cystic fibrosis
  Ehlers-Danlos syndrome
  Gaucher disease
  Homocystinuria
  Hypophosphatasia
  Hypophosphatemia
  Marfan syndrome
  Osteogenesis imperfecta
  Porphyria
  Turner's and Klinefelter's syndromes
Hematologic disorders
  Hemophilia
  Leukemia and lymphoma
  Monoclonal gammopathies
  Multiple myeloma
  Sickle cell disease
  Systemic mastocytosis
  Thalassemia
Other
  Acquired immunodeficiency syndrome/
    human immunodeficiency virus
  Ankylosing spondylitis
  Chronic obstructive pulmonary disease
  Chronic kidney disease
  Hypercalciuria
  Organ transplantation
  Renal tubular acidosis
  Rheumatoid arthritis
  Systemic lupus erythematosus

Data from AACE/ACE Guideline Table 12[16]; The Clinician's Guide Table 1[12]; AAFP Table 4.[21]

Laboratory Evaluation

The AACE/ACE Clinical Practice Guideline[15,20] recommends the following laboratory evaluation for people with osteoporosis:

Complete blood count

Comprehensive metabolic panel (including electrolytes, calcium, total protein, albumin, liver enzymes, alkaline phosphatase)

Phosphate

Serum 25-hydroxy vitamin D

Serum parathyroid hormone

24-hour urine collection for calcium, sodium, and creatinine—collect once patient has adequate vitamin D levels and calcium intake for at least 2 weeks

Additional tests if clinically indicated:

Serum thyroid stimulating hormone (patients on thyroid hormone replacement or with symptoms of thyroid disease)

Tissue transglutaminase antibodies (for suspected celiac disease)

Serum protein electrophoresis and free kappa and lambda light chains (for suspected myeloma)

Imaging

Only about 23% of vertebral fractures seen on plain radiographs come to clinical attention.[21] These often clinically silent fractures can lead to a diagnosis of osteoporosis in patients with T-scores greater than −2.5 and can affect treatment decisions. Vertebral fracture can be diagnosed with spine x-rays or by adding vertebral fracture analysis to DEXA testing. The AACE/ACE Clinical Practice Guideline recommends imaging in patients with T-scores <−1.0 and one or more of the following:[15]

Women aged ≥ 70 and men aged ≥ 80

Historical height loss >4 cm (>1.5 inches)

Self-reported but undocumented prior vertebral fracture

Glucocorticoid therapy equivalent to ≥ 5 mg of prednisone or equivalent per day for ≥ 3 months

Imaging can also be considered in patients with unexplained height loss or back pain, kyphosis, and a history of systemic glucocorticoid therapy not meeting the above criteria.

RECOMMENDATIONS TO OPTIMIZE BONE HEALTH AND DECREASE FRACTURE RISK
Combined Calcium and Vitamin D Supplementation

Combined calcium and vitamin D supplementation has been shown to reduce fracture risk in higher risk populations. A meta-analysis of randomized controlled trials that included community dwelling and institutionalized adults showed that combined calcium and vitamin D supplementation significantly reduced overall fracture risk by 15% and hip fracture risk by 30%.[22] In the included trials, participants received vitamin D3 at doses of 400 to 800 international units (IU) daily and calcium at doses of 500 to 1200 IU daily and were followed for 1 to 7 years. A Cochrane review of studies of vitamin D supplementation in postmenopausal adults found no benefit of vitamin D supplementation alone, but did find a statistically significant 5% reduction in overall fracture risk and 16% reduction in hip fracture risk with combined calcium and vitamin D supplementation.[23] This effect was greater in institutionalized participants, with a 15% reduction in overall fracture risk and a 25% reduction in major fracture risk. Current evidence does not show that calcium and vitamin D supplementation increases bone density or reduces fracture risk in healthy premenopausal women.[24] A small body of evidence shows that combined calcium and vitamin D supplementation prevents bone loss in people taking long-term glucocorticoids, who are at high risk for decreasing bone density.[25] The recommended daily calcium and vitamin D intake for adults is shown in **Table 2**.

VITAMIN D SUPPLEMENTATION

AACE/ACE guidelines recommend measuring 25-hydroxyvitamin D levels in patients who are at risk for vitamin D deficiency, especially people with osteoporosis and supplementing with vitamin D 1000 to 2000 IU to maintain 25-hydroxyvitamin D levels between 30 and 50 ng/mL in people with osteoporosis.[15] There is some concern that doses of vitamin D3 of 4000 IU daily or greater, or intermittent high-dose supplementation may not be beneficial, and some studies suggest it may actually worsen bone density and increase fall and fracture risk.[26–30]

Vitamin D3 is about 3 times more potent than equivalent doses of vitamin D2, so vitamin D3 is usually preferred; however, it may be easier to find vegetarian and vegan sources of vitamin D2 than D3.[31,32] Both can be monitored using a total 25-hydroxyvitamin D level; however some lab tests under detect vitamin D2, so consider checking 25-hydroxyvitamin D2 in patients taking D2 supplements.[32]

With vitamin D supplementation, there is a risk of mild hypercalcemia, gastrointestinal symptoms, hypercalciuria, and kidney stones, especially at higher doses.[23] The optimal interval for rechecking vitamin D levels is not known, but some suggest rechecking in about 8 weeks. https://www.nejm.org/doi/10.1056/NEJMra070553?url_ver=Z39.88-2003&rfr_id=ori:rid:crossref.org&rfr_dat=cr_pub0pubmed.[33,34]

Calcium Supplementation

Sufficient calcium intake across the lifespan is important for bone health. Guidelines recommend a dietary intake of calcium totaling 1,200 mg/day for women older than 50. Women should be encouraged to eat a variety of calcium-rich foods. Taking a dietary calcium inventory (**Table 3**) can help determine calcium intake from diet and can serve as a tool for educating patients about how to meet the recommended daily intake of calcium with calcium-rich foods.

Supplements can be added to achieve the total daily recommended calcium intake. The recommended daily intake of calcium refers to elemental calcium, so knowing how much elemental calcium is in various supplements is important for appropriate dosing (**Table 4**). Calcium is absorbed best at doses of 500 mg or less, so divided dosing may be necessary.

Table 2
Recommended calcium and vitamin D intake[12,16,28]

Age/Sex	Recommended Calcium Intake (mg/day)	Calcium Safe Upper Limit	Recommended Vitamin D Intake (mcg/day)	Vitamin D Safe Upper Limit (mcg/day)
19–50 (M + F)	1000	2500	15	100
51–70 (M)	1000	2000	15	100
51–70 (F)	1200	2000	15	100
71+ (M + F)	1200	2000	20	100

Abbreviations: F, female; IU, international unit; M, male.

Table 3
Dietary calcium intake[12,38]

Food	Calcium Per Serving (mg)	Number of Servings	Total Calcium (mg)
General diet			250
Milk (8 oz)	300	x ____ =	
Soy/almond milk (8 oz)	450	x ____ =	
Yogurt, plain (8 oz)	450	x ____ =	
Yogurt, greek, plain (8 oz)	250	x ____ =	
Yogurt, soy, plain (8 oz)	300	x ____ =	
Cheese (1 oz)	200	x ____ =	
Tofu, prepared with calcium (½ cup)	430	x ____ =	
Orange juice, calcium fortified (8 oz)	450	x ____ =	
Sardines, canned (3 oz)	325	x ____ =	
Collard greens/spinach (1 cup)	250	x ____ =	

This is not an exhaustive list; please refer to https://www.dietaryguidelines.gov/food-sources-calcium for a more comprehensive list of calcium-rich foods.

The main side effects of calcium supplementation are constipation and gastrointestinal symptoms.[35] Switching from calcium carbonate to calcium citrate or gluconate may improve symptoms. Calcium supplementation may also increase the risk of kidney stones. Some studies have raised concerns that calcium supplementation may increase the risk of cardiovascular morbidity and mortality including myocardial infarction and stroke.[36–38] However, a more recent systematic review and meta-analysis of randomized controlled trials and cohort studies concluded there is not an association between dietary calcium intake or calcium supplementation and cardiovascular events.[39]

Substance Use

Alcohol use at a level of more than 2 drinks per day is associated with an increased risk of fractures, including osteoporotic fractures and hip fractures.[40] Smoking tobacco, especially current use, also significantly increases fracture risk.[41]

Table 4
Calcium supplements[12]

	Elemental Calcium Content	Example	Dosing Considerations
Calcium Carbonate	40%	1000 mg calcium carbonate contains 400 mg elemental calcium	Requires stomach acid for absorption— take with food.
Calcium Citrate	21%	1000 mg calcium citrate contains 210 mg elemental calcium	Absorbed on an empty stomach. Preferred for patients on proton-pump inhibitors and with gastrointestinal disorders that cause malabsorption.

Exercise and Falls Prevention

A history of falls is a significant predictor of fracture risk.[42] Exercise interventions, especially those that specifically challenge balance, effectively reduce the risk of falls and rate of falls and lower quality evidence shows that they may reduce fracture risk.[43,44] The United States Preventive Services Taskforce (USPSTF) recommends exercise interventions to prevent falls in community-dwelling adults 65 years and older who are at increased risk for falls.[45] People at high risk for falls may benefit from physical therapy for an individualized exercise program and from a comprehensive clinical evaluation to identify modifiable risk factors for falls based on CDC STEADI guidelines.[19]

TREATMENT OF OSTEOPROSIS

Drugs used to treat osteoporosis are generally classified as anabolic or antiresorptive. Only alendronate, risedronate, zoledronate, and denosumab have broad-spectrum efficacy for hip, spine, and nonvertebral fracture risk reduction. Antiresorptive agents remain the preferred first-line option for most patients. Anabolic parathyroid hormone agonists, teriparatide and abaloparatide, are used for shorter duration and must be followed with an antiresorptive drug to maintain their benefit. The role of romosozumab, the newest osteoporosis drug with both anabolic and antiresorptive effects, is evolving. There remains no consensus for optimal duration of therapy or frequency of serial bone mineral density (BMD) testing; therapy decisions must be individualized.

INDICATIONS FOR PHARMACOLOGIC THERAPY AND RISK STRATIFICATION

Pharmacologic therapy is recommended when fracture risk is high. The superiority of anabolic agents over antiresorptive agents in reducing vertebral fracture risk in patients considered very high risk for fracture will guide medication selection in select patients.

High fracture risk:
- T scores between −1.0 and −2.5 and a history of fragility fracture of the hip or spine
- T score ≤ −2.5
- T-scores between −1.0 and −2.5 and an FRAX 10-year probability of major osteoporotic fracture ≥20%, or a 10-year probability of hip fracture ≥3% in the United States.

Very high fracture risk:
- Recent fracture (within the past 12 months)
- Fracture while on approved osteoporosis therapy
- Multiple fractures
- Fractures while on drugs causing skeletal harm (ie, long-term glucocorticoids)
- Very low T-scores (≤-3.0)
- High risk of falls or history of injurious falls
- Very high fracture probability by FRAX (major osteoporotic fracture ≥30%, or a 10-year probability of hip fracture ≥4.5%)

ANTIRESORPTIVE THERAPIES

Medications for osteoporosis are listed in **Table 5**.

Bisphosphonates

Bisphosphonates bind to bone mineral hydroxyapatite and reduce the activity of bone-resorbing osteoclasts. Particularly in the primary care setting, bisphosphonates

Table 5
Medications for osteoporosis

Class	Drug	Treatment Dosage/Route	Evidence for Fracture Reduction			Relevant Safety Notes	Evidence of Vertebral Fracture Reduction Superiority/Inferiority for Very High Risk Patients?	Average Annual Medicare Spending per Beneficiary in 2022 (Generic When Available)[,#98]
			Vertebral	Nonvertebral	Hip			
Bisphosphonate	Alendronate	10 mg PO daily 70 mg PO weekly	Yes	Yes	Yes	Reflux/Esophagitis Muscle Aches	Inferior to romosozumab	$42
	Risedronate	5 mg PO daily 35 mg PO weekly 150 mg PO monthly	Yes	Yes	Yes	Rare osteonecrosis of the jaw (ONJ) and atypical	Inferior to teriparatide	$473
	Ibandronate	2.5 mg PO daily 150 mg PO monthly 3 mg intravenous (IV) Q3 months	Yes	No	No	femoral fracture (AFF) Caution in renal insufficiency		$177
	Zoledronate	5 mg IV once yearly	Yes	Yes	Yes	Infusion reaction Caution in renal insufficiency		$312
RANK ligand inhibitor	Denosumab	60 mg SubQ Q6 months	Yes	Yes	Yes	Hypocalcemia Rare AFF and ONJ Risk of rebound fracture on discontinuation*		$2387
Selective Estrogen Receptor Modifier	Raloxifene	60 mg PO daily	Yes	Yes	No*	Venous thromboembolic disease risk Vasomotor symptoms		$412

(continued on next page)

Table 5
(continued)

Class	Drug	Treatment Dosage/Route	Evidence for Fracture Reduction			Relevant Safety Notes	Evidence of Vertebral Fracture Reduction Superiority/Inferiority for Very High Risk Patients?	Average Annual Medicare Spending per Beneficiary in 2022 (Generic When Available)(,#98}
			Vertebral	Nonvertebral	Hip			
Parathyroid hormone analogs	Teriparatide	20 μg SQ daily (maximum 2 y)	Yes	Yes	No*	Hypercalcemia Orthostatic hypotension Question osteosarcoma association Should be followed with antiresorptive	Superior to risedronate	$25,327
	Abaloparatide	80 μg SQ daily (maximum 18 mo)	Yes	Yes	No*			$14,032
Sclerostin inhibitor	Romosozumab	210 mg SQ monthly (maximum 1 y)	Yes	Yes	No	May increase cardiovascular risk; not for patients with myocardial infarction or stroke in the past y Requires antiresorptive after discontinuation	Superior to alendronate	$5,344

* indicates less strong data for reduction in hip fractures.

Abbreviations: PO, per os (by mouth); SubQ and SQ; subcutaneous; Q6, every 6; RANK, Receptor Activator of Nuclear Factor Kappa-B.

are the preferred initial treatment to reduce fracture risk in primary osteoporosis. The 4 available bisphosphonates in the United States—alendronate, risedronate, ibandronate, and zoledronate—have demonstrated broad reduction in fracture risk at the hip, spine, and nonvertebral fracture sites, except for ibandronate (no evidence for hip fracture reduction). The American College of Physicians (ACP) asserts that as a class, bisphosphonates maintain the most favorable balance between benefits, harms, cost, and patient value/preferences.

Oral bisphosphonates must be taken on an empty stomach, waiting at least 30 minutes before ingestion of other medications or food/beverages to help ovoid esophageal irritation, though they should be used with caution in anyone with active esophageal disease.[46] Common side effects are dyspepsia, dysphagia, abdominal pain, and musculoskeletal pain. Most gastrointestinal side effects can be avoided with intravenous (IV) zoledronate. Prescribers should counsel patients on the acute-phase reaction that occurs in as many as 30% of patients receiving their first dose of IV zoledronate, characterized by pyrexia and myalgias.[47] The incidence of this acute phase reaction typically decreases with subsequent injections.

Contraindications to oral bisphosphonates include hypocalcemia, anatomic or functional esophageal abnormalities (achalasia, stricture, dysmotility), and gastrointestinal malabsorption (gastric bypass, celiac disease, Crohn's disease, etc.). Contraindications to both oral and IV bisphosphonates include hypocalcemia or drug hypersensitivity. Renal insufficiency limits the use of bisphosphonates when glomerular filtration rate is below 30 to 35 mL/min.[48]

Safety Concerns

Osteonecrosis of the jaw (ONJ) is a rare but serious adverse event associated with antiresorptive agents. It is defined as exposed, nonhealing bone in the maxillofacial region persisting for greater than 8 weeks.[49] The risk of ONJ is estimated between 1 in 10,000 and 1 in 100,000 per year with bisphosphonates, up to 11 in 10,000 patient-years with denosumab.[50,51] Risk factors include dental pathology and poor hygiene, and delaying initiation of these antiresorptive medications until dental issues have been addressed should be considered. ONJ risk is dose and duration dependent.

Atypical femoral fracture (AFF) is a rare potential complication of all antiresorptive therapies. These fractures occur spontaneously with minimal or no trauma in the subtrochanteric region or femoral shaft. They are usually transverse, noncomminuted, and extend through both cortices. Hip or thigh pain can be the first clinical sign, and radiographs should be obtained if these symptoms occur while on therapy.[52] While rare, the risk of AFF does increase with duration of treatment. Estimates from a meta-analysis propose that treatment of 1,000 women for 3 years of bisphosphonate therapy would result in fewer than 1 AFF per 100 osteoporotic fractures prevented.[53]

Duration of Therapy

The optimal treatment durations of bisphosphonates and denosumab are unknown. Most studies evaluating bisphosphonates continued therapy for up to 5 years for oral formulations and 3 years for IV. At these intervals, antifracture benefits clearly outweigh the risks, and most guidelines agree on this duration of initial therapy.[15,54] Treatment extension to 10 years for oral bisphosphonate and 6 years for IV zoledronic acid should be considered for women initially at very high risk of fracture or in those who remain at high risk after initial treatment course, but this is based on weaker data. Those who seem to benefit most from extension of bisphosphonate treatment are those in a high-risk category, including persistently low T-score at the hip, or incident fracture during the initial study period.[55]

An algorithm for the suggested approach for long-term management of bisphosphonate therapy can be found in **Fig. 1**.

Denosumab

Denosumab is a monoclonal antibody which inhibits Receptor Activator of Nuclear Factor Kappa-B Ligand (RANKL), a major activator of osteoclastic bone resorption, reducing differentiation into mature osteoclasts and decreasing their function. Denosumab is injected subcutaneously at 60 mg every 6 months, with unclear optimal treatment duration.

Denosumab is useable in patients with renal impairment but is contraindicated in patients with hypocalcemia; calcium and vitamin D should be replete prior to starting therapy. It may also be used following treatment with an anabolic agent. Denosumab is generally well-tolerated with low incidence of side effects, which can include skin rash or skin infection. Incidence of ONJ and AFF are rare and duration dependent.[56]

An important therapeutic consideration prior to starting denosumab is that gains in BMD are lost rapidly after discontinuation—drug holidays from denosumab are not recommended. Bone turnover markers increase above baseline after 1 year of discontinuation,[57] and in that first year, there may be increased risk of multiple fractures.[58] If denosumab treatment is discontinued, transition to a bisphosphonate 6 months after the final dose can mitigate the loss of BMD.[59,60]

Selective Estrogen Receptor Modifiers

Raloxifene is Food and Drug Administration (FDA)-approved for postmenopausal osteoporosis and for the reduction of breast cancer risk. As an estrogen receptor mixed agonist and antagonist, it has an agonist effect at bone but antagonistic effect in other areas, including the uterus and breast. Raloxifene has been shown to reduce risk of fracture at the spine, though no hip or nonvertebral fracture reduction has been demonstrated.[61]

Raloxifene is associated with a 3-fold increase in venous thromboembolic disease (VTE), thus contraindications include active or past history of VTE.[62] Vasomotor symptoms contribute to increased rates of patient discontinuation of raloxifene as compared to other osteoporosis therapies. Its role in osteoporosis treatment is limited to those with less-severe osteoporosis—particularly those with discordant low BMD of the spine but not in the hip, those at especially high risk of breast cancer, or as a weaker antiresorptive for higher risk patients during drug holiday.[63]

Anabolic Therapy

Anabolic therapies are considered second line for osteoporosis treatment: they are used for failure or intolerance of previous therapies, or as initial therapy for those at very high fracture risk. The most established anabolic target is parathyroid hormone, though an emerging therapy romosozumab targets sclerostin and is currently the most potent drug available for osteoporosis.

Parathyroid hormone analogs

While high bone turnover in hyperparathyroidism results in decreased bone mass, intermittent injection of parathyroid hormone (PTH) peptides results in increased bone mass. Teriparatide is recombinant human PTH (given for 18–24 months) and abaloparatide is a modified PTH-related peptide (given for 2-year). Both agents increase BMD and prevent vertebral and nonvertebral fractures, though it remains unknown if hip fractures are reduced.

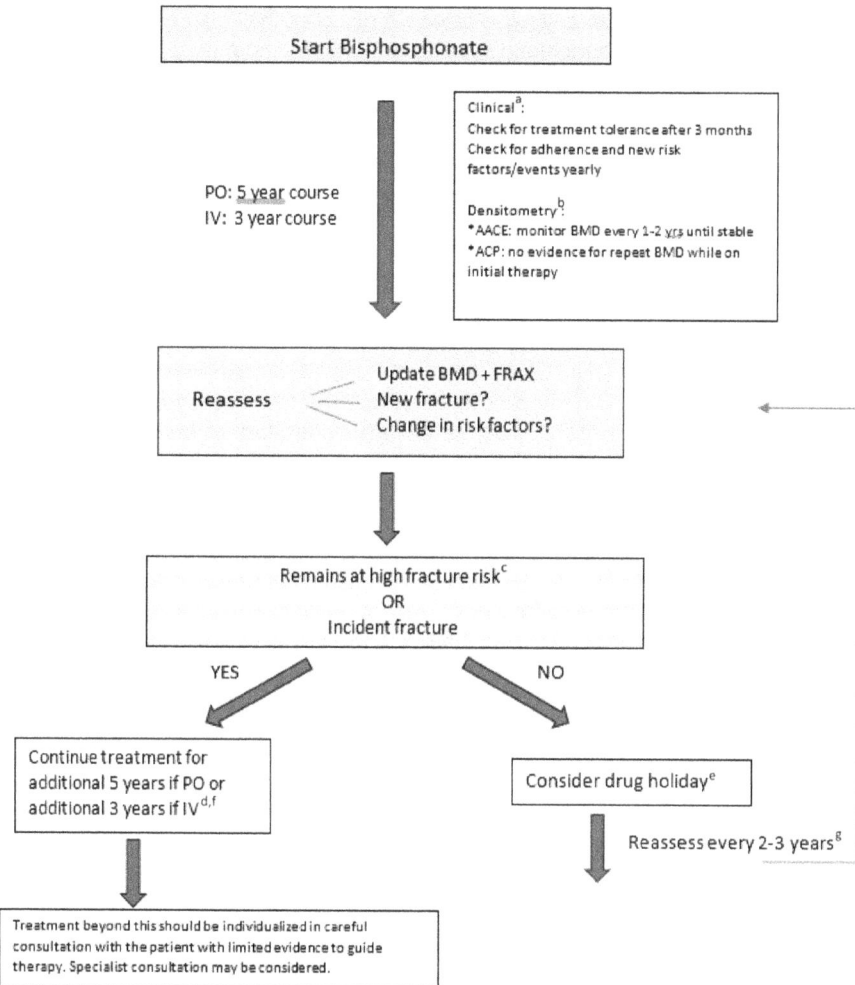

Fig. 1. Suggested approach for long-term management of bisphosphonate therapy. [a]Clinical monitoring recommendation from National Osteoporosis Guidelines Group (UK) (NOGG) guidelines.[59] [b]American Association of Clinical Endocrinologists recommends repeating bone mineral density (BMD) every 1 to 2 years until findings stabilize, whereas American College of Physicians recommends against any BMD monitoring during the first 5 years of treatment.[16,50] [c]High risk in this context includes meeting BMD threshold for pharmacotherapy, or history of hip or vertebral fracture prior to starting therapy. [d]Additional benefit of bisphosphonate extension is weaker and is limited to vertebral fracture reduction[60,61]; duration-dependent harms must be considered. The greatest benefit for extension was with persistently low T scores at the hip or those who had fractured on therapy. [e]Bisphosphonate holidays are typically no longer than 5 years; good candidates are younger than 75 years, have had no fracture in the past 2 years, no history of hip or vertebral fracture, and T scores above −2.5.[62] [f]Presently, there are no trials that have queried the antifracture efficacy of switching therapies after 3 to 5 years, extending treatment beyond 10 years, or of reinitiating therapy after drug holiday. [g]Timing depends on strength of bisphosphonate.

Contraindications include any hypercalcemic disorder, including hyperparathyroidism. Hypercalcemia and orthostatic hypotension are the most common side effects. Both abaloparatide and teriparatide have boxed warnings due to the occurrence of osteosarcomas seen in rats at high doses, though this has not been linked to human patients.

As improvements in bone density quickly decline after cessation of teriparatide or abaloparatide, each should be immediately followed by antiresorptive therapy.

Romosozumab

Romosozumab is a monoclonal antibody against sclerostin. Sclerostin inhibits the differentiation of precursor cells into bone-forming osteoblasts and increases stimulation of RANK ligand by osteocytes. By blocking sclerostin action, romosozumab has a potent anabolic effect, while also reducing bone resorption more moderately.[64] Approved for 1 year of use, romosozumab should be followed by an antiresorptive therapy as this maintains BMD gains or even provides further benefit. The role of romosozumab is summarized in **Table 5**.

Treatment Monitoring and Goals

Serial BMD testing is used to determine when to initiate treatment, as well as to monitor responses to treatment. Determining frequency of densitometry requires understanding of the inherent variability of the test measurement itself,[65] and of expected, age-related density losses: 0.5% to 1% per year beginning in the fifth decade, though more rapid bone loss (1%–2% per year) is often seen in the 3 to 5 years before and after menopause.[66]

For those with low bone density not already on treatment, the frequency of repeat testing requires individual assessment of the risk of further bone loss and how near the patient was to the treatment threshold. For those on therapy, the goal of monitoring is to identify significant bone loss despite treatment, which should prompt evaluation for medication nonadherence, secondary causes, and thorough medication review. Stable or increasing BMD at the spine and hip are considered satisfactory responses.

Current clinical guidelines give contradictory recommendations for intervals between BMD tests. Both the AACE and National Osteoporosis Foundation (NOF) recommend repeating densitometry 1 to 2 years after initiating therapy and until stable,[16] whereas the ACP recommends against any BMD monitoring during the first 5 years of bisphosphonate treatment, citing lack of evidence demonstrating benefits.[67] Repeat BMD while on therapy has not been shown to reduce fracture risk.[68]

DISCUSSION/SUMMARY

Osteoporosis is a significant chronic condition worldwide, causing morbidity and mortality that may be prevented with proper risk factor mitigation, screening, and treatment. Adequate intake of calcium and vitamin D as well as regular weight-bearing exercise are integral for bone health. Treatment options beyond the recommended first-line treatment of oral bisphosphonates exist for those who do not tolerate these medications.

CLINICS CARE POINTS

- Clinicians should address bone health risk factors in preventive visits for all women age 50 or greater.

- Bone density testing should begin at age 65 for most women, and earlier for those at higher risk for osteoporosis.
- Oral bisphosphonates are the first-line treatment for osteoporosis with use of other medications to be considered in patients with contraindications to bisphosphonates, refractory osteoporosis, or patients at very high risk for fracture at time of diagnosis.

DISCLOSURE

The authors have nothing to disclose.

REFERENCES

1. Osteoporosis. National insititute of arthritis and musculoskeletal and skin disease. 2022. Available at: https://www.niams.nih.gov/health-topics/osteoporosis. Accessed June 25, 2024.
2. Dell RM, Adams AL, Greene DF, et al. Incidence of atypical nontraumatic diaphyseal fractures of the femur. J Bone Miner Res 2012;27(12):2544–50.
3. What women need to know. Available at: https://www.bonehealthandosteoporosis. org/preventing-fractures/general-facts/what-women-need-to-know/. Accessed June 25, 2024.
4. International Osteoporosis Foundation. About osteoporosis. Available at: https:// www.osteoporosis.foundation/patients/about-osteoporosis. Accessed June 25, 2024.
5. Schnell S, Friedman S, Mendelshon D, et al. The 1-year mortality of patients treated in a hip fracture program for elders. Geriatric Orthopedic Surgery and Rehabilitation 2010;1(1):6–14.
6. Clynes M, Harvey N, Curtis E, et al. The epidemiology of osteoporosis. Br Med Bull 2020;133(1):105–17.
7. Task force issues draft recommendation on screening for osteoporosis to prevent fractures. 2024. Available at: https://www.uspreventiveservicestaskforce.org/ uspstf/sites/default/files/file/supporting_documents/osteoporosis-screening-draft-rec-bulletin.pdf.
8. FRAX calculation tool. FRAXplus. Available at: https://fraxplus.org/calculation-tool. Accessed June 25, 2024.
9. Osteoporosis to prevent fractures: screening. Website. US preventive Services Task force. 2018. Available at: https://www.uspreventiveservicestaskforce.org/ uspstf/recommendation/osteoporosis-screening;. Accessed June 25, 2024 https://fraxplus.org/calculation-tool.
10. Bone health and osteoporosis. Available at: https://transcare.ucsf.edu/guidelines/ bone-health-and-osteoporosis#:%7E:text=Transgender%20people%20. Accessed June 25, 2024.
11. LeBoff M, Greenspan S, Insogna K, et al. The clinician's guide to prevention and treatment of osteoporosis. Osteoporosis Int 2022;33:2049–102.
12. Craig K, Stevermer J. DEXA screening – are we doing too much? J Fam Prac 2012;61(9):555–6.
13. Gourlay M, Fine J, Preisser J, et al. Study of Osteoporotic Fractures Research Group. Bone-density testing interval and transition to osteoporosis in older women. N Engl J Med 2012;366(3):225–33.
14. Bone mineral density tests: what the numbers mean. 2023. Available at: https:// www.niams.nih.gov/health-topics/bone-mineral-density-tests-what-numbers-mean. Accessed June 25, 2024.

15. Camacho P, Petak S, Binkley N, et al. American association of clinical Endocrinologists/American College of Endocrinology clinical Practice guidelines for the diagnosis and treatment of postmenopausal osteoporosis—2020 update. Endocr Pract 2020;26(1):1–46.

16. Bone Health Choice Decision Aid. Mayo foundation for medical education and research. Available at: https://osteoporosisdecisionaid.mayoclinic.org/. Accessed June 26, 2024.

17. Dynamed decisions. Available at: https://decisions.dynamed.com/tools. Accessed June 26, 2024.

18. Lewiecki E, Wright N, Singer A. Racial disparities, FRAX, and the care of patients with osteoporosis. Osteoporosis Int 2020;31(11):2069–71.

19. Steadi - older adult fall prevention. US centers for disease control and prevention. Available at: https://www.cdc.gov/steadi/hcp/clinical-resources/index.html. Accessed June 26, 2024.

20. Sweet M, Sweet J, Jeremiah M, et al. Diagnosis and treatment of osteoporosis. Am Fam Physician 2009;79(3):193–200.

21. Fink H, Milavetz D, Palermo L, et al. What proportion of incident radiographic vertebral deformities is clinically diagnosed and vice versa? J Bone Miner Res 2005;20(7):1216–22.

22. Weaver C, Alexander D, Boushey C, et al. Calcium plus vitamin D supplementation and risk of fractures: an updated meta-analysis from the National Osteoporosis Foundation. Osteoporos Int 2016;27(1):367–76 [Erratum appears in Osteoporos Int 2016;27(8):2643–46].

23. Avenell A, Mak J, O'Connell D. Vitamin D and vitamin D analogues for preventing fractures in post-menopausal women and older men. Cochrane Database Syst Rev 2014;4:CD000227.

24. Méndez-Sánchez L, Clark P, Winzenberg T, et al. Calcium and vitamin D for increasing bone mineral density in premenopausal women. Cochrane Database Syst Rev 2023;1:CD012664.

25. Homik J, Suarez-Almazor M, Shea B, et al. Calcium and vitamin D for corticosteroid-induced osteoporosis. Cochrane Database Syst Rev 1998;2:CD000952.

26. Kong S, Jang H, Kim J, et al. Effect of vitamin D supplementation on risk of fractures and falls according to dosage and interval: a meta-analysis. Endocrinol Metab (Seoul) 2022;37(2):344–58.

27. Myung S, Cho H. Effects of intermittent or single high-dose vitamin D supplementation on risk of falls and fractures: a systematic review and meta-analysis. Osteoporos Int 2023;34:1355–67.

28. Anagnostis P, Bosdou J, Kenanidis E, et al. Vitamin D supplementation and fracture risk: evidence for a U-shaped effect. Maturitas 2020;141:63–70.

29. Sanders K, Stuart A, Williamson E, et al. Annual high-dose oral vitamin D and falls and fractures in older women: a randomized controlled trial. JAMA 2010;303(18):1815–22.

30. Burt L, Billington E, Rose M, et al. Effect of high-dose vitamin D supplementation on volumetric bone density and bone strength: a randomized clinical trial. JAMA 2019;322(8):736–45.

31. Heaney R, Recker R, Grote J, et al. Vitamin D3 is more potent than vitamin D2 in humans. J Clin Endocrinol Metab 2011;96(3):E447–52.

32. Kennel K, Drake M, Hurley D. Vitamin D deficiency in adults: when to test and how to treat. Mayo Clin Proc 2010;85(8):752–8.

33. Holick M. Vitamin D deficiency. N Engl J Med 2007;357(3):266–81.

34. Bordelon P, Ghetu M, Langan R. Recognition and management of vitamin D deficiency. Am Fam Physician 2009;80(8):841–6 [Erratum appears in Am Fam Physician 2009;80(12):1357].

35. Li K, Wang X, Li D, et al. The good, the bad, and the ugly of calcium supplementation: a review of calcium intake on human health. Clin Interv Aging 2018;13: 2443–52.

36. Bolland M, Avenell A, Baron J, et al. Effect of calcium supplements on risk of myocardial infarction and cardiovascular events: meta-analysis. BMJ 2010;341: c3691.

37. Bolland M, Barber P, Doughty R, et al. Vascular events in healthy older women receiving calcium supplementation: randomised controlled trial. BMJ 2008. https://doi.org/10.1136/bmj.39440.525752.

38. Li K, Kaaks R, Linseisen J, et al. Associations of dietary calcium intake and calcium supplementation with myocardial infarction and stroke risk and overall cardiovascular mortality in the Heidelberg cohort of the European Prospective Investigation into Cancer and Nutrition study (EPIC-Heidelberg). Heart 2012; 98(12):920–5.

39. Chung M, Tang A, Fu Z, et al. Calcium intake and cardiovascular disease risk: an updated systematic review and meta-analysis. Ann Intern Med 2016;165(12): 856–66.

40. Kanis J, Johansson H, Johnell O, et al. Alcohol intake as a risk factor for fracture. Osteoporos Int 2005;16:737–42.

41. Kanis J, Johnell O, Oden A, et al. Smoking and fracture risk: a meta-analysis. Osteoporos Int 2005;16:155–62.

42. Vandenput L, Johansson H, McCloskey E, et al. A meta-analysis of previous falls and subsequent fracture risk in cohort studies. Osteoporos Int 2024;35:469–94.

43. Sherrington C, Fairhall N, Wallbank G, et al. Exercise for preventing falls in older people living in the community. Cochrane Database Syst Rev 2019;1:CD012424.

44. Kemmler W, Häberle L, von Stengel S. Effects of exercise on fracture reduction in older adults. Osteoporos Int 2013;24:1937–50.

45. Falls Prevention in Community-Dwelling Older Adults: Interventions. US Preventive Services Task Force. Available at: https://www.uspreventiveservicestaskforce.org/ uspstf/recommendation/falls-prevention-community-dwelling-older-adults-interventions. Accessed June 26, 2024.

46. Crandall CJ, Newberry SJ, Diamant A, et al. Comparative effectiveness of pharmacologic treatments to prevent fractures: an updated systematic review. Ann Intern Med 2014;161(10):711–23.

47. Adami S, Bhalla AK, Dorizzi R, et al. The acute-phase response after bisphosphonate administration. Calcif Tissue Int 1987;41(6):326–31.

48. Robinson DE, Ali MS, Pallares N, et al. Safety of oral bisphosphonates in moderate-to-severe chronic kidney disease: a binational cohort analysis. J Bone Miner Res 2021;36(5):820–32.

49. Ruggiero SL, Dodson TB, Aghaloo T, et al. American association of oral and maxillofacial surgeons' position paper on medication-related osteonecrosis of the jaws-2022 update. J Oral Maxillofac Surg 2022;80(5):920–43.

50. Khan AA, Morrison A, Hanley DA, et al. Diagnosis and management of osteonecrosis of the jaw: a systematic review and international consensus. J Bone Miner Res 2015;30(1):3–23.

51. Bilezikian JP. Osteonecrosis of the jaw–do bisphosphonates pose a risk? N Engl J Med 2006;355(22):2278–81.

52. Shane E, Burr D, Ebeling PR, et al. Atypical subtrochanteric and diaphyseal femoral fractures: report of a Task force of the American society for bone and mineral research. J Bone Miner Res 2010;25(11):2267–94.

53. Black DM, Rosen CJ. Postmenopausal osteoporosis. N Engl J Med 2016;374(3): 254–62.

54. Gregson CL, Armstrong DJ, Bowden J, et al. UK clinical guideline for the prevention and treatment of osteoporosis (vol 17, pg 1, 2022). Arch Osteoporosis 2022;17(1).

55. Cummings SR, San Martin J, McClung MR, et al. Denosumab for prevention of fractures in postmenopausal women with osteoporosis. (vol 361, pg 756, 2009). N Engl J Med 2009;361(19):1914.

56. Liu FC, Luk KC, Chen YC. Risk comparison of osteonecrosis of the jaw in osteoporotic patients treated with bisphosphonates vs. denosumab: a multi-institutional retrospective cohort study in Taiwan. Osteoporosis Int 2023;34(10): 1729–37.

57. Miller PD, Bolognese MA, Lewiecki EM, et al. Effect of denosumab on bone density and turnover in postmenopausal women with low bone mass after long-term continued, discontinued, and restarting of therapy: a randomized blinded phase 2 clinical trial. Bone 2008;43(2):222–9.

58. Cummings SR, Ferrari S, Eastell R, et al. Vertebral fractures after discontinuation of denosumab: a post hoc analysis of the randomized placebo-controlled FREEDOM trial and its extension. J Bone Miner Res 2018;33(2):190–8.

59. Freemantle N, Satram-Hoang S, Tang ET, et al. Final results of the DAPS (Denosumab Adherence Preference Satisfaction) study: a 24-month, randomized, crossover comparison with alendronate in postmenopausal women. Osteoporosis Int 2012;23(1):317–26.

60. Kendler D, Chines A, Clark P, et al. Bone mineral density after transitioning from denosumab to alendronate. J Clin Endocrinol Metab 2020;105(3):E255–64.

61. Ettinger B. Reduction of vertebral fracture risk in postmenopausal women with osteoporosis treated with raloxifene: results from a 3-year randomized clinical trial (vol 282, pg 637, 1999). JAMA, J Am Med Assoc 1999;282(22):2124.

62. Barrett-Connor E, Mosca L, Collins P, et al. Effects of raloxifene on cardiovascular events and breast cancer in postmenopausal women. N Engl J Med 2006;355(2): 125–37.

63. Dennison E. Osteoporosis treatment: a clinical overview. 1st edition. Cham: Springer; 2021.

64. McClung MR, Grauer A, Boonen S, et al. Romosozumab in postmenopausal women with low bone mineral density. N Engl J Med 2014;370(5):412–20.

65. Lenchik L, Kiebzak GM, Blunt BA, International Society for Clinical Densitometry Position Development Panel and Scientific Advisory Committee. What is the role of serial bone mineral density measurements in patient management? J Clin Densitom 2002;5(Suppl):S29–38.

66. Ooms ME, Lips P, Roos JC, et al. Vitamin D status and sex hormone binding globulin: determinants of bone turnover and bone mineral density in elderly women. J Bone Miner Res 1995;10(8):1177–84.

67. Cosman F, de Beur SJ, LeBoff MS, et al. Clinician's guide to prevention and treatment of osteoporosis. Osteoporos Int 2014;25(10):2359–81.

68. Berry SD, Samelson EJ, Pencina MJ, et al. Repeat bone mineral density screening and prediction of hip and major osteoporotic fracture. JAMA 2013; 310(12):1256–62.

Effect of the Covid Pandemic on Women's Health

Monica DeMasi, MD, FAAFP[a], Laura Bujold, DO, MS[b],*

KEYWORDS

- Women's health • Coronavirus pandemic • Corona virus disease 2019

KEY POINTS

- Preventative and chronic disease care decreased during the pandemic.
- By 2023, women regained 100% of jobs lost from the pandemic. Some job categories remain below prepandemic levels, other job categories have surpassed prepandemic levels.
- Women bore more caregiving responsibilities than men during the pandemic.
- Intimate partner violence and depression increased for women during the pandemic, highlighting the importance of screening.

INTRODUCTION

The novel coronavirus disease 2019 (COVID-19) pandemic had profound repercussions on the health and wellbeing of women. This impact was across all spheres of women's lives, from increased experiences of intimate partner violence (IPV), to pausing careers in favor of caregiving for children and elders who lost access to schools and senior centers, to losing jobs. The isolation of parenting and living in quarantine, along with diminished access to routine health care and the direct health consequences of covid infections, resulted in negative impacts on physical and mental health.

PREVENTATIVE AND CHRONIC DISEASE MANAGEMENT

The pandemic impacted women's physical health in many ways. Studies have demonstrated that the physical activity of women decreased during the pandemic,[1,2] and diabetes care also decreased.[3] There were significant increases in amputations after April 2020 compared with prepandemic rates, likely because of the lack of routine care during the pandemic.[4] In addition, primary care clinicians need to be aware that

[a] Providence Family Medicine Residency Program, Portland, OR 97266, USA; [b] Department of Family Medicine, University of Connecticut School of Medicine, UCONN Family Medicine Residency Program, 99 Woodland Street, Hartford, CT 06105, USA
* Corresponding author.
E-mail address: Bujold@uchc.edu

Prim Care Clin Office Pract 52 (2025) 371–382
https://doi.org/10.1016/j.pop.2025.01.009 **primarycare.theclinics.com**

Abbreviations	
ACOG	American College of Obstetricians and Gynecologists
CDC	Centers for Disease Control and Prevention
COVID-19	corona virus disease 2019
FDA	US Food and Drug Administration
IPV	intimate partner violence
OR	odds ratio
PTSD	post-traumatic stress disorder
SNRI	serotonin and noroepinephrine reuptake inhibitor
SSRI	selective serotonin reuptake inhibitor
WHO	World Health Organization

preventative care was decreased during the pandemic, and this could have a significant effect on the diagnosis and prevention of coronary vascular disease, diabetes, hyperlipidemia, and other diseases.

In 2020, an estimated 9.4 million fewer screening tests were performed in the United States compared with what would have been expected.[5] Screening mammograms decreased among all racial/ethnic and age groups during the pandemic., and this was especially pronounced for older women and Asian women.[6,7] Asian women also had the lowest rate of rebound of mammograms, and the rate of mammography for women overall had not returned to baseline by May 2021.[7] To improve screening and decrease this deficit, primary care clinicians can get involved with the local community groups, create support networks, and question why their patients are not returning to routine screening (**Figs. 1** and **2**).

The Return-to-Screening Study used quality improvement methodology across 786 cancer screening programs with the goal of accelerating the return to baseline cancer screening and making up for the deficit in screening during the height of the pandemic.[8] The methods used to increase screening rates fell into 3 main categories: increasing patient demand, increasing delivery of screening, and increasing community access. Seventy-nine percent of these programs reached prepandemic screening volumes plus 10% or more growth in their cancer screening.

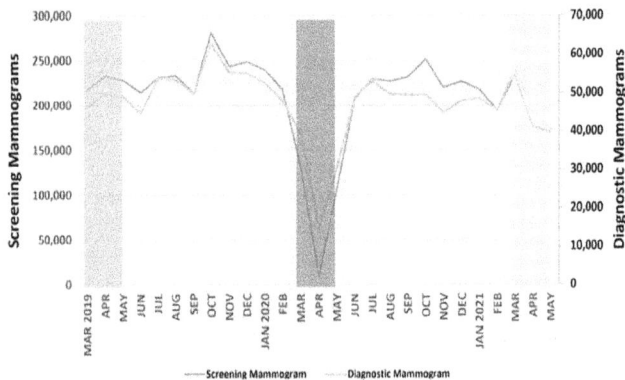

Monthly volume of screening and diagnostic mammographic examinations from the National Mammography Database from March 1, 2019, through May 31, 2021. The green, red, and yellow boxes refer to the 3-month-long pre-COVID-19, peak COVID-19, and COVID-19 recovery periods, respectively, used for analysis. COVID-19 = coronavirus disease 2019.

Fig. 1. Monthly volume of screening and diagnostic mammograms before, during, and after COVID-19.[7]

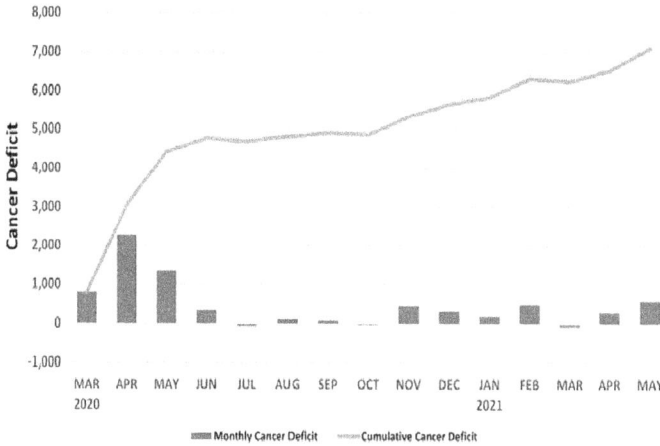

Monthly and cumulative cancer deficits from March 2020 to May 2021 on the basis of the average monthly cancer diagnoses from March 2019 to February 2020.

Fig. 2. Monthly and cumulative cancer deficits from March 2020 to May 2021.[7]

Primary care access during the pandemic affected some subgroups of women more than others. Women who identified as lesbian or bisexual, women with cancer, and women with incomes less than $75,000 per year had more difficulty accessing primary care.[9]

REPRODUCTIVE HEALTH

Birth rates in the United States have been slowly trending down since 2000.[10] Even given this trend, from August 2020 to February 2021, there were about 100,000 fewer births than would have been expected in prepandemic times.[10] There was a rebound of births from March 2021 to April 2022, with 80,000 more births than expected.[10] However, it is difficult to continue to relate the number of births to the COVID-19 pandemic as one gets further away from the pandemic.

Reproductive health care in particular was affected from the direct impact of COVID infections, leading to pregnancy loss and complications, increased rates of pre-eclampsia, preterm births, increased rates of cesarean sections, increased maternal mortality, as well as less access to anesthesia during birth, and birthing in isolation.[11,12] Although many women chose to delay pregnancy during the pandemic, access to contraception and abortion care was also decreased (**Tables 1** and **2**).

American College of Obstetricians and Gynecologists (ACOG) and World Health Organization (WHO) strongly recommend COVID vaccination in pregnancy and lactation.[13] The COVID vaccine is widely regarded as safe for pregnant women and their fetuses by the medical community.[14–16] However, studies have demonstrated that the uptake of the vaccine among pregnant women at the peak of the pandemic was only about 30% in the United Kingdom[14] and ranged from 3% to 58%in the United States.[17] Acceptance of vaccination for COVID 19 during pregnancy was lower in historically under-represented communities of color because of a combination of health disparities (eg, access to health care, transportation, or housing) and justified historic distrust and fear of being experimented upon by the health care community.[13] Vaccination rates also varied by state and rural versus urban communities, largely based on

Table 1
Association between corona virus disease 2019 and preeclampsia (patients with corona virus disease 2019 vs patients without corona virus disease 2019)[12]

	Pre-eclampsia	Total Pregnancies	Percent of Patients Affected
With COVID-19 infection in pregnancy	665	7866	8.5%
Without COVID-19 infection in pregnancy	24,406	417,491	5.8%

Odds ratio (OR) 1.82 (1.38–2.39).
From meta analysis adapted from Ref.[12]

misinformation campaigns. These fears have been compounded by intentional disinformation widely spread on social media.[18]

As for the COVID-19 booster vaccine, the Vaccine Safety Datalink in July 2023 showed 16% of pregnant people received a COVID booster vaccine. Rates of booster vaccination were lower in people of color, with only 8.3% of Black pregnant women and 9.6% of Latina pregnant women receiving the COVID booster[19]

Clinicians caring for pregnant women should discuss vaccine safety with their preconception and pregnancy visits using a collaborative motivational interviewing approach. The Centers for Disease Control and Prevention (CDC) has a toolkit[20] that outlines a basic approach of discussing vaccines in pregnancy, including presenting vaccination as a standard part of prenatal care, providing a strong recommendation, tailoring the vaccine benefits to the specific needs of the pregnant patient, listening and responding to patient concerns and fears, and explaining the risks of not receiving the vaccine.

MENTAL HEALTH

The pandemic brought mental health consequences for people across the world, including isolation in the setting of quarantine, misinformation and political divisiveness, social stigma, loss of kin and friends, and health fears increased post-traumatic stress disorder (PTSD), depression and anxiety.[21] These impacts were more severe for women.[22] Women also experienced higher levels of intimate partner violence during the pandemic.[23]

The experiences surrounding reproductive health, pregnancy, and childbirth during the pandemic had effects on women's mental health also.[20] For example, in Canada, moderate to severe anxiety was experienced by 72% of pregnant and postpartum women during the pandemic, versus 29% before the pandemic. Other studies showed a similar increase in anxiety and depression. Social support and exercise were protective factors.[23] Access to mental health care including physician visits, therapy, and addiction services was limited during the pandemic.[24] Although the increase in

Table 2
The association between coronavirus disease 2019 and stillbirth[12]

	Stillbirths	Total Births	Percent of Patients Affected
With COVID-19 infection in pregnancy	40	7590	0.05%
Without COVID-19 infection in pregnancy	1318	405,532	0.03%

OR 2.11 (1.14–3.90).
From meta analysis adapted from Ref.[12]

depression, anxiety, and PTSD remained elevated in late 2020,[25] there are few data about the sustained impacts of the pandemic on mental health.

Suggestions for treatment of pandemic-related PTSD are similar to those for PTSD from any source of trauma, and include therapeutic modalities such as cognitive behavioral therapy, eye movement desensitization and reprocessing, and medication such as selective serotonin reuptake inhibitors (SSRIs) and serotonin and noroepinephrine reuptake inhibitors (SNRIs). Paroxetine and sertraline are the only US Food and Drug Administration (FDA)-approved medications for PTSD.[21] Universal screening for intimate partner violence, depression, and substance abuse should be part of standard primary care visits. Patients who screen positive should be asked about their pandemic experiences. In order to improve the availability and flexibility of mental health care after the pandemic, access to telehealth should be maintained and continue to evolve (**Fig. 3**).[26]

LONG CORONA VIRUS DISEASE

In addition to the short-term health and social consequences of acute covid infections and the longer-term impacts of pandemic obstacles to access to health care and mental health sequelae of the pandemic, many women have struggled with chronic impacts of

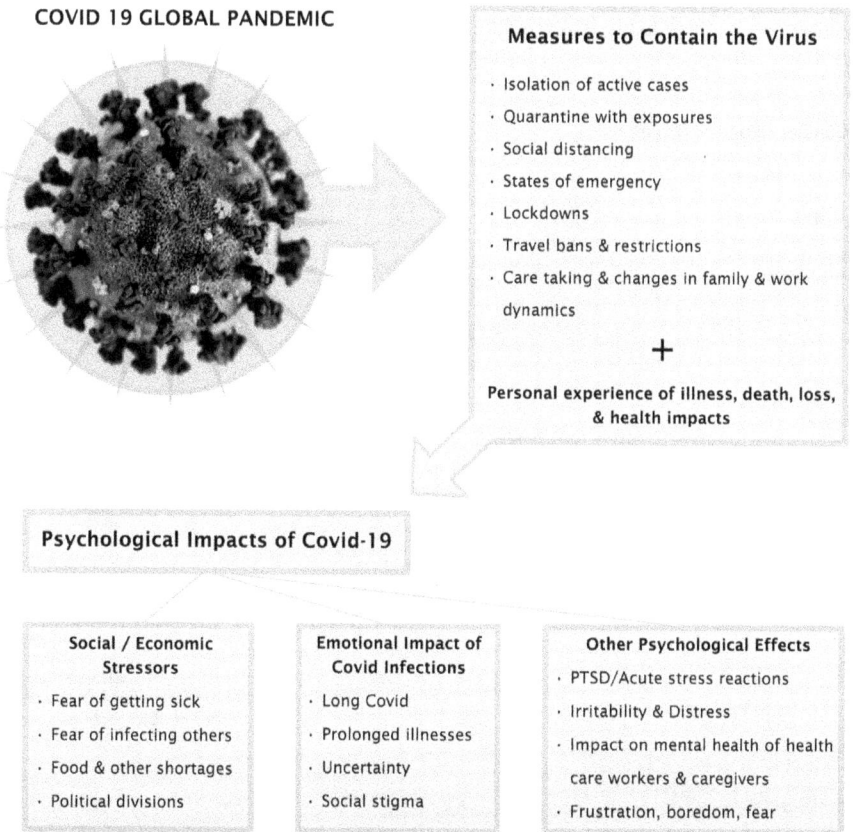

Fig. 3. Psychological impacts of COVID-19.[27] (*Adapted from* https://www.ncbi.nlm.nih.gov/pmc/articles/PMC9185760/figure/F1/.[27])

long COVID. Long COVID can cause chronic fatigue, muscle aches, palpitations, cognitive impairment, sleep disturbance, and other symptoms. It can have a long-lasting impact on health and the ability to function in society. Long COVID can involve various organ systems, including the respiratory, neurologic, and cardiovascular systems. Long COVID also seems to impact women's reproductive health, including menstrual irregularities, fertility, and pregnancy outcomes.[28] A study from 2022 demonstrated that women who had contracted COVID exhibited a higher incidence of long COVID (8.5%) than men (5.2%).[28] Because many symptoms of long COVID can have overlap of symptoms associated with perimenopause, long COVID prevalence in women might be underestimated[29] (**Fig. 4**).

ECONOMIC IMPACT

Although many people experienced economic impacts during the COVID-19 pandemic, the most profound economic impacts were encountered by women. Mothers of school-aged and younger children, Black and Hispanic women, single mothers, and adult women caring for their parents were the most affected. Childcare demands for women increased by 250 percent, and were much higher than for men in 2 custodial parent households. However, the decrease of employment during the pandemic was greater based on educational disparities than gender, with noncollege graduate workers losing access to employment or not having caregiving support. Employed women were more likely to experience an enormous increase in caregiving burdens while simultaneously working, often from home.[30]

General signs and symptoms

Specific symptoms in female

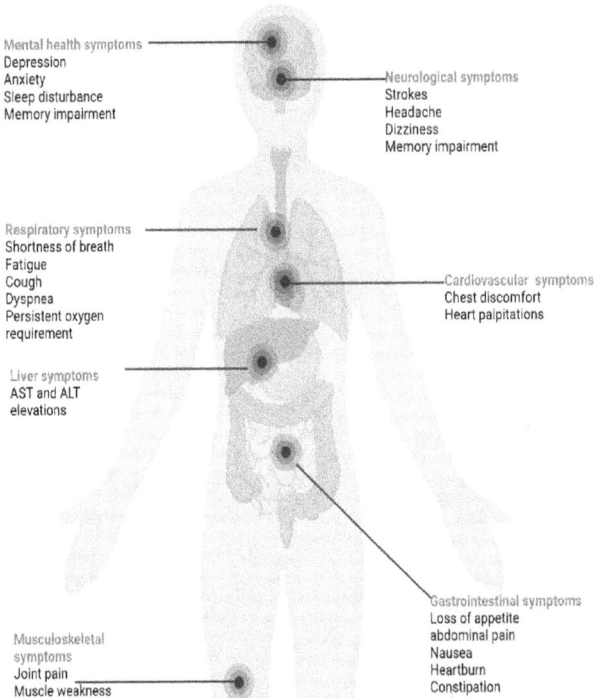
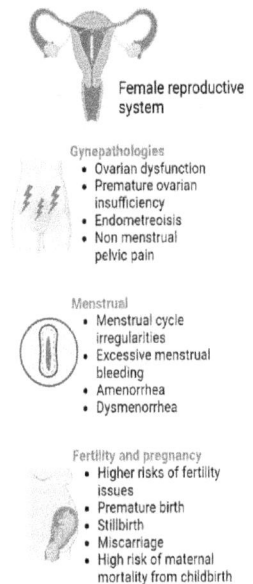

Fig. 4. Long COVID symptoms and pathology.[28]

CAREER

The COVID-19 pandemic affected women's work status and careers. Women had steeper job losses than men during the pandemic. From quarter 4 of 2019 to quarter 2 of 2020, women had −12.7% job loss and men had −11.9% job loss. By quarter 3 of 2020, both men and women recovered jobs; however, more men than women recovered jobs. Full recovery of employment for women did not occur until late in 2023[31] (**Table 3**).

The industries that had the most job losses were accommodations, food services, and arts and entertainment; thus, several industries that have a majority of female employees had significant job losses during the pandemic. The jobs that are majority male dominant, had less job losses during the pandemic such as construction, manufacturing, mining, quarrying and oil, and utilities. Women had a larger share of lost jobs and slower recovery than men in some but not all industries. Women's jobs recovered well in transportation and warehousing, manufacturing, professional, scientific and technical services, and construction (**Table 4**).[31]

Other work career gaps also occurred during the pandemic. One study looked at first authorship, last authorship, and any author within a COVID-19 medical paper. It compared the number of papers in March and April 2020 with all papers in 2019. There were 14 percent fewer women first authors for papers in March and April 2020 compared with all 2019 papers and 3% fewer women last authors for papers in March and April 2020 compared with all 2019 papers; however the decrease in last authors was not statistically significant.[32] A second study showed that during the first 2 months of the pandemic, women had a significant decrease of first author and coauthor submissions.[33] Unfortunately, no studies have measured whether the factors listed have affected women's careers, promotion, or financial status.

There have been other changes in career status following the COVID-19 pandemic. A study by the Pew Research Center[34] shows that men are working fewer hours since the COVID pandemic, while women's work hours have stayed the same; this change is consistent among different educational backgrounds. For women in the workforce who had less than a high school degree, there was an almost 13% decrease of people in the workforce from 2019 to 2021 compared with an almost 5% decrease in men with the same education.[34] The number of women with a high school degree in the workforce decreased 6%, and men with a high school degree decreased 1.8% from 2019 to 2021. College-educated women and men had similar declines in the workforce during this timeframe.[34] These data show a pattern of women with lower educational status being at more risk of losing employment during the pandemic, and it is not known whether their employment status has since recovered.

Although more women have been seeking out leadership positions, the COVID-19 pandemic resulted in fewer women in the workforce.[35] More women than men took

Table 3
Gender employment gap

Quarter of Calendar Year	Men	Women
2019 Q4	83.3 million jobs	78 million jobs
2020 Q2 (pandemic)	73.4 million jobs	68 million jobs
2020 Q3	77.7 million jobs	71 million jobs
2022 Q3	83.6 million jobs	78 million

Data from Ref.[31]

Table 4
Lost jobs at the peak of the pandemic and rebound of jobs for men and women

Job Category	Share of Lost Jobs - Men 2019Q4-2020Q2	Share of Lost Jobs - Women 2019Q4-2020Q2	Rebound of Jobs for Men by 2022Q3	Rebound of Jobs for Women by 2022Q3
Other services	14%	21%	97%	78%
Retail trade	14%	16%	94%	78%
Health care and social assistance	7%	8%	156%	89%
Accommodation and food services	36%	37%	96%	97%
Transportation and warehousing	9%	10%	152%	194%
Manufacturing	9%	10%	103%	122%
Professional, scientific and technical services			233%	309%
Construction			131%	257%

Data from Ref.[31]

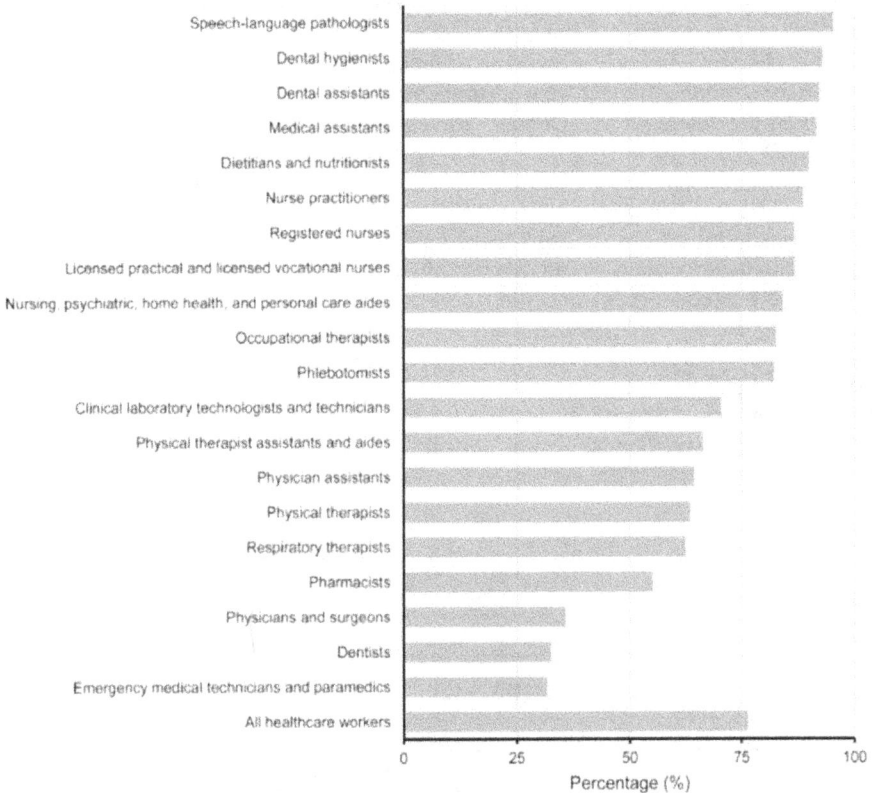

Fig. 5. Percent of women employees by health care occupation.[38]

leave during the pandemic for caregiving.[36] In medicine, men and women faculty both had increased stress levels during COVID-19 at home and at work.[37] Women reported more stress with work-related items such as teaching, patient care, and scholarly activity than men. Parents who had children between the ages of 0 and 5 years had the biggest decrease in work hours during the pandemic, and parents with children between 0 and 5 years old submitted fewer first author articles. Recommendations to support women in the workforce and keep them in the workforce include having women be a part of leadership teams that decide on hazard pay, childcare, hiring processes, and work shift scheduling.[36]

Women make up 76 percent of the health care workforce and were more likely to encounter workplace exposures and work burnout during the height of the crisis. During the COVID pandemic, women reported that their personal protective equipment was difficult to find and when found, it did not fit well.[36] It is also notable that women were under-represented in research in clinical trials combating the disease, particularly women who were pregnant or breastfeeding. The pandemic highlighted existing structural inequities that exacerbated these impacts for women from historically minoritized or disadvantaged communities (**Fig. 5**).

SUMMARY

The COVID-19 pandemic impacted all spheres of the lives of women, including access to and utilization of routine and reproductive health care, careers and advancement of careers, caregiving, and mental health and wellbeing. Although the crisis point of the pandemic has passed, there is a lasting impact on the lives and health of women. This pandemic revealed opportunities for clinical and policy changes that could better prepare medicine for the next pandemic.

CLINICS CARE POINTS

- Cancer screening deficits from the COVID-19 pandemic are ongoing; however, interventions to increase screening have been shown to be effective.
- Physical activity and chronic disease management were decreased during the pandemic.
- Personal protective equipment that fits women needs to be created and ready for the next pandemic.
- Policies need to be created for working women for the next pandemic, and expanding leadership to include women will help tailor policies appropriately.
- Parents of 0- to 5-year-olds were more likely to decrease the work hours during the pandemic; however male versus female was not studied, and the downstream effects have not been studied.
- Vaccine counseling and combating misinformation is an important ongoing discussion especially for pregnant women.

DISCLOSURE

The authors have nothing to disclose.

REFERENCES

1. Wegner L, Mendoza-Vasconez AS, Mackey S, et al. Physical activity, well-being, and priorities of older women during the COVID-19 pandemic: a survey of Women's

Health Initiative Strong and Healthy (*WHISH*) intervention participants. Transl Behavior Med 2021;11(12):2155–63.

2. Lum KJ, Simpson EEA. The impact of physical activity on psychological well-being in women aged 45-55 years during the COVID pandemic: a mixed-methods investigation. Maturitas 2021;153:19–25.

3. Van Grondelle SE, Van Bruggen S, Rauh SP, et al. The impact of the COVID-19 pandemic on diabetes care: the perspective of healthcare providers across Europe. Prim Care Diabetes 2023;17(2):141–7. Epub 2023 Feb 16. PMID: 36822977; PMCID: PMC9933343.

4. University of Maryland Medical Center. COVID 19 Impact on limb loss and techniques to improve outcomes. 2024. Available at: https://www.umms.org/ummc/pros/physician-briefs/heart-vascular/limb-preservation/covid-19-impact-on-limb-loss-and-techniques-to-improve-outcomes#:~:text=TheCOVIDD19pandemic resulted,comparedtopreCOVIDD19rates. Accessed August 5, 2024.

5. Wang L, Working to close the cancer screening gap caused by COVID, 2022, National Cancer Institute, Available at: https://www.cancer.gov/news-events/cancer-currents-blog/2022/covid-increasing-cancer-screening (Accessed 25 June 2024).

6. Richman I, Tessier-Sherman B, Galusha D, et al. Breast cancer screening during the COVID-19 pandemic: moving from disparities to health equity. J Natl Cancer Inst 2023;115(2):139–45. PMID: 36069622; PMCID: PMC9494402.

7. Grimm LJ, Lee C, Rosenberg RD, et al. Impact of the COVID-19 pandemic on breast imaging: an analysis of the national mammography database. J Am Coll Radiol 2022;19(8):919–34. Epub 2022 Jun 8. PMID: 35690079; PMCID: PMC9174535.

8. Joung RH, Mullett TW, Kurtzman SH, et al. Return-to-screening quality improvement collaborative. Evaluation of a national quality improvement collaborative for improving cancer screening. JAMA Netw Open 2022;5(11):e2242354. https://doi.org/10.1001/jamanetworkopen.2022.42354. PMID: 36383381; PMCID: PMC9669819.

9. Turner K, Brownstein NC, Whiting J, et al. Impact of the COVID-19 pandemic on women's health care access: a cross-sectional study. J Womens Health (Larchmt) 2022;31(12):1690–702. Epub 2022 Oct 31. PMID: 36318766; PMCID: PMC9805885.

10. Kearney M and Levine P, US births are down again, after the COVID baby bust and rebound, 2023, Brookings, Available at: https://www.brookings.edu/articles/us-births-are-down-again-after-the-covid-baby-bust-and-rebound/ (Accessed 25 June 2024).

11. Connor J, Madhavan S, Mokashi M, et al. Health risks and outcomes that disproportionately affect women during the COVID-19 pandemic: a review. Soc Sci Med 2020;266:113364.

12. Wei SQ, Bilodeau-Bertrand M, Liu S, et al. The impact of COVID-19 on pregnancy outcomes: a systematic review and meta-analysis. CMAJ (Can Med Assoc J) 2021;193(16):E540–8.

13. Hsu AL, Johnson T, Phillips L, et al. Sources of vaccine hesitancy: pregnancy, infertility, minority concerns, and general skepticism. Open Forum Infect Dis 2022;9(3):ofab433. US: Oxford University Press.

14. Blakeway H, Prasad S, Kalafat E, et al. COVID-19 vaccination during pregnancy: coverage and safety. Am J Obstet Gynecol 2022;226(2):236-e1.

15. Fell DB, Dhinsa T, Alton GD, et al. Association of COVID-19 vaccination in pregnancy with adverse peripartum outcomes. JAMA 2022;327(15):1478–87.

16. Shafiee A, Kohandel Gargari O, Teymouri Athar MM, et al. COVID-19 vaccination during pregnancy: a systematic review and meta-analysis. BMC Pregnancy Childbirth 2023;23(1):45.

17. Rawal S, Tackett RL, Stone RH, et al. COVID-19 vaccination among pregnant people in the United States: a systematic review. Am J Obstet Gynecol MFM 2022;4(4): 100616.
18. Pierri F, Perry BL, DeVerna MR, et al. Online misinformation is linked to early COVID-19 vaccination hesitancy and refusal. Sci Rep 2022;12:5966.
19. Williams JTB, Kurlandsky K, Breslin K, et al. Attitudes toward COVID-19 vaccines among pregnant and recently pregnant individuals. JAMA Netw Open 2024;7(4): e245479.
20. Maternal vaccine information for healthcare providers, Pregnancy and vaccination, 2024. Available at: https://www.cdc.gov/vaccines-pregnancy/hcp/?CDC_AAref_Val=https://www.cdc.gov/vaccines/pregnancy/hcp-toolkit/index.html (Accessed 10 June 2024).
21. Chamaa F, Bahmad HF, Darwish B, et al. PTSD in the COVID-19 era. Curr Neuropharmacol 2021;19(12):2164.
22. Devoto A, Himelein-Wachowiak M, Liu T, et al. Women's substance use and mental health during the COVID-19 pandemic. Wom Health Issues 2022;32(3):235–40.
23. Ahmad M, Laura V. The psychological impact of COVID-19 pandemic on women's mental health during pregnancy: a rapid evidence review. Int J Environ Res Publ Health 2021;18(13):7112.
24. Liese BS, Monley CM. Providing addiction services during a pandemic: lessons learned from COVID-19. J Subst Abuse Treat 2021;120:108156.
25. Gonzalez O, Alexander A, et al. Depressive symptomatology in adults during the COVID-19 pandemic. J Invest Med 2022;70(2):436–45.
26. Shaver J. The state of telehealth before and after the COVID-19 pandemic. Prim Care Clin Off Pract 2022;49(4):517–30.
27. Chamaa F, Bahmad HF, Darwish B, et al. PTSD in the COVID-19 era. Curr Neuropharmacol 2021;19(12):2164–79.
28. Maham S, Yoon M-S. Clinical spectrum of long COVID: effects on female reproductive health. Viruses 2024;16.7:1142.
29. Stewart S, Newson L, Briggs TA, et al. Long COVID risk-a signal to address sex hormones and women's health. Lancet Reg Health Eur 2021;11:100242.
30. Goldin C. Understanding the economic impact of COVID-19 on women. No. w29974. National Bureau of Economic Research; 2022.
31. Chmura Economics and Analytics, The disproportionate impact of the COVID-19 pandemic on women in the workforce, 2024. Available at: https://www2.census.gov/about/training-workshops/2023/2023-02-14-women-in-workforce-presentation.pdf (Accessed 27 June 2024).
32. Andersen JP, Nielsen MW, Simone NL, et al. COVID-19 medical papers have fewer women first authors than expected. Elife 2020;9:e58807. PMID: 32538780; PMCID: PMC7304994.
33. Krukowski RA, Jagsi R, Cardel MI. Academic productivity differences by gender and child age in science, technology, engineering, mathematics, and medicine faculty during the COVID-19 pandemic. J Womens Health (Larchmt) 2021;30(3):341–7. Epub 2020 Nov 18. PMID: 33216682; PMCID: PMC7957370.
34. Fry R, Some gender disparities widened in the US workforce during the pandemic, 2022, Pew Research Center, Available at: https://www.pewresearch.org/short-reads/2022/01/14/some-gender-disparities-widened-in-the-u-s-workforce-during-the-pandemic/ (Accessed 27 June 2024).
35. Dempere J, Grassa R. The impact of COVID-19 on women's empowerment: a global perspective. J Glob Health 2023;13:06021. PMID: 37325883; PMCID: PMC10273027.

36. Morgan R, Tan HL, Oveisi N, et al. Women healthcare workers' experiences during COVID-19 and other crises: a scoping review. Int J Nurs Stud Adv 2022;4:100066. https://doi.org/10.1016/j.ijnsa.2022.100066. Epub 2022 Jan 30. PMID: 35128472; PMCID: PMC8801061.

37. Kotini-Shah P, Man B, Pobee R, et al. Work-life balance and productivity among academic faculty during the COVID-19 pandemic: a latent class analysis. J Womens Health (Larchmt) 2022;31(3):321–30. Epub 2021 Nov 25. PMID: 34846927; PMCID: PMC8972018.

38. Connor J, Madhavan S, Mokashi M, et al. Health risks and outcomes that disproportionately affect women during the Covid-19 pandemic: a review. Soc Sci Med 2020;266:113364.

Moving?

Make sure your subscription moves with you!

To notify us of your new address, find your **Clinics Account Number** (located on your mailing label above your name), and contact customer service at:

Email: journalscustomerservice-usa@elsevier.com

800-654-2452 (subscribers in the U.S. & Canada)
314-447-8871 (subscribers outside of the U.S. & Canada)

Fax number: 314-447-8029

Elsevier Health Sciences Division
Subscription Customer Service
3251 Riverport Lane
Maryland Heights, MO 63043

*To ensure uninterrupted delivery of your subscription, please notify us at least 4 weeks in advance of move.

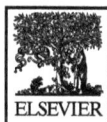

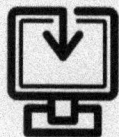

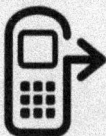

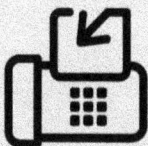

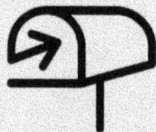

ELSEVIER